DERMATOLOGY

for the small animal practitioner

exotics

feline

canine

Edited by

Gene H. Nesbitt, DVM, MS
Diplomate, American College of Veterinary Dermatology
Veterinary Referral Associates, P.C.
West Caldwell, New Jersey

Lowell J. Ackerman, DVM
Diplomate, American College of Veterinary Dermatology
Mesa Veterinary Hospital, Ltd. Dermatology Service
Mesa, Arizona

CONTENTS

CONTRIBUTORS

Gene H. Nesbitt, DVM, MS
Diplomate, American College of Veterinary Dermatology
Veterinary Referral Associates, P.C.
West Caldwell, New Jersey

Lowell J. Ackerman, DVM
Diplomate, American College of Veterinary Dermatology
Mesa Veterinary Hospital, Ltd. Dermatology Service
Mesa, Arizona

R. Dean Axelson, DVM
The Links Road Animal and Bird Clinic
Willowdale, Ontario
Canada

Petra Burgmann, BSc, DVM
High Park Animal Clinic
Toronto, Ontario
Canada

Elliott R. Jacobson, DVM, PhD
Department of Small Animal Clinical Sciences
College of Veterinary Medicine
University of Florida
Gainesville, Florida

PREFACE

Dermatologic diseases in dogs and cats represent a significant percentage of the cases seen by small animal practitioners. The proliferation of knowledge in the field of veterinary dermatology has made the diagnosis of dermatoses more difficult for the clinician. To further complicate the daily life of the veterinarian, other species of animals, including birds, small mammals, and reptiles, are being examined in increasing numbers for dermatologic disease. The dissemination of knowledge concerning these latter species is still in its infancy.

The precursor to this book, written by one of the authors (GHN), emphasized a logical approach to diagnosis and treatment of canine and feline dermatoses. The basic format, using diagnostic keys as a basis for the systematic approach to the dermatoses of dogs and cats, has been continued. The addition of Dr. Lowell Ackerman as co-author has added much depth and experience. This book is written by active dermatology referral practitioners for fellow general practitioners and students.

We are most grateful to our three colleagues, Drs. Dean Axelson, Petra Burgmann, and Elliot Jacobson, for their major contributions of the avian, small mammal, and reptile chapters, respectively. The addition of these species gives the general practitioner a complete practical reference book.

The most commonly encountered dermatologic entities receive the most detailed attention. This book is not meant to be an exhaustive review of veterinary dermatology and clinical allergy; therefore, it should be supplemented when necessary with other more detailed or specific references, which are listed at the end of each chapter.

Chapter 1

STRUCTURE AND FUNCTION OF THE SKIN

Lowell Ackerman, DVM
Gene H. Nesbitt, DVM, MS

To understand the pathologic mechanisms associated with diseases of the skin, the clinician must have a basic knowledge of the skin's structure and function. This background is essential before the clinical skills of observation, interpretation, and correlation of history, clinical findings, and diagnostic tests can be used best to arrive at a diagnosis and to formulate a therapeutic plan.

Skin is usually considered in terms of two principal layers—the *epidermis* and the *dermis*—not only in association with their development and functional morphologic factors, but also in terms of disorders and disease processes. These two layers are intimately related functionally and remain mutually interdependent throughout life. The epidermis is a composite of cells of different types, function, and developmental origin. The dermis is a dense, fibroelastic, connective tissue stroma that encloses the extensive vascular and neural networks as well as the specialized glands and appendages derived from the epidermis. Beneath the dermis is a subcutaneous layer or *panniculus* of variable thickness. The skin is normally thickest over the dorsal anterior trunk, becoming progressively thinner posteriorly and ventrally. The integration of structure and function of canine and feline skin is summarized in Table 1-1.

EPIDERMIS

The epidermis is an organized, stratified epithelium with appendages, including hair follicles and apocrine and sebaceous glands, all of which project deep into the dermis (Fig. 1-1). The major cellular epidermal component is the keratinocyte, which is of ectodermal origin. Other cellular components include melanocytes, derived from the neural crest, and Langerhans' cells, of reticuloendothelial origin.

The primary function of the epidermis is protection from the external environment. The epidermis forms the barrier layer of the skin which prevents the entrance of toxic substances and microorganisms and the loss of water and electrolytes. The epidermal keratinocyte produces keratin, a highly resistant, insoluble, fibrous protein that is largely responsible for the mechanical protective function of the epidermis.

Most of the canine and feline epidermis is divided histologically into four layers (Fig. 1-2): (1) the *germinal basal cell layer*; (2) the *stratum spinosum*, which is composed of several strata of polyhedral cells lying above the germinal layer; (3) the *stratum granulosum*, a layer of flattened nucleated cells containing distinctive keratohyaline granules, which marks the transition to the overlying keratinized lamellae of the fourth layer; and (4) the *stratum corneum*. The stratum granulosum is not prominent in many microscopic sections of feline skin. A fifth layer, the *stratum lucidum* or clear layer, is present only in the footpads between the granular and corneal layers.

Although the exact structural components of the epidermal barrier have not been agreed upon, it is generally accepted that the stratum corneum constitutes the major protective barrier. Recent evidence suggests that the stratum granulosum or granulosum-corneum junction is also an important element of the epidermal barrier. Evidence shows that together with the transformation of viable nucleated cells into cornified cells, there is also complete sealing of the intercellular environment, which provides absolute control of the passage of aqueous solvents from both within and outside the epidermis.

A chemical and structural interface between the basal cell layer and the dermis is referred to as the *basal lamina* or the *basement membrane zone*. The specific function of the basal lamina embryologically or postnatally is not well understood. Known or presumed functions of the basal lamina include anchoring the epidermis to the underlying dermis, providing a substrate for the epidermis, maintaining normal tissue structure, and acting as a barrier to the exchange of cells and large molecules.

Melanocytes are pigment-producing cells of neural crest origin found in the basal cell layer. The only known function of melanocytes is the synthesis of pigment granules or melanosomes, which are subsequently transferred to the surrounding keratinocytes. The melanin released from the granules acts as a screen against solar ultraviolet radiation.

Langerhans' cells are dendritic cells of reticuloendothelial origin seen in the upper layers of the stratum spinosum. Their function in humans is immunologic, and they are involved with the uptake and processing of antigenic material. It has been suggested that Langerhans' cells are special macrophages that function as the initial receptors for the cutaneous response to external antigens. These cells can be identified with certainty only by electron microscopy.

DERMIS

The dermis is located between the epidermis and the subcutaneous panniculus (Fig. 1-3). It consists of a matrix of loose connective tissue composed of the fibrous proteins (collagen, elastin, and reticulin) embedded in an amorphous ground substance. The matrix is traversed by blood vessels, nerves, and lymphatics and is penetrated by the epidermal appendages, including the apocrine glands and pilosebaceous units.

Arrector pili muscles are the major muscles in the dermis. Variable numbers of smooth muscle fibers are present.

Collagenous fibers are the largest and most numerous type of fiber in the dermis, constituting approximately 90% of all fibers. The appearance of the fibers varies according to their depth in the dermis as well as the function of the dermis. The *reticular fibers*, or *precollagen*, are finely branched; these fibers are present throughout the ground substance at birth and gradually decrease in number within four weeks postnatally. They become concentrated around blood vessels, hair follicles, glands, and arrector pili muscles, and beneath the basal cell layer of the epidermis. With age, the reticular fibers closely approximate collagen fibers.

Elastic fibers, composed of single fine branches, are not abundant in the deeper part of the dermis. An inverse relationship exists between the abundance of terminal hairs in an area and the quantity of elastic fibers. Elastic fibers stretch easily with little loss of energy and resume their original shape when the stress is relieved. Fine elastic fibers in the upper dermis most likely function to anchor the epidermis to the dermis. The fiber content of the dermis plays a role in determining the

TABLE 1-1

Integration of Structure and Function of Canine and Feline Skin

Anatomic Structure	*Principal Functions*	*Biologic Process*	*Description*
Epidermis			
Stratum corneum	Protection, permeability to entrance of toxic substances and microorganisms and to loss of water and electrolytes	Desquamation	Dead, flattened keratinocytes in lamellar pattern
Stratum lucidum	Unknown	Unknown	Fully keratinized compact, thin layer of nonnucleated dead cells; present only in footpads
Stratum granulosum	Permeability barrier to prevent loss of water and electrolytes	Keratinization	Flattened nucleated cells containing keratohyaline granules
Stratum spinosum	Synthesis of keratin precursors	Keratinogenesis and keratinization	Several layers of polyhedral nucleated cells; no blood vessels or nerves; not mitotically active
Germinal or basal cell layer	Precursor cells for keratinocytes		
Melanocytes	Synthesis of melanin resulting in pigmentation and protection from sunlight	Melanogenesis and transfer of melanosomes	Neural crest derivation; dendritic cells that lie on the basal lamina packed between basal cells
Langerhans' cells	Involved in cell-mediated immune reactions	Antigen recognition and processing	Dendritic cells in upper stratum spinosum usually identified by electron microscopy
Dermis			
Fibrous portion Collagen Reticulin Elastin	Passively protects body from external injury; main support structure of skin	Synthesis and maturation of fibers	Matrix of loose connective tissue compound of fibrous proteins embedded in a ground substance
Ground substance	Water binding; barrier to bacterial penetration; provides reservoir and diffusion for regulating the distribution of water and salts	Undefined	Amorphous matrix of connective tissue derived from blood elements and metabolic products of parenchymal and connective tissue cells
Cells			
Fibroblasts	Precursors for collagen, elastin, and ground substance; wound healing	Collagenogenesis	Mesenchymal origin; most numerous cells in connective tissue; flat elongated cell with cytoplasmic processes and elongated oval nucleus
Macrophages	Phagocytosis	Immune defense mechanism	Transformed blood monocytes or lymphocytes; eccentrically located in dented nucleus, often with concentration of chromatin at periphery and one or two nucleoli
Mast cells	Release of vasoactive amines (histamine and heparin)	Inflammation	Round nucleus with prominent nucleolus; prominent cytoplasm with spherical basophilic and metachromatic granules
Subcutis	Heat insulation; mechanical protection	Fat synthesis and storage	Connective tissue with collagen and elastin, nerves, blood vessels, and lipocytes
Vasculature	Thermoregulation; reducing heat loss by vasoconstriction; delivers nutrients and oxygen to the skin	Inflammation and wound healing	Simple and mixed cutaneous arteries and vascular plexus
Lymphatics	Drainage system; transports capillary transudates	Inflammation and circulation	Arise from capillary networks in superficial dermis

TABLE 1-1 (continued)

Integration of Structure and Function of Canine and Feline Skin

Anatomic Structure	*Principal Functions*	*Biologic Process*	*Description*
Nerves			
Somatic sensory	Sensory perception; mediation of touch, pain, temperature, and itch	Afferent impulse transmission	Lie in subcuticular area and continue by a nerve plexus that extends through dermis to epidermis innervating epidermis, glands, muscles, and hair follicles
Autonomic	Secretomotor; control of blood vessels, glands, and pilosecretion	Efferent impulse transmission	Motor nerves to blood vessels, arrector pili muscles, and myoepithelial cells around apocrine glands
Appendages			
Hair follicle	Precursor for hair	Formation of hair	Invagination of epidermis into the dermis; usually compound
Sebaceous glands	Lubrication	Secretion of lipids	Simple alveolar holocrine glands
Apocrine sweat glands	No known function in normal conditions; minor heat regulation in abnormal conditions	Secretions of proteins	Coiled secretory tubule extending deep into dermis and subcutis; may be globoid shaped in cats
Eccrine sweat glands	Possible lubrication	Gland secretions	Found only in footpads; small, tightly coiled, and tubular; located deep in the skin; secretory duct to the surface

presence and direction of tension lines in the skin.

The *ground substance* of the dermis is the structureless portion of connective tissue that lies outside the cells, fibers, blood vessels, and nerves. All other dermal components are embedded in this amorphous matrix. The ground substance appears to be a system of multiple components: substances derived from the blood, such as water, inorganic ions, blood sugars, blood proteins, and urea; metabolic products of parenchymal cells; and metabolic products of connective tissue cells. The ground substance thus is considered the immediate environment of the cells and fibers of the dermis and an extension of the vascular system.

The cellular components of the dermis include *fibroblasts*, *macrophages*, and *mast cells*. Fibroblasts, the most numerous cells in connective tissue, are responsible for the formation of collagenous and elastin fibers and the amorphous ground substance. These cells develop from tissue mesenchymal cells.

Macrophages, or histiocytes, appear early in embryonic development. The phagocytic activity of these cells increases progressively throughout fetal and neonatal life. Controversy still exists about the origin and fate of tissue macrophages.

Mast cells vary in number among species as well as in different regions of the same animal. They are often arranged around the walls of small blood vessels. These cells probably have a hematogenous origin or arise from perivascular connective tissue cells. Mast cells degranulate under physical conditions such as cold, heat, and ultraviolet light, and in the presence of chemicals or various bacterial or animal toxins. Heparin and histamine contained within the granules are released. Mast cells are believed to participate in the regulation of lipid metabolism because of the accelerating effect of heparin on lipid transportation or clearance. Histamine increases capillary permeability, causes smooth muscle fibers to contract, stimulates the phagocytic activity of blood and connective tissue cells, and promotes secretion by various glands. It is thus responsible for the onset of inflammation, hyperemia, and the early increase in capillary permeability during the inflammatory process.

Several changes occur in the dermis with aging. In the fetal dermis, collagen fibers are fine and fibrillar, whereas in mature individuals they form coarse bundles. Collagen is synthesized continually, although its metabolic activities, including both synthesis and degradation, sharply decrease with age. Elastic fibers increase in

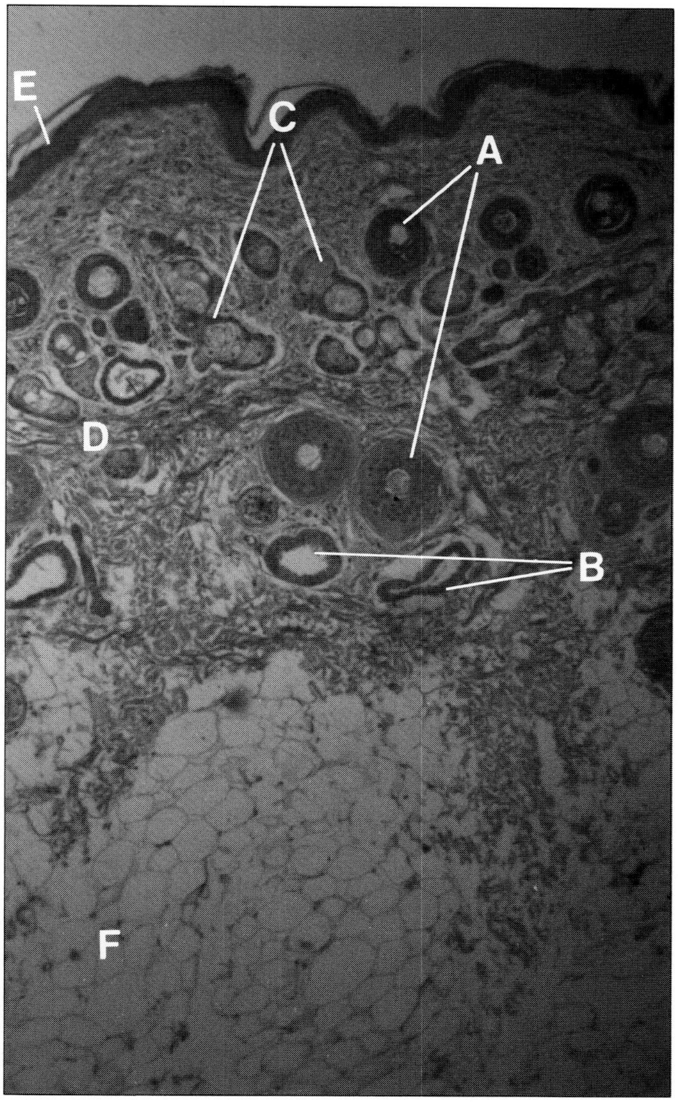

Figure 1-1. Microscopic section of normal canine skin. Note epidermis (*E*), multiple appendages (hair follicle, *A*), apocrine glands (*B*), and sebaceous glands (*C*) in the dermis (*D*) and subcutis (*F*) (low power).

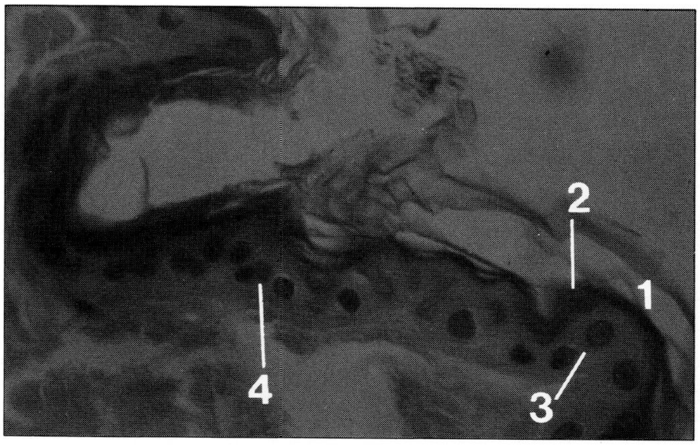

Figure 1-2. Microscopic section of normal feline skin. Note the four layers: (1) stratum corneum, (2) stratum granulosum, (3) stratum spinosum, and (4) basal cell layer (high power).

number and diameter during aging. Dermal ground substance undergoes little histologic change.

The biologic functions of the dermis are many and complex. A primary function is to protect the body from external injury. The dermis is uniquely constructed to resist tearing, shearing, and localized pressure, but is also flexible enough to allow joint movement and local stretch. Both the amount and architecture of collagen determine the tensile strength of the dermis. It plays an important role as a substratum for the epidermis. The hyaluronic acid of the ground substance acts as a barrier to bacterial penetration. Hyaluronic acid also binds water and maintains dermal turgor in the tissues; thus, the dermis can function as a water storage organ. The dermis plays a minor role in cation exchange; it has a homeostatic function in maintaining proper levels of blood cat-

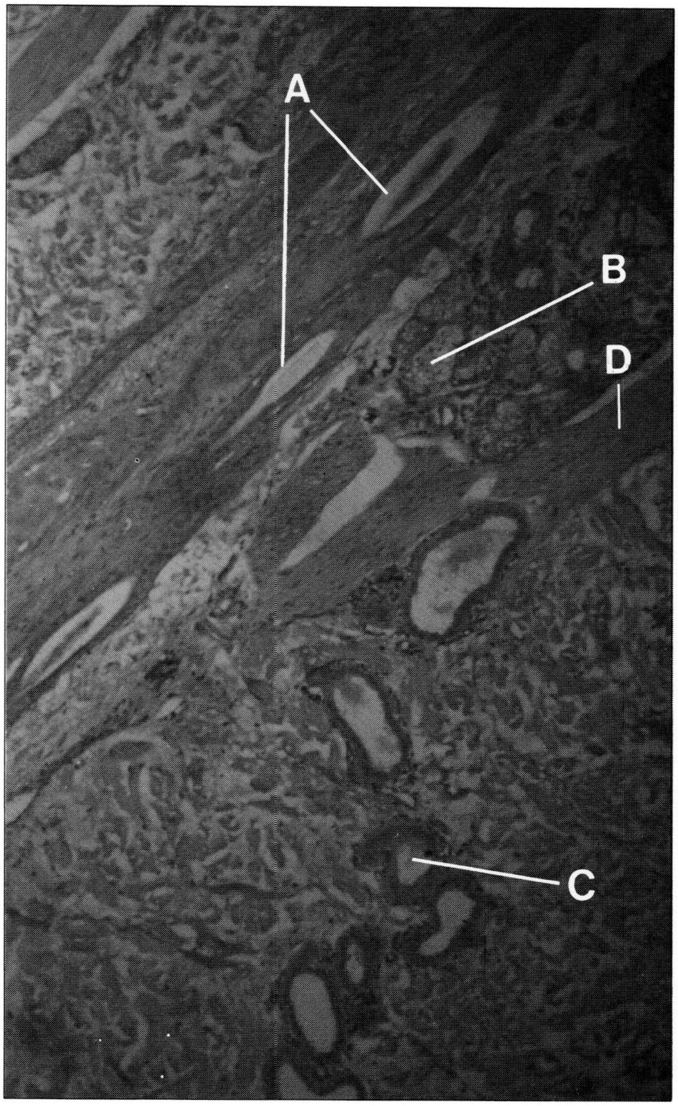

Figure 1-3. Microscopic section of dermis of normal canine skin. Note hair follicle unit (compound hair follicle, *A*), sebaceous glands (*B*), apocrine glands (*C*), and arrector pili muscle (*D*) surrounded by connective tissue matrix (low power).

ions and in supplying mineral metabolism in general. Finally, the dermis is involved in thermal regulation by providing the supporting bed for the vasculature.

SUBCUTIS

The subcutis is composed of connective tissue, nerves, blood vessels, and lipocytes. The connective tissue consists of loose collagenous trabeculae that contain many elastic fibers that cross each other to form a meshwork; the spaces of the meshwork are further subdivided by smaller bundles. The adipose tissue can serve as a cushion or shock absorber, a filler, a sheath for easily injured parts such as nerves and vessels, and an insulator to protect the body from excessive heat loss. The degree to which the skin can be folded or displaced depends on the development of the subcutis and the extensibility, length, and thickness of the fiber bundles.

VASCULAR SYSTEM

The kinds of cutaneous vascular beds are determined by the areas of skin they perfuse, the thickness of the various dermal and hypodermal layers, the types and numbers of appendages present, and the specific relation of the skin to the bones and muscle fascia under it. The primary function of the cutaneous vascular system is to deliver nutrients to the skin. The sources of the arteries and their large primary branches in the subcutaneous fascia are generally constant in all animals. The divisions and subdivisions of these arteries all run parallel to the skin surface, with no constancy in the arrangement of the smaller vessels and no pattern common to all dogs and cats.

The two types of primary cutaneous vasculature are simple and mixed cutaneous arteries. The simple cutaneous arteries reach the skin by running between muscle masses and giving off small branches to the muscle tissue. The mixed cutaneous arteries pass through muscle beds with large branches, supplying the muscle before terminating in the skin.

The three vascular plexuses are the subcutaneous or deep, the cutaneous (middle or intermediate), and the superficial (subepidermal or subpapillary). These plexuses lie parallel to the surface of the skin. The extensive microscopic plexus of the skin vessels appear to ensure a continuous and complete blood supply to the skin, even when there is temporary blockage of the main vessels coming from the deeper layers.

LYMPHATICS

Lymphatics of the skin arise from capillary networks that lie in the superficial area of the dermis and surround the follicles and glands. Their main function is to transport the capillary transudate.

NERVES

Nerves of the skin serve as sensory receptors and also control the sweat glands and arrector pili muscles. The nerves lie in the subcutaneous area and are continuous with a nerve plexus that extends through the dermis to the epidermis, with branches from these plexuses innervating the epidermis, glands, muscles, and hair follicles. Sensory nerve fibers have three types of terminal receptors: the dermal nerve network, the hair follicle network, and specialized end organs. The density of dermal nerve networks in the skin varies inversely with the hair coverage of the area. The dermal nerve network functions in pain perception and temperature variation.

The principal organ for touch perception is made up of sensory nerve fibers that form a double network around the primary hair. Every hair has a nerve ending associated with it. The nerve penetrates the follicle below the sebaceous gland duct, divides, and then lies parallel to the long axis of the hair. The mechanism of touch perception is more refined in the sinus or tactile hairs, where engorgement of the vascular sinus surrounding the base of the hair follicle enhances sensory acuity.

In addition to the dermal and follicular networks, the hairless skin also contains many encapsulated nerve endings that make up the specialized receptors. These special end organs are found primarily at the mucocutaneous junctions and in the footpads. The skin also is supplied with adrenergic sympathetic motor nerves to blood vessels, arrector pili muscles, and myoepithelial cells around the apocrine sweat glands.

PILIARY APPARATUS

The pilosebaceous unit consists of the *hair follicle*, which is an epidermal appendage that penetrates the dermis, and the *sebaceous glands* that originate from the sides of the follicle. Hairs consist of compactly cemented keratinized cells produced by the hair follicles.

Hair Follicle

The basic unit of hair production is the hair follicle (Fig. 1-4), which is made up of a peripheral connective tissue portion and an inner epithelial part or root sheath. The connective tissue portion is derived from the dermis; the epithelial portion has an epidermal origin. The epithelial portion is divided into the outer root sheath, which is a continuation of the basal cell layer of the epidermis, and the inner root sheath, which grows upward with the hair from the hair bulb.

At birth the hair follicles are simple or primary, with one hair per follicle. As the animal ages, accessory hairs develop in accessory or secondary follicles, which arise as buds from the original single follicle, forming a compound follicle (Fig. 1-4). There is a single follicular ori-

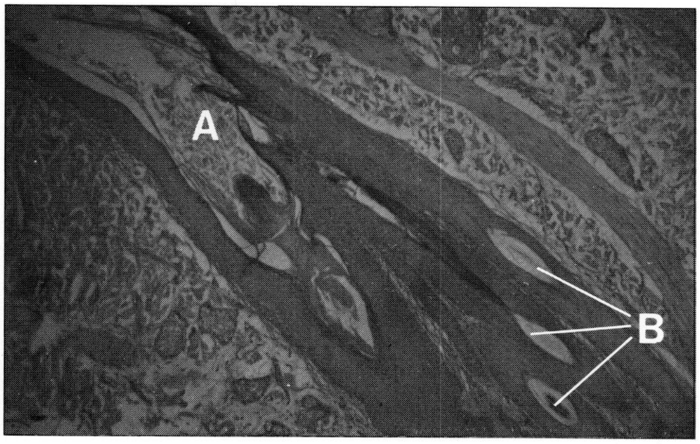

Figure 1-4. Microscopic section of compound hair follicle in normal canine skin. Note multiple hair follicles with larger primary follicle (*A*) and several accessory follicles (*B*) (low power).

fice with one primary cover or guard hair and a number of secondary hairs. The follicle and hair bulb of the guard hair in the compound follicle are larger and penetrate deeper into the subcutaneous tissue than those of the secondary hairs. Each secondary hair is also accompanied by sebaceous glands and an arrector pili muscle.

Hair

Hairs are epidermal structures. The free portion is called the ***hair shaft*** and the proximal portion is called the *root*. The root is usually set obliquely to the skin. The root is attached to the underlying dermal papilla. The shaft is composed of medulla, cortex, and cuticle. The cortex is composed of tightly packed keratin cells that form the major portion of the hair. Hair color is determined by pigment in these cells.

Several classifications exist for hair types in dogs but they may be generally referred to as normal, short, or long. Two types of haircoats are described for cats: Persian or long hair, and domestic or short hair. The gene for short hair is dominant.

Hair has several functions, including the first line of external defense against physical, chemical, and ultraviolet or actinic trauma. It also performs sensory functions and plays a significant role in the thermoregulatory mechanism.

Hair Cycle

The hair grows cyclically, with alternating periods of growth and quiescence. During the growth phase, follicles are in the anagen stage; during the subsequent resting phase, they contain club hairs and are in the telogen state. The catagen stage is the transition period when the follicles are reorganizing into an inactive state.

Several factors affect the hair growth cycle. The photoperiod plays a significant role. As the daylight hours increase, the rate of shedding increases and the haircoat becomes coarser and less dense. As the photoperiod decreases, the coat is again shed and there is a stimulation of hair growth that produces a dense haircoat accompanied by decreased sebum production. Poor health or generalized disease shortens the anagen period and results in a larger percentage of body hairs being in telogen at one time. Anagen is stimulated by thyroxine, adrenocorticotropic hormone (ACTH), and testosterone, while estrogens have an inhibitory effect on anagen.

Sebaceous Glands

Sebaceous glands are simple, alveolar holocrine glands associated with the pilosebaceous apparatus (Figs. 1-1 and 1-3). There are a few body regions where these glands are not associated with the hair follicle, including the external ear canal, anus, prepuce, vulva, and the tarsal glands of the eyelids. These glands tend to be larger and more numerous along the dorsal part of the neck, back, and tail.

Sebaceous glands are evaginated from the hair follicle and are connected to the upper part of the follicle by a short duct. These glands have a peripheral basal cell layer with the central part of the gland consisting of large, foamy, lipid-filled cells.

Apocrine Glands

Apocrine glands are large, loosely coiled sweat glands that are distributed over the entire skin as an appendage of the hair follicles. Greater numbers are found on the face and between the toes. Specialized apocrine glands are also present in the external ear canal (ceruminous glands), in the eyelids in association with the cilia (glands of Moll), and in the mammary glands. One apocrine gland is associated with each follicle complex in the form of a coiled secretory tubule that extends deep into the dermis and subcutaneous tissue. The apocrine secretory duct empties into the follicle above the opening of the sebaceous gland duct.

The apocrine sweat glands do not appear to function under normal conditions; however, they do respond to the application of local heat and to circulating catecholamines. The apocrine sweat glands of dogs do not actively participate in the central thermoregulatory mechanism; they serve mainly to protect the skin from an excess temperature rise. The apocrine secretion is a proteinaceous, white, odorless, milky fluid that is slowly and continuously formed.

Eccrine (Merocrine) Sweat Glands

These glands are found only in the footpads of dogs and cats and are located deep in the dermis at its junction with the hypodermis. The excretory duct follows a tortuous path through the dermis and epidermis to a pore on the surface of the pad. The secretion of the eccrine sweat gland is watery. These glands have no thermoregulatory function.

Tail Glands

The tail gland area of a dog is located on the dorsal surface of the tail about 2 inches (5 cm) from the base of the tail. The haircoat over the glands is composed of coarse hairs emerging from single follicles. Numerous large sebaceous and apocrine glands composing the tail glands extend deep into the dermis and subcutaneous tissue.

Circumanal and Perianal Glands

These glands are complexes found near the anal orifice. The circumanal glands are superficial sebaceous glands whose secretory ducts empty into hair follicles and onto the mucocutaneous anal surface. Perianal or deep circumanal glands make up the deeper, nonsebaceous part of the complex. The perianal glands do not have any secretory activity.

FOOTPADS

The footpads are characterized by a thick stratum corneum and a prominent stratum lucidum or clear layer. There are numerous eccrine (merocrine) sweat glands in the lower dermis and hypodermis.

TABLE 1-2

Factors Influencing or Regulating Keratinization

Factor	*Effect*	*Target*
Intrinsic		
Epidermal chalone and epinephrine	Antimitotic	Basal cells
Prostaglandins	Proliferation	Epidermal cells
Extrinsic		
Dermis	Substrate for proliferation	Epidermal cells
Epidermal growth factor	Proliferation	Basal cells
Vitamin A		
Normal	Proliferation	Basal cells
Excessive	Inhibition of keratinization	Epidermis
Deficient	Stimulation	Epidermis
Corticosteroids	Inhibition of keratinization	Epidermis
Copper deficiency	Weak hair	Hair
Estrogens	Stimulation of keratinization	Epidermis
Zinc deficiency	Lack of maturation of keratinocytes	Epidermis

NASAL SKIN

Nasal skin (planum nasale) is characterized by only three layers in the epidermis: stratum corneum, stratum spinosum, and basal cell layer. There is an absence of hair and glandular structures in the dermis. Pigment granules are usually prominent in the lower epidermis.

BIOLOGIC OR PHYSIOLOGIC PROCESSES OF SKIN

Five biologic or physiologic processes have great impact on clinical veterinary dermatology: keratinization, pigmentation, sebum production, pruritus, and alopecia. The veterinary clinician must be familiar with the mechanisms involved and the factors influencing these processes to appreciate the historical, clinical, and diagnostic findings of many cutaneous diseases or syndromes.

Keratinization

Three distinct phases occur in the life cycle of keratinocytes: mitosis in the basal cell layer; differentiation in the stratum spinosum and stratum granulosum; and exfoliation of the corneal layer.

Because the surface layers are continuously being shed, the constant thickness of the epidermis depends upon a consistent rate of mitotic reproduction in the basal layer. The regulation of basal cell proliferation involves both intrinsic and extrinsic factors, which are summarized in Table 1-2.

Intrinsic factors are not well delineated at this time. In human and in pig skin, a tissue substance called an *epidermal chalone* has demonstrated antimitotic activity on basal cells; epinephrine is required to produce this effect. Prostaglandins can stimulate epidermal cell proliferation.

Extrinsic factors that influence basal cell proliferation include the dermis, which provides a substratum of suitable texture and produces factors that promote basal cell proliferation. An epidermal growth factor and vitamin A have been shown to stimulate mitosis, although hydrocortisone inhibits epidermal mitotic activity. Trauma, such as radiation, scraping, or incision on the surface of the epidermis, results in a sudden burst of mitotic activity in the basal cell layer. There must be a complex interplay of these many intrinsic and extrinsic regulatory factors to ensure that the epidermis maintains the proper proportion of proliferating and differentiating cells sufficient to maintain a constant thickness in relation to the rate of surface desquamation. Several factors that affect the desquamation process are summarized in Table 1-2.

Pigmentation

The process of pigment development and the regulation of pigmentation in the hair and skin is not fully understood. The melanocytes are the basic structural units of the melanin pigmentary system. They lie on the basal lamina tightly packed between basal cells. Dendrites from the melanocytes project into the epidermis. The melanocytes synthesize melanosomes or pigment granules. In a manner not completely understood in humans or animals, the melanosomes are transferred to keratinocytes. Some evidence from studies in humans shows that keratinocytes actively phagocytize the dendrites containing melanin.

Melanin pigmentation depends on the interaction between melanocytes and keratinocytes, the rate of pigment production (melanogenesis), the transfer to keratinocytes, and the final disposition of melanosomes within the keratinocytes. A functional epidermal-melanin unit consists of a melanocyte and a constant population of satellite keratinocytes. An example of the interaction of the components of this unit is the pigmentation of hair, in which melanocytes synthesize and transfer pigment to the keratinocytes of the hair shaft only during the anagen stage of the hair cycle.

Genetic and hormonal factors are thought to be the major regulators of melanocyte activity. Melanocyte-stimulating hormone (MSH) from the intermediate lobe of the pituitary gland causes increased pigmentation in humans by influencing a greater dispersion of melanosomes and an increase in the number of melanosomes in the keratinocytes. Increases in estrogen, progesterone, and MSH are associated with hyperpigmentation during pregnancy and with hyperestrogenism or ovarian imbalance I syndromes. The mode of action is unknown. Pigmentation also is increased by ACTH.

The role of melatonin from the pineal gland in pigmentation is unclear. Conditions of darkness stimulate melatonin production. It may be an antagonist to MSH.

Hyperpigmentation is a clinical entity associated with an increase in melanin pigment in the basal layer of the epidermis and in the upper dermis. The intensity of hyperpigmentation depends on the amount of melanosomes produced and the number of melanosomes transferred to the keratinocytes. Two general categories of hyperpigmentation are defined: *melanosis* develops without preceding inflammatory skin disease; *melanoderma* is associated with or follows inflammatory disorders or lesions. Lentigo is a clinical finding characterized by focal hyperpigmented macules.

Clinical hypopigmentation, vitiligo, is also observed. Albinism is associated with a genetic trait causing a lack of tyrosinase to synthesize melanin. Hypopigmentation is associated with discoid lupus erythematosus, nasal solar dermatitis, burns, trauma, and ionizing irradiation, presumably as a result of depression or destruction of the melanocytes.

Sebum Production

Sebum is an oily secretion composed of the products of the degenerated and disrupted cells of the sebaceous gland. Sebum tends to keep the skin and hair soft and pliable by forming an emulsion (lipid film) on the skin and hair surface to retain moisture. Approximately 90% of the lipid film results from sebum production, and 10% is derived from cytoplasmic contents of the epidermal cells and the apocrine sweat glands. The flow of sebaceous glands is thought to be continuous and the quantity of sebum released in a given time per unit area is proportional to the total glandular volume.

Both the size and the rate of maturation of sebaceous glands are regulated by hormones. Human studies have shown that androgens are the primary trophic hormone, estrogens have a suppressive effect, and progesterone and glucocorticoids have little direct effect on sebaceous gland secretion. In women, sebum production is thought to be stimulated by ovarian and adrenal androgens. The apparent decrease of sebum production in women after prednisone administration is possibly the result of suppression of ovarian androgens. Large doses of exogenous progesterone have a stimulatory effect on the sebaceous glands.

Pruritus

Pruritus is defined as an irritating, nonadapting cutaneous sensation that evokes the impulse to scratch. A wide variety of stimuli and noxious agents are believed to liberate peripheral chemomediators. The major mediators of pruritus in dogs and cats are thought to be proteolytic enzymes. Proteases are released by both fungi and bacteria, by mast cell degranulation following an antigen-antibody reaction, and by leukocytes in inflammatory infiltrates. Extracellular proteases, such as plasmin, are released as a result of capillary dilatation. Cathepsin from epidermal cells has proteolytic activity. This may account for the persistence of the itch sensation after epidermal damage induced by scratching. The role of kinins and prostaglandin E_1 has not been well defined. Pruritus may be initiated or potentiated by boredom and neuroses. Factors such as foreign bodies, insect bites, parasitism, allergic reactions, infections, inflammation, or vasodilation may facilitate access to proteases and thus potentiate pruritus.

The mediators of pruritus act on a finely arborizing, complex network of myelinated and nonmyelinated nerve endings, believed to be the fundamental cutaneous sensory receptor organ. In humans, itch perception is lo-

TABLE 1-3

Etiologic Factors and Mechanisms of Reversible or Potentially Reversible Alopecia

Etiologic Factors	*Mechanisms*
Endocrine disorders Hypothyroidism Hyperadrenocorticism Growth hormone deficiency Ovarian imbalance Estrogen excess in male dogs	Direct suppressive effect on hair follicle in a resting (telogen) state
Bacterial infection	Superficial folliculitis with neutrophilic exudate and hyperkeratosis of the infundibular portion of hair canal alters intrafollicular environment resulting in shedding of hair from the infected follicle
Dermatophytes	Fungal hyphae invade and proliferate within the hair shaft, weakening its structure and causing subsequent fracture of hair shaft
Parasitic infestation	
Nematode (*Pelodera strongyloides*)	Hyperkeratosis of hair canal and displacement of hair; facilitation by self-trauma resulting from irritation and inflammation associated with the presence of larvae
Fleas (hypersensitivity)	Self-trauma and immunologic mechanisms
Sarcoptic mange	Self-trauma associated with mites burrowing through the epidermis
Demodicosis	Stimulation of hyperkeratosis within the hair canal by proliferating mites with subsequent displacement and dislodgement of hair shafts, inflammation, and immunologic responses
Chemical and drug-induced alopecia	
Antimitotic drugs	Inhibit hair synthesis in anagen follicles; hair shaft becomes constricted and breaks off
Thallium	Converts follicles from anagen to telogen with subsequent shedding, inflammation, and parakeratotic hyperkeratosis
Nonscarring cutaneous disease	
Seborrheic syndrome	Faulty keratinization with increased epidermal turnover time and parakeratotic hyperkeratosis, edema, and perivascular infiltration
Acanthosis nigricans	Faulty keratinization resulting from increased epidermal turnover time, direct or indirect suppression of hair follicles by hormone influences
Alopecia areata	Antitissue antibodies directed against hair follicles resulting in follicular atrophy and hair shedding
Telogen effluvium	Variety of stress factors (fever, fright, parturition, shock, and other traumatic episodes)

calized in the area of the dermoepidermal junction and is independent of the presence of the epidermis. These sensory or "itch points" are specific areas that vary in number from animal to animal and from site to site. After skin damage, they may change in number and respond to a lower threshold of stimulation.

Two types of pruritus described are *physiologic itch*, which is a spontaneous, well-localized itch believed to be conducted by myelinated, rapid-conducting delta A fibers; and *pathologic itch*, which is an unpleasant, poorly localized itch conducted by unmyelinated, slow-conducting C fibers. The itch perception travels from the subepidermal nerve plexus by way of the dorsal root and the anterolateral spinothalamic tract to the thalamus and then through the internal capsule to the sensory cortex.

The predisposition to pruritus by neuroses and bore-

TABLE 1-4

Etiologic Factors and Mechanisms of Irreversible Alopecia

Etiologic Factors	*Mechanisms*
Genetic alopecia Hypotrichosis Epitheliogenesis imperfecta Hereditary black hair follicular dysplasia Congenital ectodermal defect Color-mutant alopecia	Genetically controlled faulty growth and development (dysplasia), or complete absence (defect) of some, many, or all hair follicles
Necrotizing processes	
Physical or chemical injury	Destruction of dermal tissue including hair follicles with subsequent lack of piloglandular appendages and replacement of normal dermal tissue with scar tissue
Deep bacterial and fungal infection	Excessive inflammatory response, which destroys hair follicles by necrosis; intrafollicular bacteria or fungi attract leukocytes that are liberating proteolytic enzymes which destroy the follicular epithelium with subsequent scarring
Nasal solar dermatitis	Repeated necrotizing inflammatory response and scar tissue formation
Lupus erythematosus	Inflammatory response and subsequent scar tissue formation
Cutaneous neoplasms and granulomas	Replacement of the follicular and glandular appendages by proliferating neoplastic cells or granulation tissue

dom in humans has been attributed to the modification of the perception of itching at the higher cortical levels of the nervous system. Mental distraction may depress consciousness of itching, although boredom may greatly intensify pruritus.

Alopecia

Alopecia is defined as the loss or lack of hair in any amount up to complete baldness. The causes of alopecia can be divided into external and internal factors. Internal factors are further classified as primary (genetic) and secondary (consequence of other internal disease). Conroy has categorized the external factors as nutrition, biologic agents (parasites, microorganisms), physical and chemical factors, stress, inappropriate therapy, and trauma. The external factors, acting alone or in combination, can alter the external or internal environment to produce or enhance susceptibility.

Alopecias can be classified on the basis of permanence of the hair loss: irreversible (permanent), and reversible or potentially reversible (temporary).

The pathomechanism operative in alopecias is related to causative factors and can involve faulty development, suppression of the hair follicle, destruction and displacement, acute loss of telogen hairs, irritation and self-trauma, leukocytic activity, invasion and weakening of the hair shaft, necrosis and fibrosis of tissue, and immune-mediated responses. Tables 1-3 and 1-4 summarize the causative factors and mechanisms associated with reversible and irreversible alopecias.

SELECTED READINGS

Conroy JD: The etiology and pathogenesis of alopecia. *Compend Contin Educ Pract Vet* 1:806, 1979.

Soter NA, Baden HT: Pathophysiology of dermatologic diseases. New York, McGraw-Hill, 1984, pp 1–466.

Chapter 2

FUNDAMENTALS OF DERMATOLOGIC DIAGNOSIS

Gene H. Nesbitt, DVM, MS
Lowell Ackerman, DVM

The skin has a relatively limited number of pathologic responses to injury that are manifested by various lesions consisting of either single or multiple types, superficial or deep, and may have a distribution pattern that is localized, regionalized, or generalized. Some lesions may be of primary concern to the pet owner even though they do not alter the normal physiologic functions of the skin.

The component of the skin that is primarily affected—the epidermis, dermis, or hair follicle—should first be identified; thus, the clinician must be familiar with the anatomy and function of the skin. One must also be able to recognize types of skin lesions based on the morphologic structure and the arrangement and distribution of lesions as they relate to specific or general disease patterns. A working knowledge of these basic facts makes it easier to arrive at a definitive diagnosis and a specific therapeutic plan.

Steps for a systematic approach to a dermatologic diagnosis are outlined in Table 2-1.

TABLE 2-1

Steps for a Systematic Approach to Dermatologic Diagnosis

1. Obtain an adequate history.
2. Complete a thorough physical examination.
3. Correlate the historical and clinical findings.
4. List all possible general etiologic classifications (differential diagnoses) based on Dermatologic Diagnostic Key.
5. Complete screening diagnostic tests to rule in or rule out the etiologic classifications listed in step 4.
6. Make a new differential diagnosis list based on step 5.
7. List possible specific etiologic classifications based on the individual etiologic diagnostic keys (history and clinical findings).
8. Complete the definitive diagnostic tests to rule in or rule out specific etiologic classifications or diagnoses.

TABLE 2-2

Interpretation of Key Historical Points

	Differential Diagnosis	
History	*Include*	*Exclude*
Pruritus	Allergic Parasitic Bacterial Fungal Immune-mediated Neoplastic Seborrheic Endocrine	None
External parasites	Parasitic	None
100% Response to corticosteroids	Allergic Immune-mediated (if high dose) Neoplastic Seborrheic Panniculitis	Endocrine Fungal Bacterial (primary) Parasitic
100% Response to antibiotics	Bacterial (primary)	Parasitic Fungal Endocrine Neoplastic Immune-mediated
100% Response to parasiticides	Parasitic Allergic	Endocrine Bacterial (primary) Fungal Immune-mediated Neoplastic

HISTORY

The initial dermatologic history includes age, sex, and breed; the owner's complaint (how the problem is perceived); date of onset of signs; original location of lesions; and the course of disease. Previous treatment administered and the clinical response elicited (drug history) often have diagnostic value. The intensity and frequency of pruritus, observation of external parasites, and history of possible contagion to other animals or humans also should be noted.

The three historical points most useful in making the initial list of differential diagnoses are absence of pruritus, presence of external parasites, and the drug history. The interpretation of these key historical points is given in Table 2-2. Pruritus must be considered in conjunction with other historical and clinical findings in order to be of initial diagnostic value. Although endocrine diseases are generally nonpruritic, mild pruritus may be related to other primary diseases (for example, allergy) or secondary to complication of a primary disease (for example, pyoderma). There is a wide variation in frequency and intensity of pruritus in most etiologic classifications.

Although a history of external parasites indicates parasitic disease, failure of the pet owner to observe them does not rule out this diagnosis. History of a previous response to corticosteroids may have been a result of dosage and/or type of drug used. All animals in a given etiologic classification do not respond equally to the same drug. A complete failure of clinical response to corticosteroids suggests endocrine, fungal, neoplastic, and bullous skin diseases. A good response to a high dose (2 to 4 mg/kg/day) suggests autoimmune disease. A good clinical response to antibacterial therapy does not differentiate between primary or secondary infection. History of partial response to antibiotics or parasiticides indicates the possibility of concurrent disease.

PHYSICAL EXAMINATION

A complete physical examination should be performed that includes all organ systems. Systemic signs are commonly seen with some endocrine, bullous, neoplastic, and fungal diseases, whereas systemic signs are not characteristic of allergic and bacterial diseases.

When examining the skin all areas of the body should be included. Primary and secondary morphologic lesions, as well as miscellaneous skin lesions, should be identified and recorded. The various types of lesions and their pathogenesis are defined in Tables 2-3 (primary), 2-4 (secondary), and 2-5 (miscellaneous) and some of these lesions are illustrated in Figure 2-1. The distribution pattern and extent of alopecia and erythema should be noted and carefully correlated with other historical and clinical findings. The morphologic classification of cutaneous lesions and differential diagnoses are summarized in Table 2-6. The interpretation of key clinical findings is given in Table 2-7.

TABLE 2-3

Primary Gross Morphologic Lesions

Lesion	*Definition*	*Pathogenesis*
Macule	Circumscribed, flat discoloration of the skin up to 1 cm in diameter	Hypopigmentation, hyperpigmentation, or permanent vascular abnormalities of the skin
Patch	Circumscribed, flat discoloration of the skin > 1 cm	Same as above
Papule	Circumscribed, elevated, superficial, solid lesion up to 1 cm in diameter	Metabolic deposits, localized hyperplasia of cellular components of the epidermis or dermis, or localized cellular infiltrates in the dermis
Wheal	Rounded or flat-topped elevation in the skin of any size	Dermal edema
Nodule	Palpable, solid, rounded or ellipsoidal lesion in the dermis or subcutis that is deeper than a papule	Neoplasia, inflammation, or metabolic deposits
Vesicle	Circumscribed, elevated lesion up to 1 cm in diameter containing fluid	Separation of epidermal cells or of cells at the dermoepidermal junction and infiltration with fluid
Bulla	Circumscribed, elevated lesion > 1 cm that contains fluid	Enlargement of a vesicle or confluence of vesicles
Pustule	Circumscribed elevation of the skin that contains purulent fluid	Inflammation
Tumor	Neoplastic mass of any structure at any depth	Neoplastic growth
Petechia	Circumscribed deposit of blood or blood pigment up to 1 cm in diameter	Hemorrhage
Purpura	Circumscribed deposit of blood or blood pigment > 1 cm in diameter	Hemorrhage

SCREENING DIAGNOSTIC TESTS

Screening diagnostic tests are those tests that are easily completed as part of a routine office procedure, or for which samples are obtained on an outpatient basis and sent to a reference laboratory. These tests may also be definitive, yielding confirmation of a specific diagnosis. The screening diagnostic tests include skin scraping, Wood's lamp (ultraviolet lamp), potassium hydroxide (KOH) preparation, fungal and bacterial cultures, direct smear, hematologic and biochemical testing, hormonal assays, cutaneous biopsy, and therapeutic trial. Interpretations of positive findings of screening diagnostic tests are given in Table 2-7.

Skin Scrapings

This simple procedure is indicated in all dermatologic diagnostic workups. A scalpel blade (dulled), coated with mineral oil, is used to scrape the skin surface. Superficial scrapings are sufficient for surface-dwelling parasites (such as *Cheyletiella* and *Sarcoptes*) and scrapings that draw blood are necessary for deeper dwellings parasites (such as *Demodex* and *Pelodera*).

Wood's Lamp (Ultraviolet Light, Black Light)

The diagnostic value of the Wood's lamp is limited to a screening and definitive test for *Microsporum canis.* The lamp must be used in a totally darkened room. The characteristic fluorescent color of areas positive for dermatophyte infection is a bright apple green. Individual broken hairs are examined; both the extrafollicular and intrafollicular portions of the hair shaft will fluoresce. Scales and many topical medications have a diffuse, dull white or blue color under the Wood's lamp. Negative fluorescence does not rule out *M. canis* because fewer than 50% of these infections routinely fluoresce.

KOH Preparations

Potassium hydroxide–dimethyl sulfoxide (KOH-DMSO) and/or chlorazo dye preparations are occasionally used to identify fungal arthrospores and/or hyphae. Much experience is necessary to accurately interpret a KOH preparation. Material from skin scrapings and plucked hairs are cleared with one of the solutions with 30 minutes' contact at room temperature or a few seconds with gentle heating. The cleared material is examined microscopically for arthrospores and hyphae. A negative KOH-DMSO preparation does not rule out fungal disease.

Fungal Culture

Two types of media are used routinely for fungal cultures: dermatophyte test medium (DTM) and Sabouraud's medium.

TABLE 2-4

Secondary Gross Morphologic Skin Lesions

Lesion	*Definition*	*Pathogenesis*
Scale	Accumulation of loose fragments of the stratum corneum	Abnormal keratinization
Crust	Dried exudate on the surface of a lesion	Results when serum, blood, or purulent exudate dries on the skin surface
Excoriation	Superficial punctate or linear excavations of epidermis	Trauma, such as scratching, biting, or rubbing (friction)
Erosion	An excavation in the skin limited to the epidermis not breaking the integrity of the dermoepidermal junction	Ruptured vesicle or mild trauma
Ulcer	Cavitation in the skin of irregular size and shape extending into the dermis	Trauma, tissue infarction, or parasites
Fissure	Linear break in the skin, sharply defined with abrupt walls	Excessive drying of the skin or trauma
Sclerosis	Circumscribed or diffuse hardening of the skin with nearly transparent epidermis	Dermal or subcutaneous edema, cellular infiltration, or collagen proliferation
Scar	Area of connective tissue replacing normal tissue lost through injury or disease	Healing process following an ulceration
Induration	Palpable thickening of the skin	Edema or cellular proliferation or infiltration
Lichenification	A diffuse area of thickening and scaling, with an exaggeration of the superficial skin markings	Chronic irritation
Hyperpigmentation	Excessive coloration of the skin	Increased melanin deposition or melanin incontinence

A sample for fungal culture is obtained by selecting individual, representative hairs or scale. Broken hair shafts, fluorescent hairs, or scale from nails are satisfactory specimens. Large amounts of hair should be avoided. There should be minimal preparation of the skin before sampling because the fungal spores and hyphae are in the keratin layers of the epidermis and hair. A light disinfection with alcohol can be used to remove surface contamination. For best results the hair or scales should be lightly embedded in the culture medium by cutting the specimen into the medium with a sterile scalpel blade.

Dermatophyte test medium is Sabouraud's medium with cycloheximide and chloramphenicol added to inhibit selected fungal and bacterial growth and phenol red added to act as a pH indicator. The pathogenic fungi utilize protein initially, producing alkaline metabolic products which turn the medium red. Nonpathogenic fungi usually use carbohydrates first and then use protein after the carbohydrates are used up; thus, there is a larger amount of growth before the medium turns red. The DTM is a useful medium if used correctly. A culture positive for dermatophyte growth must show colony growth and color change from yellow to red simultaneously (see Plate V-4), which can occur from 1 to 14 days but usually occurs within the first 7 days. Therefore, the cultures must be observed daily. The three common dermatophytes of dogs and cats all have white colonies. Contaminant fungi show colony growth, which is usually dark in color before a medium color change (see Plate V-5). All DTM culture media that have fungal growth, whether contaminant or pathogenic, change from yellow to red over time.

TABLE 2-5

Miscellaneous Gross Skin Lesions

Lesion	*Definition*	*Pathogenesis*
Furuncle	Deep necrotizing form of folliculitis with pus accumulation	Deep bacterial infection
Carbuncle	Coalescing of several furuncles	Deep bacterial infection
Abscess	Localized accumulation of purulent material so deep in the dermis or subcutis that the pus is not visible on the surface of the skin	Deep bacterial infection
Sinus	Tract leading from a suppurative cavity to the surface, or between cystic or abscess cavities	Chronic deep infection
Cyst	Sac that contains liquid or semisolid material	Plugging of an orifice

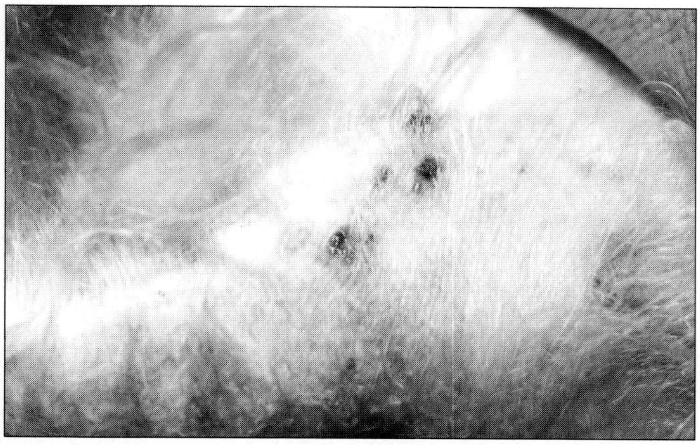

A

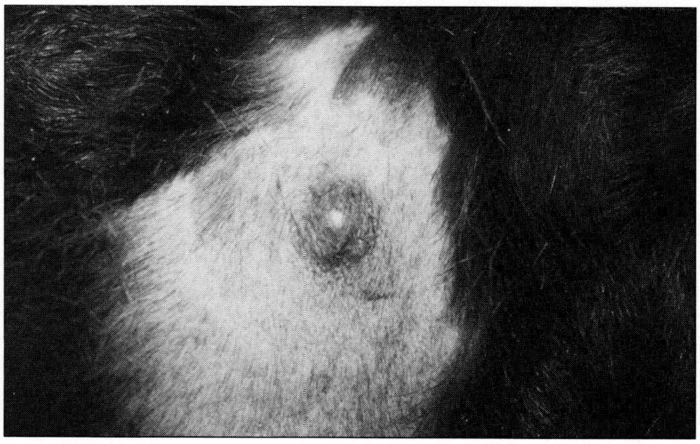

B

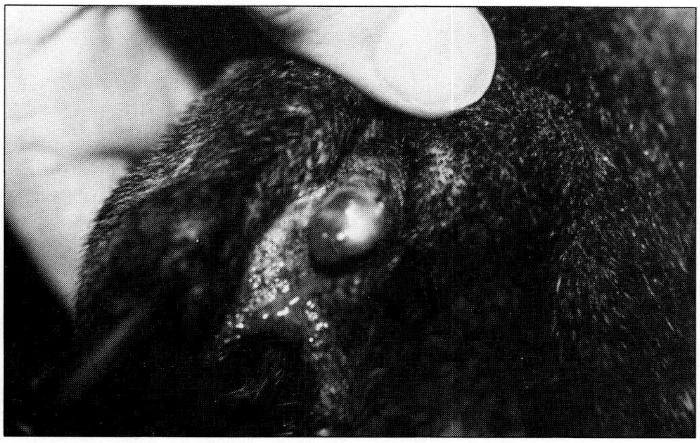

C

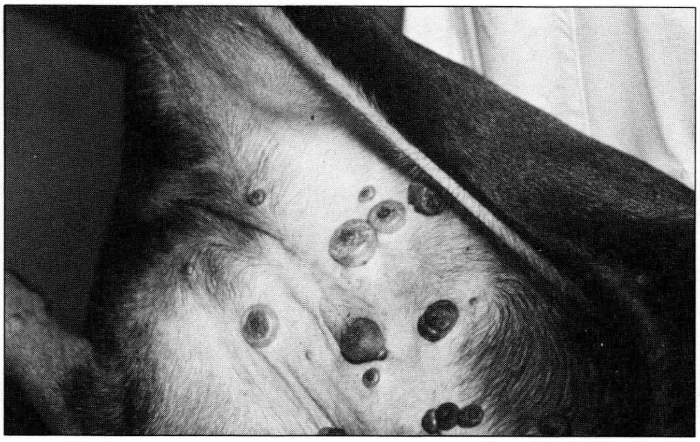

D

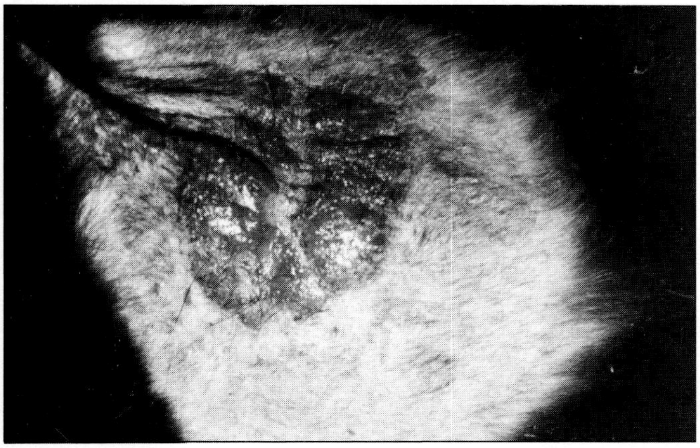

E

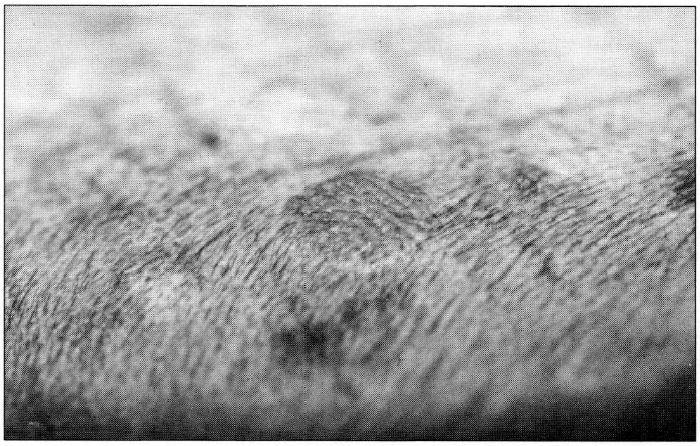

F

Figure 2-1. Primary and secondary lesions. **A**, Maculopapular eruption on the ventrum associated with fleabite dermatitis. **B**, Pustular eruption consisting of a fluid-filled structure containing purulent material. **C**, Nodule, a palpable solid mass. **D**, Tumor, a nodule containing neoplastic cells; these are papillomas. **E**, Plaque, a large, flat-topped lesion; erythematous in this case. **F**, Wheal, a superficial elevation with a smooth rounded surface resulting from edema; this one is an allergy test site. **G**, An erosive to ulcerative dermatosis seen in association with pyotraumatic dermatitis. **H**, Pronounced scaling in a dog with epidermal dysplasia. **I**, Facial crusting in a puppy with dermatomyositis.

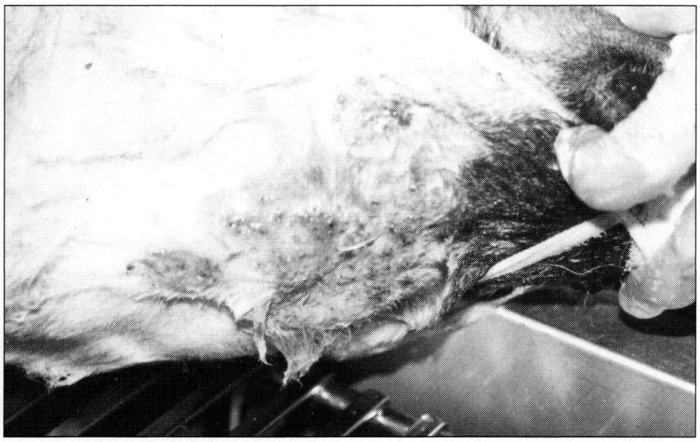

G

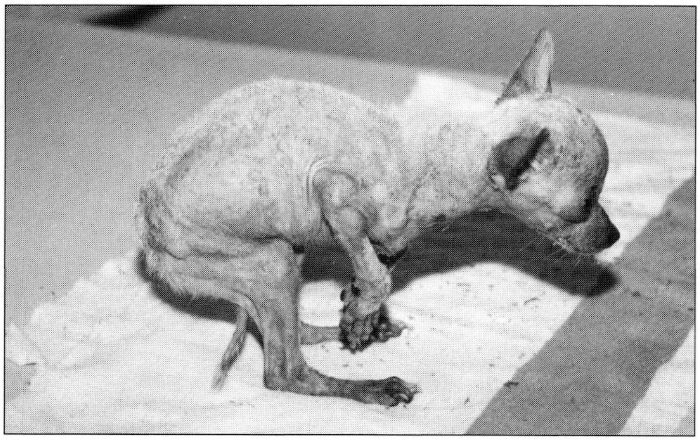

H

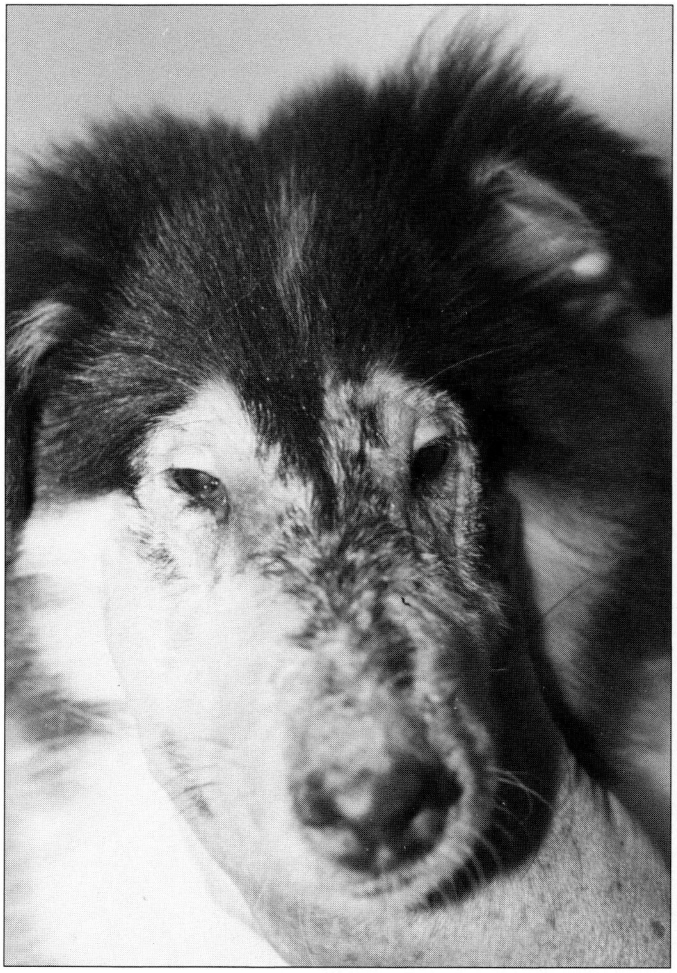

I

Sabouraud's medium without color indicator also can be used. Each pathogenic and contaminant fungus has characteristic surface colony growth. The reverse side (bottom of plate) also shows characteristic color changes. Gross colony appearance and growth characteristics often are sufficient to make a specific genus and species identification on both Sabouraud's medium and DTM if the technician has had sufficient experience. The pathogens can be easily differentiated from contaminant growth by microscopic examination. Specific details of fungal identification are given in Chapter 8.

An acetate tape technique is a simple method for obtaining a satisfactory mount for microscopic examination. The steps for performing this test are described in Figure 2-2. The microscopic appearance of several fungi can be found in Chapter 8.

Bacterial Culture and In Vitro Antibiotic Sensitivity Testing

Pyoderma is a frequently encountered dermatologic problem associated with many different diseases and syndromes. Whether the pyoderma is superficial or deep and primary or secondary, identification of the causative organism and determination of sensitivity of the bacteria to specific antibiotics often is important to the successful diagnosis and/or treatment of the condition. Specific indications for bacterial cultures are discussed in Chapter 7.

The proper technique of obtaining a specimen for bacterial culture is important. An intact superficial pustule is sampled differently than a crusty lesion or deep pyoderma. The clinician and technician should be familiar with the various techniques that are used to obtain a representative sample from different types of bacterial lesions. These techniques are outlined in Table 2-8. Commercially available transport media make possible the preservation of bacterial specimens to be sent to a reference laboratory.

Culturing of bacteria has been simplified by commercially available culture plates that contain several selective media. Pathogenic bacteria can be tentatively identified by their characteristic behavior on these selective media. In addition, Gram stains and microscopic examination can be used to help identify bacterial growth. The

TABLE 2-6

Morphologic Classification of Cutaneous Lesions

		Differential Diagnosis		
Category		*Canine/Feline*	*Canine Only*	*Feline Only*
Maculopapular	Macular	Allergic inhalant dermatitis Food allergy Allergic contact dermatitis Irritant contact dermatitis Drug eruption Erythema multiforme Lupus erythematosus Alopecia areata Endo/ectoparasitism	Acanthosis nigricans	
	Papular	Parasitic dermatoses Bacterial folliculitis Drug eruption Food allergy Dermatophytosis Comedones/acne Erythema multiforme	Vitamin A-responsive dermatosis Dermatitis herpetiformis Hormonal hypersensitivity	Miliary dermatitis Hypereosinophilic syndrome
Papulonodular	Nodular	Parasitic Deep pyoderma Atypical pyoderma Dermatophytosis Intermediate mycoses Deep mycoses Lupus profundus Neoplastic Dermoid cyst Nodular panniculitis Juvenile cellulitis Mucinosis Eosinophilic granuloma Periappendageal dermatitis Sterile pyogranuloma Calcinosis circumscripta	Superficial pyoderma	Abscess Acne Panniculitis
	Plaques	Dermatophytosis Urticaria Lymphoma	Bacterial hypersensitivity Lupus profundus Viral papillomatosis Calcinosis cutis Calcinosis circumscripta Histiocytoma Histiocytosis Keratoses Nevi Lichenoid dermatoses Mucinosis Erythema multiforme Acanthosis nigricans Dermatitis herpetiformis	Sporotrichosis Eosinophilic plaque Mast-cell tumor Linear granuloma Vitamin E deficiency Mucopolysaccharidosis Xanthomatosis Tumoral calcinosis
	Vegetative		Pemphigus vegetans Mast-cell tumor Cutaneous papilloma Sebaceous gland hyperplasia Squamous-cell carcinoma Transmissible venereal tumor Fibroma Nevi	
Vesiculopustular	Vesicular	Pemphigus Pemphigoid Erythema multiforme	Dermatomyositis Epidermolysis bullosa simplex Dermatitis herpetiformis	Lupus erythematosus

TABLE 2-6 (continued)

Morphologic Classification of Cutaneous Lesions

Category		Differential Diagnosis		
		Canine/Feline	*Canine Only*	*Feline Only*
	Pustular	Demodicosis Bacterial pyoderma Dermatophytosis	Subcorneal pustular dermatosis Sterile eosinophilic pustules Lupus erythematosus pustulosis	Abscess Acne Feline immunodeficiency virus (FIV) infection
Alopecia	Focal/ multifocal	Demodicosis Bacterial pyoderma Dermatophytosis Alopecia areata Cutaneous asthenia	Scleroderma	
	Patchy	Demodicosis Lice infestation Cheyletiellosis Dermatophytosis Drug eruption Lupus erythematosus Telogen defluxion	Protein deficiency Bronzing syndrome Color-mutant alopecia Spiculosis	Hyperadrenocorticism
	Regional	Discoid lupus erythematosus Hypothyroidism Hyperadrenocorticism	Growth hormone responsive Hyperestrogenism Hypoestrogenism Pattern baldness Testicular neoplasia Dermatomyositis Follicular dysplasia Toxicity	Feline endocrine alopecia Psychogenic alopecia
	Generalized	Dermatophytosis Systemic lupus erythematosus Drug eruption	Demodicosis	Alopecia universalis Hypotrichosis
Erosive-ulcerative	Parasitic		Fleas Demodicosis Sarcoptic mange	
	Microbial		Skin-fold pyoderma Pyotraumatic dermatitis Perianal pyoderma Bacterial granuloma	Superficial pyoderma Systemic mycosis Cat pox infection FIV infection Mycetoma Atypical mycobacteriosis
	Immune-mediated	Pemphigus Pemphigoid Cutaneous vasculitis Toxic epidermal necrolysis Drug eruption		
	Miscellaneous			Indolent ulcer Squamous-cell carcinoma Fleabite reactions
Exfoliative	Patchy	Ectoparasitism Dermatophytosis Drug eruption Pemphigus foliaceus Fatty acid deficiency	Pagetoid reticulosis Sjögren's syndrome Color-mutant alopecia Hyperestrogenism Vitamin A–responsive dermatosis Periappendageal dermatosis Generic dog food disease Subcorneal pustular dermatosis Chronic maculopapular dermatoses Parapsoriasis Food hypersensitivity Hypothyroidism	Protein deficiency Vitamin A deficiency Vitamin E deficiency Biotin deficiency Lynxacariasis

TABLE 2-6 (continued)

Morphologic Classification of Cutaneous Lesions

Category		*Differential Diagnosis* *Canine/Feline*	*Canine Only*	*Feline Only*
	Regional	Pemphigus foliaceus Pemphigus erythematosus Discoid lupus erythematosus	Hypothyroidism Zinc-responsive dermatosis Tyrosinemia Nasodigital hyperkeratosis	Cheyletiellosis
	Generalized	Dermatophytosis Drug eruption Systemic lupus erythematosus Pemphigus foliaceus Keratinization disorders	Demodicosis Hypothyroidism Vitamin E deficiency Ichthyosis Lymphoma Metabolic disorders	Cheyletiellosis Hypereosinophilic syndrome Lynxacariasis
Indurated	Turgid	Urticaria Angioedema	Myxedema Mucinosis Juvenile cellulitis	Growth hormone–secreting tumor Mucopolysaccharidosis
	Solid	Cellulitis Bacterial granuloma Fungal granuloma Calcinosis cutis Tumoral calcinosis Neoplasia	Scar Amyloidosis Intermediate mycoses Scleroderma Periappendageal dermatitis Chronic maculopapular dermatoses (lichenification)	
Pigmented	Red	Drug eruption Petechiae Purpura Vasculitis Contact dermatoses Lupus erythematosus Photodermatitis Erythema multiforme	Fold pyoderma Pyotraumatic dermatosis Histiocytoma Demodicosis	Eosinophilic plaque Linear granuloma
	White	Systemic lupus erythematosus Albinism	Vogt-Koyanagi-Harada syndrome Scleroderma Vitiligo Tyrosinase deficiency	Waardenburg syndrome Chédiak-Higashi syndrome
	Dark	Basal cell tumor Melanoma	Postinflammatory Hypothyroidism Hyperadrenocorticism Growth hormone responsive Acanthosis nigricans Lentigines Melanoma Vascular nevi Hemangioma Hemangiosarcoma Organoid nevus Melanocytic nevus	
	Skin-colored	Scleroderma Papilloma Sebaceous gland hyperplasia Callus Epidermal nevus Sebaceous nevus		

Adapted with permission from Ackerman LJ: *Practical Canine Dermatology*, ed 3.
Goleta CA, American Veterinary Publications, 1989, pp 12–19; and from Ackerman LJ: *Practical Feline Dermatology*, ed 3. Goleta, CA, American Veterinary Publications, 1989, pp 13–16.

TABLE 2-7

Interpretation of Routine Screening Diagnostic Tests

Screening Diagnostic Test (Positive)	*Differential Diagnosis* — *Include*	*Suggestive*
Skin scrapings	Parasitic	
Wood's lamp	Fungal	
KOH-DMSO preparation	Fungal	
Fungal culture	Fungal	
Direct smear	Neoplasia Bacterial	Neoplasia Bacterial Immune-mediated
Bacterial culture	Bacterial	
Blood screens (CBC, biochemical profiles)		Endocrine Neoplasia
Hormonal assays		
Thyroid	Endocrine (thyroid disease)	
Cortisol	Endocrine (hyperadrenocorticism)	
Sex hormones		Endocrine (gonadal dermatoses)
Cutaneous biopsy	Parasitic Bacterial (primary/secondary) Fungal Immune-mediated Neoplasia Panniculitis	Allergic Seborrheic Endocrine Immune-mediated Neoplasia

	Clinical Response					
	Complete		***Partial***		***None***	
	Include	*Exclude*	*Include*	*Exclude*	*Include*	*Exclude*
Therapeutic trial						
Corticosteroid	Allergic Parasitic Immune-mediated Neoplasia Panniculitis	Endocrine Fungal Bacterial (primary)	Allergic Seborrheic Bacterial Parasitic Immune-mediated Neoplasia Acral lick granuloma		Endocrine Fungal Bacterial Immune-mediated Parasitic Seborrheic Neoplasia	Allergic
Antibiotic	Bacterial (primary)	Endocrine Fungal Neoplasia Immune-mediated Seborrheic (primary) Parasitic	Fungal Endocrine Immune-mediated Neoplasia Parasitic Panniculitis Allergic			
Parasiticide	Parasitic Seborrheic (secondary) Allergic Bacterial (secondary)	Endocrine Fungal Immune-mediated Neoplastic	Allergic Parasitic Bacterial Seborrheic	Neoplastic Bullous Endocrine Fungal	Endocrine Immune-mediated Neoplasia Fungal Parasitic Bacterial Allergic Seborrheic	

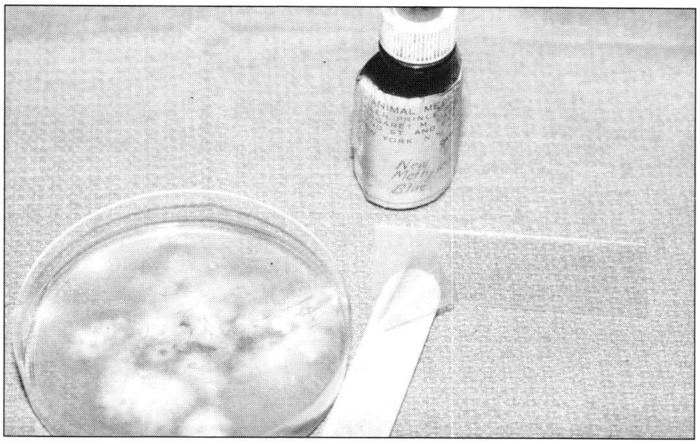

A

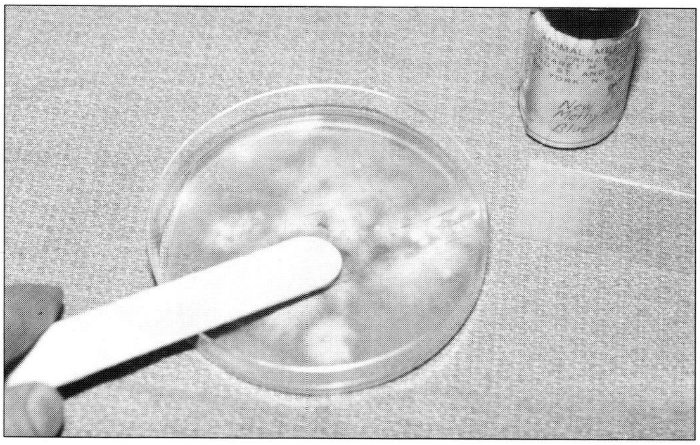

B

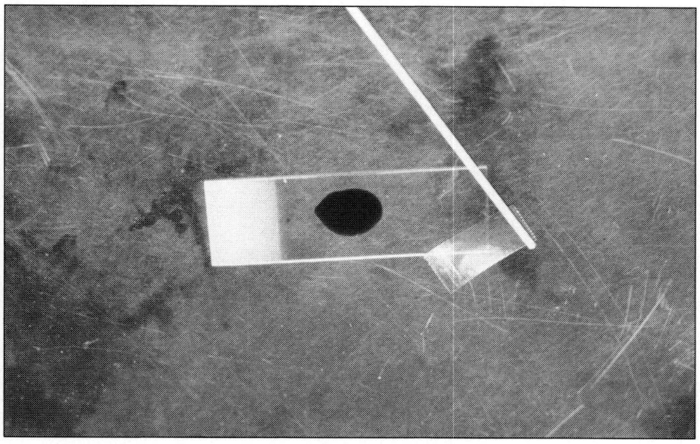

C

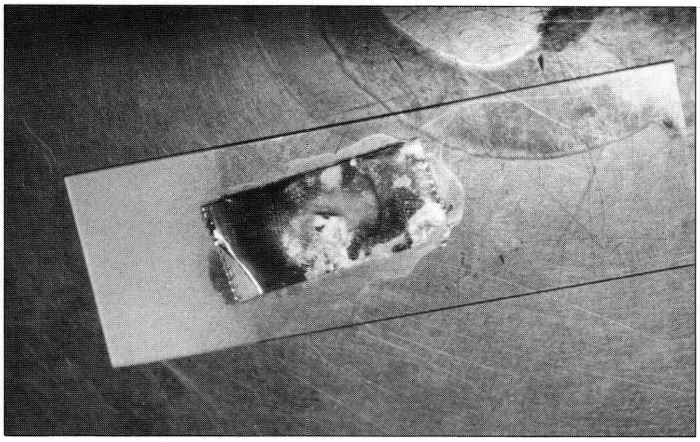

D

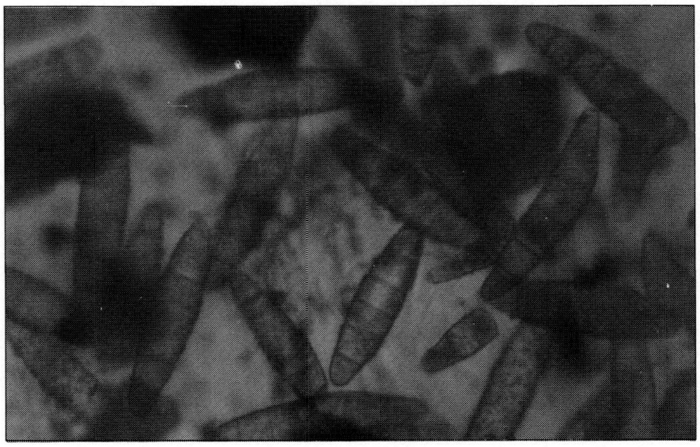

E

Figure 2-2. Acetate tape technique for fungal identification. **A**, Materials include fungal culture, applicator, acetate tape, microscope slide, lactophenol cotton blue, or new methylene blue. **B**, Gently touch tape, which is attached to the end of the applicator with the sticky tape surface outside, to the surface of the culture. **C**, Place tape with sticky surface down onto glass slide over drop of stain. **D**, Smooth tape on glass slide and examine under microscope. **E**, Macroconidia of *Microsporum gypseum* (low power).

manuals that accompany commercially prepared multimedia culture plates should be referred to for guidelines on identification.

Antibiotic sensitivity disks and dispensers also are readily available. Most of the multimedia plates are adapted for use with these disks. Refer to the laboratory manuals accompanying the plates and disks for specific techniques and interpretations. In vitro antibiotic sensitivity testing should be done only on single isolates, not on mixed bacterial growth. This diagnostic test is often reserved for staphylococcal isolates. Remember that sensitivity to antibiotics in vitro does not assure they will be effective in vivo.

Blood Screens

Hematologic testing, including a differential white blood cell count and serum biochemical testing, is helpful for some differential diagnoses but there are no general etiologic classifications in which these screening blood tests are definitive. In the majority of conditions in both dogs and cats with primary skin disease, the blood cell indices and biochemical profiles are within the normal range if they are not influenced by therapy, such as the administration of glucocorticoids. More abnormali-

TABLE 2-8

Bacterial Sampling Techniques

Type of Lesion	*Technique*
Superficial pustule	1. Clip hair around lesion, if necessary, avoiding trauma to surface of pustule. 2. Gently wipe surface of pustule with alcohol and let dry. 3a. Open pustule with No. 10 or No. 11 sterile scalpel blade. b. Force exudate to surface by carefully squeezing open pustule. c. Touch sterile swab to the exudate avoiding contact with surrounding skin or hair. or 4a. Aspirate exudate from pustule using a fine needle and syringe. b. Place exudate from syringe and needle onto sterile swab. 5. Streak directly onto agar plate or place in transport medium.
Crusty lesion	1. Clip hair around lesion, if necessary, leaving crust intact. 2. Gently wipe surface of crust and surrounding area with alcohol and let dry. 3. Remove crust with forceps using as aseptic a technique as possible. 4. Rub sterile swab over the moist surface directly beneath the crust avoiding contact with surrounding area. 5. Streak directly onto agar plate or place in transport medium.
Deep pyoderma with tract but no pustule	1. Clip hair from site of lesion. 2. Wipe surface of lesion with alcohol and let dry. 3. Apply pressure to deeper layers of skin, forcing the exudate onto the surface. 4. Touch sterile swab to exudate avoiding contact with surrounding skin or hair. 5. Streak directly onto plate or place in transport medium.
Deep pyoderma with unruptured pustule	1. Clip hair from area, if necessary, avoiding trauma to pustule. 2. Gently wipe surface with alcohol and let dry. 3a. Open pustule with No. 10 or No. 11 sterile scalpel blade. b. Insert swab into cavity and rub vigorously. or 4a. Aspirate exudate from pustule using a fine needle and syringe. b. Place exudate from syringe and needle onto sterile swab. 5. Streak directly onto agar plate or place in transport medium.
Deep pyoderma with ulcerated skin	1. Clean area of lesion with soap and water. 2. Swab area with alcohol. 3. Infiltrate lesion subcutaneously with local anesthetic. 4. Use 6-mm biopsy punch to obtain plug of skin at the site to be cultured. 5. Carefully split the plug longitudinally, cutting from the bottom to the surface with a No. 10 or No. 11 sterile scalpel blade. 6. Place sterile swab into the midsection of the split biopsy and rub vigorously avoiding contact with the surface. 7. Streak directly onto agar plate or place in transport medium.

ties are associated with endocrine diseases than most other disease classifications. Borderline anemia and hypercholesterolemia are sometimes associated with canine hypothyroidism. Hyperadrenocorticism is characterized by lymphopenia, eosinopenia, neutrophilia, and elevated alkaline phosphatase. A T-lymphocyte immunodeficiency is suspected if the absolute lymphocyte count is less than 1000 cells/mm^3.

Cutaneous Biopsies

Indications. Biopsies are indicated in any skin condition characterized by nodules, tumors, vesicles, bullae, or any lesions that are unresponsive to symptomatic therapy, or in those lesions in which specific causative factors have not been identified. Biopsies can help deny or confirm the presence of some parasites and fungi.

Cutaneous biopsies are diagnostically valuable if they provide a definitive diagnosis or deny or suggest a clinical diagnosis. The latter two indications require the clinician to correlate the history, clinical findings, and other laboratory data with histologic findings.

Contraindications. There are only a few absolute contraindications for cutaneous biopsies, such as animals that have uncontrollable hemorrhage. Sepsis should be

TABLE 2-9

Cutaneous Biopsy Techniques

Biopsy Technique	*Procedure*	*Indications*
Punch	1. Equipment and supplies: 4-mm or 6-mm disposable biopsy punch, needle holder, skin suture, smooth thumb forceps, fine sharp-sharp scissors, 2 × 2 gauze sponges, formalin. 2. Carefully clip (not close) lesion only if needed, avoiding removal of scale or crust on surface. 3. Do not wash or disinfect the biopsy site because the diagnostic value of the specimen may be on the surface. 4. Inject 0.3 to 0.5 ml of local anesthetic subcutaneously. 5. Place biopsy punch on exact site to be biopsied and drill into tissue with rotary motion in one direction, applying moderate pressure. There will be less resistance when punch reaches subcutis. 6. Withdraw punch. The plug should follow punch to surface if cut to an adequate depth. 7. Carefully lift plug with fine smooth forceps or a fine needle and cut all base of plug including some fat with scissors or scalpel blade. 8. Close wound with one or two skin sutures. 9. Place specimen in 10% buffered formalin and submit to laboratory.	All types of solid skin lesions if total excision is not indicated All small lesions, up to 5 mm, that can be totally excised
Needle aspiration	1. Equipment and supplies: syringe (6 ml to 12 ml), hypodermic needle (25 to 20 gauge), clean glass slides, stain, microscope. 2. Carefully clip hair from lesion, avoiding trauma to surface. 3. Prepare biopsy site with surgical scrub. 4. Insert sterile needle attached to syringe into the lesion while creating a firm vacuum with syringe. (Needle and syringe sizes depend on size of lesion and density of tissue or content.) When material is aspirated into the syringe, withdraw the needle after allowing the pressure to equalize. 5. If initial aspiration is nonproductive, carefully move needle back and forth several times within the tissue while aspirating. 6. Place aspirate in the needle and syringe on the clean glass slides; spread it to make a thin film. 7. Select appropriate stain or send to reference laboratory.	To characterize cell type or contents of a mass (tumor, nodule) or cavity (cyst, vesicle, pustule) without surgical invasion
Excisional	1. Equipment and supplies: sterile surgical pack (drape, scalpel handle and blade, hemostats, needle holder, suture needles, smooth thumb forceps, scissors, gauze sponges, suture), formalin. 2. Carefully clip hair from lesion and surrounding area avoiding trauma to skin. 3. Clean surgical site with soap and water, rinse, apply 70% alcohol avoiding vigorous scrubbing. 4. Inject local anesthetic subcutaneously, using ring block, or use general anesthesia. 5. Make an elliptical excision of the full depth of skin to the subcutis. 6. Close the wound in a routine manner. 7. Submit specimen in 10% buffered formalin.	Total removal of small nodules, cysts, vesicles, and tumors
Incisional	Steps 1, 2, 3, and 4 are same as excisional biopsy technique. 5. Select a biopsy site on basis of a representative tissue, access to biopsy site, and minimal postsurgical complications. 6. Be prepared to control excessive hemorrhage on large or active lesions. 7. Make a full-thickness incision to subcutis in form of wedge or ellipse, removing a section at least 5-mm wide. 8. Close the wound in a manner to prevent postsurgical complications. 9. Submit specimen in 10% buffered formalin.	To obtain a specimen for histopathologic examination from a large mass which cannot be totally excised because of size, location, or for cosmetic reasons.
Direct impression smear	1. Equipment and supplies: microscope, glass slides, cover slips, stain, sterile cotton-tipped applicator sticks, and scalpel blade (optional). 2. Carefully clean the area of debris and blot away excessive blood, serum, or contaminating exudate. 3. Obtain sample by (1) pressing a clean slide firmly against lesion to transfer cells to slide or (2) gently scraping the lesion with scalpel blade and transfer material to glass slide, or (3) collecting material on a sterile cotton-tipped applicator and then rolling it onto slide. 4. Select appropriate stain or submit to laboratory.	To characterize cell type or debris on the surface of any lesion

TABLE 2-10

Glossary of Dermatopathologic Terms

Term	*Definition*	*Correlation with Gross Morphologic Structure*
Acantholysis	Loss of coherence between epidermal cells as a result of degeneration of intercellular cement substance and intercellular bridges	Vesicles, bullae
Acanthosis	Increase in thickness of the stratum spinosum	Lichenification, plaque
Bulla-vesicle	Cavity formed either within or beneath the epidermis and filled with fluid	Vesicles, bullae
Crust	Coagulated tissue fluid and blood plasma intermingled with degenerated inflammatory cells and epithelial cells	Crust
Dyskeratosis	Faulty keratinization of individual epidermal cells	Keratinization disorder
Atrophy		
Epidermal	Thin epidermis with a decrease in the number of epidermal cells	Thin skin
Dermal	Decrease in the upper dermal connective tissue	Thin skin
Erosion	Superficial loss of epithelium; dermis is intact	Erosion
Granulation tissue	Newly formed, edematous collagenous tissue arising in wounds, healing ulcers, or inflammatory processes	Scar, sclerosis
Hyperkeratosis	Excessive thickness of the stratum corneum	Scale
Intercellular edema (spongiosis)	Edema between squamous cells causing an increase in the width of the space separating them	Edema
Liquefaction degeneration of basal cells	Type of degeneration causing vacuolation of basal cells	Vesicles, erosion, ulceration
Microabscess	Small accumulations of cells in the epidermis	Pustule, papule
Parakeratosis	Incomplete keratinization, showing retention of nuclei in the horny layer and absence of a granular layer	Scale
Ulcer	Area in which the epidermis and also part of the dermis are absent	Ulcer
Hyperpigmentation	Increase in melanin pigment in the epidermis, dermis, or both	Hyperpigmentation

considered in debilitated animals or in those receiving immunosuppressive drugs, although this is rarely a problem and is not a valid reason for not performing a biopsy.

Choice of Biopsy Site. A small specimen taken from a carefully chosen site can yield more information about the dermatosis than a large piece of skin removed from a poorly chosen site. If the site chosen has clinically diagnostic features, the histologic features are more likely to be diagnostic.

General guidelines to follow for selection of the biopsy site include (1) in generalized dermatoses, select a lesion that is typical, not subjected to trauma, not encrusted, and not modified by treatment; (2) select a fully developed lesion, but if there are stages in the evolution of a lesion, multiple biopsies of the different stages should be obtained; (3) avoid scarred lesions; and (4) remove small vesicles or bullae intact.

Biopsy Techniques. Five methods are commonly used to obtain cutaneous biopsies, including excisional, incisional, needle aspiration, direct impression smear, and cutaneous punch. Each type of biopsy procedure is outlined in Table 2-9.

An *excisional biopsy* is a complete surgical excision of the lesion, which has the advantage of diagnosis and treatment in one procedure. A large sample can be obtained for a histologic examination. This technique is used routinely for removing small nodules, cysts, vesicles, and tumors.

An *incisional biopsy* is the partial excision of a lesion. This technique is used when the lesion is too large to totally excise easily. It also is indicated in those lesions that do not lend themselves to surgical removal. Both excisional and incisional biopsies may require general sedation or anesthesia if the lesion is large or in a difficult location.

Needle aspiration biopsy is the technique of removing cells or their contents from a lesion by negative pressure in a syringe. This is a simple, nonsurgical method of characterizing many cysts, nodules, tumors, and pustules. The staining and examining of cells or their contents may yield a diagnosis or suggest one, often directing the clinician to another diagnostic procedure.

The *impression smear* is most helpful when there is potentially diagnostic material (cells or their contents) on the surface of a lesion. It also can be used in conjunction with excision of larger masses by making a direct smear from a cut surface of the excised mass.

The *punch biopsy* technique is the most commonly used cutaneous biopsy procedure. In many instances, only a local anesthetic is required. Trauma, hemorrhage, and postbiopsy problems are minimal. Disposable biopsy punches have made this procedure a routine diagnostic test in many hospitals.

Handling the Biopsy Specimen. Care must always be exercised when handling biopsy specimens. The microscopic architecture of the tissue can be disrupted by injecting the anesthetic intradermally, by crushing the tissue, or by stretching the tissue. The tissues should be placed in individual containers and carefully labeled. Cutaneous biopsies submitted to the pathologist should be accompanied by the following information: age, sex, and breed; history; description of gross lesions(s); duration of lesion; clinical diagnostic test data; treatment; and clinical diagnosis or impressions (a list of differential diagnoses).

Interpretation of Histopathologic Findings. Familiarity with the common dermatopathologic terms (Table 2-10) can be invaluable when interpreting the histopathology report and attempting subsequent correlation with the history, clinical findings, and laboratory data.

All histopathology reports should include information concerning the depth of the lesion and the specific structures involved and what microscopic pathologic process was found, including description, distribution, and, if possible, the interpretation of the pathogenesis of the process. It is the clinician's responsibility to read the pathology report and to correlate the pathologic findings with the history, clinical findings, and therapeutic responses. Only then will the biopsy have the most diagnostic value.

Therapeutic Trials

Therapeutic trial is often the most valuable screening diagnostic test used for differential diagnoses based on history and clinical signs (Table 2-2). Corticosteroids are widely used to differentiate between etiologic classifications of pruritus (see Table 3-9). Only the short-acting corticosteroids should be used. Clinical response must be carefully evaluated, taking into consideration the dosage used, the duration of therapy, and any concurrent diagnostic or therapeutic procedures.

Antibiotic therapeutic trials must also be carefully evaluated. The antibiotic of choice (see Table 3-11) for the test must be selected on the basis of the history of previous antibiotic therapy, the respective clinical response, the dosage and the duration of antibiotics used, the clinical signs, and the concurrent diagnostic and therapeutic procedures.

Therapeutic trials with parasiticides (see Table 3-5) are indicated if a specific parasitic disease (for example, sarcoptic mange, fleas) is suspected on the basis of history and/or clinical signs and has not been identified with other screening diagnostic tests.

The clinician must have the systematic approach clearly defined before initiating any therapeutic trial. Concurrent use of corticosteroids and antibiotics does not allow differentiation of allergic disease from primary bacterial disease. Similarly, concurrent administration of corticosteroids and parasiticides does not differentiate between primary parasitic and allergic disease; however, these drugs may be helpful diagnostic tests if used singularly.

General Classifications of Dermatologic Disease (Diagnostic Key 1) should be used as a guide for the initial history, physical examination, and selection of diagnostic tests, as well as for making a list of differential diagnoses based on general etiologic classifications of skin disease. If the steps and procedures discussed in this chapter are understood and implemented, a definitive diagnosis will often be determined. Therapeutic trials frequently become the treatment of choice as well as diagnostic tests. If the specific causative factor has not been defined and the problem is not resolved, a more definitive diagnostic workup using the specific diagnostic disease keys (Diagnostic Keys 2 through 13) is indicated.

THE GENERAL DERMATOLOGIC DIAGNOSTIC KEY

General Classifications of Dermatologic Disease (Diagnostic Key 1) places all canine and feline skin diseases into etiologic classifications.

Dermatologic diagnostic keys (Diagnostic Keys 2 through 13) can be the most important aid in achieving maximum efficiency when working up any skin disease. The diagnostic keys assist the clinician by focusing on pertinent history, clinical signs, and screening diagnostic tests that will help to establish a list of differential diagnoses in a minimal amount of time. The diagnostic keys can also serve as a basis for an organized in-depth discussion with the pet owner about the various aspects of the differential diagnoses.

SELECTED READINGS

Ackerman L: A new approach to dermatologic diagnosis in the dog. *Vet Focus* 1(1):6–11, 1989.

Griffin CE: Diagnostic approach to dermatologic disease, in Nesbitt GH (ed): *Contemporary Issues in Small Animal Practice. Dermatology.* New York, Churchill Livingstone, 1987, pp 1–19.

DIAGNOSTIC KEY 1

General Classifications of Dermatologic Disease

Etiologic Classification	*History*	*Clinical Signs*	*Screening/Definitive Tests*
Allergic	Pruritus; responsive to corticosteroids; cats responsive to megestrol acetate	Variable erythema, excoriation, ulcers, plaques, crusts	Skin scrapings; therapeutic trials with parasiticides and corticosteroids; diet testing; intradermal (ID) skin testing; ELISA allergy test
Parasitic (external including *Demodex*)	Parasites observed; responsive to parasiticides; variable contagion	Evidence of parasites (fleas, lice, *Cheyletiella, Otodectes*)	Skin scrapings; parasiticide therapeutic trial
Bacterial	Responsive to antibiotics: variable pruritus	Pustules, papules, crusts, hyperpigmented macules, focal alopecia	Skin scrapings; bacterial culture; direct smear; antibiotic therapeutic trial
Fungal	No response to antibiotics and corticosteroids; slowly progressive alopecia	Scales, crusts, alopecia—focal or generalized; broken hairs	Skin scrapings; Wood's lamp; fungal culture; KOH preparation; biopsy
Endocrine	Pruritus—none to mild; slowly progressive alopecia; slow regrowth of hair after clipping	Alopecia—partial to complete and focal to generalized; no inflammation; scaling—variable	Skin scrapings; fungal culture: biochemical profile; complete blood count (CBC); T_3/T_4 TSH stimulation; ACTH stimulation: low- or high-dose dexamethasone suppression; estrogen assay
Immune-mediated	Poor response to antibiotics and low-dose corticosteroids; variable pruritus	Bullae, vesicles, ulcers, erosions, crusts, hypopigmentation; distribution—often facial and pinnae initially	Skin scrapings; biopsy; direct immunofluorescence; therapeutic trial with high-dose corticosteroids
Neoplastic	Poor response to antibiotics and corticosteroids; variable pruritus	Nodules, scales, crusts, ulcers, excoriation	Skin scrapings; biopsy; direct smear
Keratinization disorders (seborrhea)	Partial response to antibiotics, corticosteroids, and shampoos; progressive and/or persistent; often concurrent disease; variable pruritus	Scales; oily or dry skin; variable inflammation; alopecia—partial, focal, regionalized or generalized	Skin scrapings; T_3/T_4, TSH stimulation; fungal culture; biopsy; ID skin test; diet test
Miscellaneous Physical and chemical disorders Congenital/hereditary disorders Diseases of unknown/multiple causes Diseases of anal sacs Diseases of the ear	Variable; dependent upon specific disease entity	Variable	Skin scrapings; biopsy; therapeutic trials

DIAGNOSTIC KEY 2

Allergic Disease

Etiologic Classification	*History*	*Clinical Signs*	*Screening/Definitive Tests*
Canine atopy (atopic dermatitis)	Seasonal or nonseasonal pruritus; progressively worse with age; familial history; face, feet, axillary predilection; age of onset 1 to 4 years; low-dose cortisone responsive	Maculopapular eruptions; mild to severe erythema, excoriation, scales, crusts, papules, pustules; variable alopecia; salivary stain of feet	Intradermal skin test; ELISA test
Feline atopy	Seasonal or nonseasonal pruritus: methylprednisolone acetate responsive	Signs are variable including miliary dermatitis, alopecia, indolent ulcer, eosinophilic or linear granuloma; feline asthma	Intradermal skin testing
Allergic contact dermatitis	Nonseasonal pruritus; age of onset often > 2 years; cortisone responsive; contact distribution	Maculopapular eruptions; ventral distribution most common; mild to severe excoriation, erythema, alopecia, crusts	Isolation and provocative exposure; open patch test
Food allergy	Nonseasonal pruritus; age of onset often > 2 years; variable response to corticosteroids	Maculopapular eruptions; mild to severe erythema, papules, crusts, excoriation, and alopecia; variable distribution in dogs; often head and neck lesions in cats	Diet testing
Flea allergy dermatitis	Fleas observed; seasonal or nonseasonal pruritus with lesions on dorsal caudal back and abdomen; often dorsal neck (cats); often concurrent atopy; partial or complete response to parasiticides; responsive to corticosteroids	Maculopapular eruptions. Dog: erythemic papules on ventral abdomen; erythema and crusts on dorsal, caudal back; alopecia; superficial pyoderma; secondary seborrhea; acute moist dermatitis. Cats: miliary dermatitis on dorsal neck, shoulders, and trunk	Intradermal skin testing; therapeutic trial with parasiticides
Tick bite hypersensitivity	Marked pruritus or skin reaction associated with presence of tick	Marked erythema/ granulomatous reaction at site of tick attachment	No diagnostic test available
Ear mite hypersensitivity	Severe pruritus associated with ear mite infestation	Marked pinneal erythema and crusting; ear mite infestation	Otoscopic examination and direct smear of debris
Hormonal hypersensitivity	In females recurrence of pruritus at the same stage of the estrous cycle; often worse with each recurrence In males chronic, nonseasonal pruritus	Pruritus with or without dermatitis over lower back, perineum, and posteromedial thighs	Intradermal skin testing with hormones; neuter

DIAGNOSTIC KEY 3

Immune-Mediated Disease

Etiologic Classification	*History*	*Clinical Signs*	*Screening/Definitive Tests*
Lupus erythematosus			
Systemic	Systemic disease concurrent with skin lesions; lesions exacerbated with sunlight; poor response to antibiotics; partial response to low-dose steroids	Maculopapular eruptions; papules, ulcerations, and crusts on face and ears; variable erythema and alopecia; may be scaling, scarring, purpura, lymphedema, hypopigmentation, and secondary pyoderma	Antinuclear antibody (ANA); biopsy; direct immunofluorescence
Discoid	Facial dermatitis; poor response to antibiotics; partial response to low-dose steroids; lesions exacerbated by sunlight	Scales, crusts, erosions, and ulcerations on nasal planum and dorsal muzzle; hypopigmentation; variable erythema	Biopsy; direct immunofluorescence
Pemphigus			
Pemphigus vulgaris	Poor response to antibiotics and low-dose steroids; may be systemic signs	Oral and mucocutaneous vesicles and ulcerations; nail bed lesions with sloughing of nails; focal or multifocal truncal ulcerations and crusts	Biopsy; direct immunofluorescence
Pemphigus vegetans	Rare; generalized proliferative dermatitis not involving mucocutaneous junctions; poor response to antibiotics and low-dose steroids	Crusts, alopecia, and erythema; multifocal or diffuse, verrucose superficial lesions; some erosions and ulcerations; pustules common	Same as above
Pemphigus foliaceus	Facial and generalized proliferative dermatitis not involving mucocutaneous junctions; poor response to antibiotics and low-dose steroids; variable pruritus	Bullae, scales, crusts, erosions, variable erythema and alopecia, and pustules on face, ears, and trunk; hyperkeratotic footpads	Sames as above
Pemphigus erythematosus	Lesions localized to face; otherwise nondistinguishable from pemphigus foliaceus	Scale, crusts, and exudative lesions of nose, pinnae, and periorbitally; hypopigmentation	Same as above
Pemphigoid			
Bullous pemphigoid	Usually mucocutaneous and oral lesions; poor response to antibiotics and steroids; variable pruritus; collies, Shetland sheep dogs predisposed	Vesicles, pustules, ulcers, crusts, and variable erythema; oral, periorbital, neck, axillae, ventral abdomen, and footpads	Same as above
Cicatricial pemphigoid	Primarily affects mucous membranes; very rare; chronic	Vesicles; erosions; scarring	Same as above
Drug eruption	Skin lesions following administration of drug; remission upon withdrawal of drug	Variable lesions including vesicles, erosions, ulcers, crusts, papules, and pustules	Provocative exposure to drug (usually done inadvertently)
Erythema multiforme	Most often associated with drug reaction or pyoderma	Macules, papules, urticarial plaques, vesicles/bullae, erosions, and ulcerations of limbs and ventrum; usually symmetric; "target" lesions	Biopsy
Toxic epidermal necrolysis	Painful ulcerative lesions; slow healing; concurrent systemic disease	Diffuse, deep focal or multifocal ulceration	Biopsy
Cutaneous vasculitis	Usually secondary to other diseases, but may be idiopathic	Elevated bruise (palpable purpural) on dependent parts of body, feet, and ears; erosions and ulcers; depressed area with scarring	Biopsy; various tests to identify primary cause

DIAGNOSTIC KEY 3 (continued)

Immune-Mediated Disease

Etiologic Classification	*History*	*Clinical Signs*	*Screening/Definitive Tests*
Juvenile cellulitis (puppy strangles)	Dachshund, golden retriever, Labrador retriever, pointers at highest risk; puppies (< 4 months)	Facial edema, ulceration, nodules, induration with scarring; submandibular lymphadenopathy; draining tracts	Biopsy
Sterile pyogranuloma	Nonbacterial pododermatitis; Great Dane, St. Bernard, shar pei, pit bull terrier, English bulldog predisposed	Firm, erythematous nodules interdigitally; frequent ulceration and drainage	Biopsy
Uveodermatologic syndrome (Vogt-Koyanagi-Harada-like)	Granulomatous panuveitis and hypopigmentation; Akita, Samoyed, Siberian husky predisposed	Hypopigmentation of nose, lips, eyelids	Biopsy
Alopecia areata	Patches of asymptomatic, noninflammatory alopecia	Focal to multifocal, noninflammatory alopecia; usually asymmetric on head, neck, or trunk	Biopsy
Scleroderma	Asymptomatic, focal alopecic plaques	Smooth, alopecic areas which are thickened on palpation (plaque); trunk and limbs	Biopsy
Sjögren's syndrome	Syndrome with keratoconjunctivitis sicca, dry mouth (xerostomia), and connective tissue disease	Variable clinical signs including keratinization disorders, erythroderma, and hypothyroidism may be present; keratoconjunctivitis sicca; lupus erythematosus, rheumatoid arthritis, etc.	Biopsy of lacrimal gland; ANA; rheumatoid factor
Dermatitis herpetiformis	Rare, pruritic, papulocrustaceous disease of dogs; poor response to antibiotics and steroids	Papules, pustules, scaling, and erythema; generalized distribution	Biopsy
Sterile eosinophilic pustulosis	Acute onset; poor response to antibiotics	Papules and pustules; scales, crusts, alopecia, and hyperpigmentation; peripheral eosinophilia	Biopsy; complete blood count

DIAGNOSTIC KEY 4

Parasitic Disease

Etiologic Classification	*History*	*Clinical Signs*	*Screening/Definitive Tests*
Fleas			
Ctenocephalides felis *Pulex irritans*	Fleas or flea excrement observed; responsive to parasiticides; pruritus variable	Maculopapular eruption; caudal, dorsal distribution of alopecia and scale; fleas or flea excrement	Parasiticide therapeutic trial
Mites *Sarcoptes scabiei* (dog)	Severe pruritus, nonresponsive to low-dose steroids; contagion to humans and other animals	Maculopapular eruptions; crusting of ear margins and elbows; excoriation, papules on ventral abdomen	Skin scrapings; parasiticide therapeutic trial
Notoedres cati (cat)	Intense pruritus, poor response to low-dose steroids and megestrol acetate; contagion to humans or animals	Maculopapular eruptions; crusts, scales, excoriation of ears, face, and neck	Skin scrapings; parasiticide therapeutic trial
Cheyletiella yasguri (dog) *C. blakei* (cat)	Usually young animal; dorsal dandruff; pruritus—none to moderate; contagion to humans and animals	Exfoliative dermatosis; excessive dorsal scaling; minimal inflammation	Skin scrapings; parasiticide therapeutic trial
Demodex canis (dog) *D. cati* (cat)	Nonpruritic if no pyoderma; progressive focal or generalized alopecia; may resolve without treatment, pyoderma common with poor response to antibiotics	Maculopapular, exfoliative or erosive-ulcerative dermatosis; focal, alopecic, hyperpigmented macules or patch on face, feet, or trunk; may be generalized distribution; variable erythema; pyoderma common	Skin scrapings; biopsy
Otodectes cynotis	Pruritus of ears; head shaking; waxy discharge from external ear canal	Mites, wax, and debris in external ear canal; excoriation at base of ear; occasional focal alopecia, erythema, and excoriation on head, neck, or back	Otoscopic examination; skin scraping
Ticks *Rhipicephalus sanguineus* *Dermacentor andersoni* *D. variabilis* *Amblyomma americanum* *Ixodes dammini*	Observed ticks; history of exposure to endemic tick area; pruritus—none to minimal	Ticks seen on head, neck, trunk, or feet; focal crust and erythema at site of tick attachment	None required
Otobius megnini	Head shaking, pain, and pruritus of ear region	Mites and wax in ear canal; excoriation at base of ear	Otoscopic examination
Lice *Trichodectes canis* (dog) *Heterodoxus spiniger* (dog) *Linognathus setosus* (dog) *Felicola subrostratus* (cat)	Parasites of all stages observed; mild pruritus or asymptomatic	Exfoliative or maculopapular eruption; lice present on haired areas of body; mild, focal alopecia and inflammation	None required
Pelodera strongyloides	Exposure to straw bedding and damp soil; intense ventral pruritus	Maculopapular eruptions; ventral erythema, papules, crusts, scales	Skin scrapings; larvae in washed bedding
Trombiculiasis *Eutrombicula alfreddugesi*	Pruritus; orange-red larvae observed	Maculopapular eruptions; scaling, erythematous papules, alopecia on head, neck, axilla, and feet; parasites observed	Skin scrapings; parasiticide therapeutic trial
Myiasis Calliphorid flies Sarcophagid flies	Fly larvae–infested wound; foul odor from lesion; systemic toxic signs	Erosive-ulcerative dermatitis; ulcerated lesion with larvae; signs of toxicity	None needed
Hookworm dermatitis (dog) *Ancylostoma caninum* *Uncinaria stenocephala*	Intense pruritus of all feet; history of hookworm exposure or infestation	Erythema, edema, and pain in all feet if acute; hyperkeratotic footpads if chronic; may have paronychia	Fecal examination; anthelmintic therapeutic trial
Cutaneous dirofilariasis *Dirofilaria immitis* (dog)	Skin lesions concurrent with positive heartworm test or with heartworm disease	Erythema, alopecia, papules or ulcerating nodules of head, neck, trunk, and limbs	Microfilariae test; skin scrapings; biopsy; therapeutic trial with dirofilaricide

DIAGNOSTIC KEY 5

Canine Bacterial Disease

Etiologic Classification	*History*	*Clinical Signs*	*Screening/Definitive Tests*
Surface pyodermas			
Pyotraumatic dermatitis	Predisposed by ectoparasites, trauma, grooming, otitis, anal sacculitis; most common in thick-coated dogs; acute onset; intense pruritus; painful	Maculopapular or erosive-ulcerative dermatosis; discrete, edematous erythematous, alopecic patch	Skin scrapings; bacterial culture if refractory to symptomatic treatment; parasiticide therapeutic trial
Skin-fold pyoderma			
Lip fold	Anatomically predisposed; common in Cocker spaniel, setter breeds, springer spaniel; halitosis common	Erosive-ulcerative dermatitis; ulcers, erythema, crusting of lip folds	Same as above
Vulvar fold	Predisposed by obesity and anatomical factors; constant licking of vulvar region	Erosive-ulcerative lesions; erythema and crusting of vulvar margins and perivulvar area	Same as above
Facial fold	Anatomical predisposition in brachycephalic breeds; variable facial pruritus; foul odor	Erosive, moist surface; debris accumulation in facial folds	Same as above
Tail fold	Boston terrier and English bulldog anatomically predisposed; minimal pruritus	Debris accumulation in tail folds; moist, erosive surface	Same as above
Superficial pyodermas			
Impetigo (juvenile pustular dermatitis)	Predisposed by unsanitary environment and crowding; puppy 4–12 weeks of age; distribution of lesions on nonhaired areas	Maculopapular or vesiculopustular lesions; pustules and papules in groin and axillae	Skin scrapings; direct smear; antibiotic therapeutic trial
Superficial folliculitis	Often secondary to parasitic, allergic, and endocrine diseases; variable pruritus; most common in young dogs	Maculopapular or vesiculopustular lesions; acute stage—pustules, papules, crusts, variable erythema; chronic stage—alopecia, hyperpigmented macule	Skin scrapings; direct smear; antibiotic therapeutic trial; bacterial culture if refractory to treatment; thyroid function tests
Dermatophilosis	Predisposed by chronic moist skin and concurrent flea dermatitis, seborrhea, or chronic folliculitis	Dorsal and medial thigh distribution; papules, pustules, crusts; hyperpigmentation and alopecia in chronic lesions	Direct smear
Deep pyodermas			
Furunculosis	Predisposed by demodicosis; immune deficiency; often young dog <1 year of age; predilection for muzzle, dorsum of nose, pressure points; German shepherds—high incidence and usual recurrence	Maculopapular and erosive-ulcerative dermatosis; fistulas with exudate; erythematous pustules and papules; scarring	Skin scrapings; biopsy; bacterial culture from biopsy; thyroid function tests; direct smears
Cellulitis	Commonly seen with furunculosis of German shepherds and other chronic deep pyodermas; lethargy and anorexia may be reported	Warm, diffuse, edematous, erythematous weeping lesions most common on rear limbs; commonly associated with fistulous tracts	Same as above
Interdigital pyoderma	Often secondary to demodicosis, allergy, immune deficiency; most common in Great Danes, English bulldogs, German shepherds, boxers, and dachshunds; often chronic or recurrent; poor or partial response to antibiotics commonly observed; lameness observed	Moist interdigitally; pustules; hemorrhagic bullae; pyogranulomas; ventral feet often erythematous and edematous with pustules; often peripheral lymphadenopathy	Same as above
Callous pyoderma	Common on elbows and hocks of large breeds (Great Dane, St. Bernard) and sternum (dachshund, Doberman pinscher); secondary to pressure and trauma	Pustules; pyogranulomas; ulcers; occasional fistulous tract	Same as above

DIAGNOSTIC KEY 5 (continued)

Canine Bacterial Disease

Etiologic Classification	*History*	*Clinical Signs*	*Screening/Definitive Tests*
Pyonychia	Usually chronic; variable foot licking and pain; one or more nails may separate or fall off; often resistant to treatment	Exudate and crusting around nail bed; variable erythema; nail may be split or separate easily from nail plate	Same as above
Perianal pyoderma	Associated with anal sacculitis and perianal fistulas; most common in German shepherd and Irish setter breeds	Fistulous tracts perianally; variable erythema and ulceration	Biopsy; bacterial culture

DIAGNOSTIC KEY 6

Feline Bacterial Disease

Etiologic Classification	*History*	*Clinical Signs*	*Screening/Definitive Tests*
Surface pyodermas	Associated with "mouthing" by the queen; young kittens; no systemic signs	Alopecia, papules, pustules, and crusts on dorsal neck	Direct smear
Superficial pyoderma (folliculitis)	Associated with feline acne; variable pain and pruritus; antibiotic responsive	Alopecia, erosions, ulcers, crusts	Culture; biopsy; direct smear
Deep pyoderma			
Folliculitis	Associated with feline acne; variable pain and pruritus	Alopecia, erosions, ulcers, crusts; fistulous tracts; peripheral lymphadenopathy	Same as above
Subcutaneous abscess	Recent cat bite; acute onset of fluid-filled lesion; may notice after rupture; pyrexia; often painful	Fever; subcutaneous abscess; focal erythema; alopecia and crusts variable	Aspiration; direct smear; culture
Cellulitis	Recent cat bite or trauma; painful; acute, diffuse, soft-tissue swelling; painful; often anorexic	Diffuse soft-tissue swelling; usually one extremity; erythema; fever; peripheral lymphadenopathy; alopecia or easy epilation of hair	Direct smears; culture
Miscellaneous pyodermas			
Cutaneous tuberculosis	Young adult cats; occurs in bovine tuberculosis–endemic areas; often no systemic signs	Single or multiple ulcers, abscesses, plaques and nodules; thick yellow to green exudate; head, neck, and extremity distribution	Culture; biopsy with acid-fast stain
Feline leprosy (atypical mycobacterial granuloma)	Usually young cat (1–3 years); subcutaneous nodules; poor response to antibiotics	Solitary or multiple nodules or abscess in subcutis; may be ulcerative	Same as above
Actinomycotic mycetoma			
Actinomycosis	Chronic nonhealing wound; no systemic signs; poor response to antibiotics	Subcutaneous abscess; ulceration; draining tracts	Direct smear; culture; biopsy
Nocardiosis	Chronic subcutaneous nodules with concomitant lung disease	Ulcerated nodules; cellulitis; draining abscesses	Direct smears; culture; biopsy

DIAGNOSTIC KEY 7

Fungal Disease

Etiologic Classification	*History*	*Clinical Signs*	*Screening/Definitive Tests*
Superficial mycoses			
Microsporum canis	Nonresponsive to antibiotics and steroids; variable pruritus; may be human or animal contagion	Focal or diffuse alopecia of head, neck, extremities, or trunk; variable scaling; cats frequently asymptomatic	Wood's lamp; KOH preparation; fungal culture; biopsy
M. gypseum	Nonresponsive to antibiotics and steroids; history of soil contact; variable pruritus	Heavy scales and crusts; focal alopecia; head and extremities most common distribution	KOH preparation; fungal culture; biopsy
Trichophyton mentagrophytes	Nonresponsive to antibiotics or steroids; often large areas of body involved; usually pruritic	Focal or diffuse alopecia, erythema, and hyperpigmentation; scaling or crusting moderate to severe	KOH preparation; fungal culture; biopsy
Intermediate mycoses			
Aspergillosis	Secondary to immune suppression; respiratory signs usually predisposed to skin lesions	Nodules or ulcers of skin or nasal membranes; nasal discharge; systemic signs	KOH preparation; fungal culture (Sabouraud's agar); biopsy
Eumycotic mycetoma	Predisposed by trauma to extremities; nonresponsive to antibiotics	Nodule with draining tract; granules (grains) in exudate; swelling; abscessation; lesions predominantly on feet	KOH preparation of crushed granules; fungal culture (Sabouraud's agar); biopsy
Phaeohyphomycosis	Solitary nodule occurs at site of penetrating wound; nonpainful	Solitary nodule; may see exudate; usually on extremities	Fungal culture (Sabouraud's agar); biopsy
Pythiosis (Oomycosis)	Exposure to warm climates with stagnant water; trauma predisposes to infection	Papulonodular dermatitis: induration; ulceration; draining tracts	Biopsy; fungal culture (Sabouraud's agar)
Sporotrichosis	Often lymph node and cutaneous lesions; poor response to antibiotics and steroids; tender draining nodules	Subcutaneous, firm nodules; crusted ulcers; thick brownish-red exudate; regional lymph nodes swollen and ulcerative	Direct smear of aspirate; fungal culture (Sabouraud's agar); impression smears; biopsy
Zygomycosis	May have both gastrointestinal and cutaneous signs; poor response to all therapy	Nodules; ulceration; draining tracts; often regional extremities	Fungal culture (Sabouraud's agar); biopsy
Systemic mycoses			
Blastomycosis	Chronic debilitation; primary respiratory signs with later onset of skin lesions; poor response to antibiotics and steroids	Cutaneous and subcutaneous nodules, abscesses, ulcers, and fistulous tracts; marked lymphadenopathy; usually multiple lesions	Direct smear; biopsy; serology
Coccidioidomycosis	Intermittent respiratory signs prior to onset of skin lesions; poor response to antibiotics and steroids	Granulomatous nodules; abscesses with draining tracts; ulcers	Serology
Cryptococcosis	Cats more commonly affected; chronic course of multiple facial lesions; poor response to antibiotics and steroids	Ulcers or granulomatous nodules; occasional abscesses with mucoid exudate on the face; may have CNS signs	Direct smear of exudate; biopsy
Histoplasmosis	Chronic respiratory or large bowel disease with late onset of skin lesions; poor response to antibiotics and steroids	Subcutaneous nodules, ulcers, and fistulous tracts	Serology; direct smear; biopsy

DIAGNOSTIC KEY 8

Endocrine Disease

Etiologic Classification	*History*	*Clinical Signs*	*Screening/Definitive Tests*
Hypothyroidism	Nonpruritic to mildly pruritic; slowly progressive alopecia; lethargic; sensitive to cold; rare in cats; slow regrowth of hair	Symmetric alopecia of trunk or extremities; mild to marked scaling; often dry, lusterless haircoat; secondary folliculitis is common	Baseline T_3/T_4; TSH response test; complete blood count
Hyperadrenocorticism (Cushing's disease)	Polyuria and polydipsia (85%); polyphagia; progressive thinning of truncal haircoat; rare in cats	Symmetric truncal alopecia; mild to moderate hyperpigmentation; thin skin; pendulous abdomen; comedones on ventrum; may have calcinosis cutis; ecchymotic hemorrhages associated with venipuncture	Complete blood count; absolute eosinophil count; biochemical screen; ACTH response test; dexamethasone suppression tests; ACTH serum level
Growth hormone–responsive dermatosis (dog)	Breed predilection for keeshonds, chow chows, pomeranian, airedale, samoyed, and American water spaniel; age of onset 1–3 years; males predominantly; nonpruritic; normal thyroid and adrenal function tests	Multifocal areas of alopecia with marked hyperpigmentation on neck, trunk, and perineum	Growth hormone stimulation test; biopsy
Hyperestrogenism (dog)	Intact middle- to older-aged; abnormal estrous cycle; pruritus—none to moderate	Lichenification and hyperpigmentation with variable alopecia of posterior abdomen, perineum, and perivulvar areas; gynecomastia; vulvar hyperplasia	Clinical response to ovariohysterectomy
Estrogen-responsive dermatosis (dog)	Middle-aged to older female; ovariohysterectomy at young age; progressive alopecia	Infantile haircoat or alopecia on abdomen, ventral neck, and ears; infantile vulva and nipples	Therapeutic trial with estrogens
Testicular tumors	Breeds at risk (Chihuahua, boxer, pomeranian, miniature schnauzer, miniature and standard poodle, shetland sheepdog, Siberian husky, Yorkshire terrier); age of onset >7 years; often cryptorchid; pruritus with advanced clinical signs	Often unilateral cryptorchid; if scrotal testicles, one large and one small; alopecia and hyperpigmentation of perineum, ventral-abdomen, and posterolateral trunk	Serum estrogen levels; testicular biopsy

DIAGNOSTIC KEY 9

Keratinization Disorders (Seborrhea)

Etiologic Classification	*History*	*Clinical Signs*	*Screening/Definitive Tests*
Primary idiopathic seborrhea	Cocker spaniel, springer spaniel, Irish setter, basset hound, West Highland white terrier, Doberman pinscher, shar pei, Labrador retriever have highest incidence; partial response to antibiotics, steroids, and baths	Variable—dry to greasy coat, minimal to marked inflammation periocular, interdigital, axillae, and perineum; variable multifocal or diffuse scaling and crusting; often secondary pyoderma and ceruminous otitis	Rule out all other primary causes
Secondary keratinization defects	Identification of a primary disease; partial response to symptomatic treatment	Dog: scaling, crusting, greasiness, and alopecia; variable inflammation and pruritus Cat: generalized dry skin and coat with excessive scaling	Skin scrapings; fungal culture; therapeutic trials with parasiticides, antibiotics, shampoos; thyroid function tests; allergy tests; biopsy
Epidermal dysplasia	Congenitohereditary defect in West Highland white terriers; early age of onset; pruritic	Scaling with variable erythema, alopecia, hyperpigmentation and lichenification; lesions most common on extremities, axillae, perineum, and medial thighs	Biopsy
Ichthyosis	Hereditary disease; age of onset <6 months; progressive scaling and hyperkeratosis with age	Generalized scaling with tightly adhered tannish-gray scales with feathered keratinous projections; hyperkeratotic margins of footpads	Biopsy
Fatty acid deficiency	Feeding poor quality food or food stored at high temperatures; slow onset of lusterless coat	Dry, lusterless coat; prominent scaling; secondary pyoderma	Therapeutic trial with fatty acid supplementation
Zinc-related dermatoses			
Syndrome I	Siberian husky, malamute, Doberman pinscher, and Great Dane predisposed; age of onset about one year; clinical signs may be precipitated by stress	Erythema, crusting, scaling, and alopecia around mouth, chin, surface of joints of extremities, scrotum, prepuce, or vulva; variable hyperpigmentation	Biopsy; therapeutic trial with zinc supplementation
Syndrome II	Rapidly growing puppy fed zinc-deficient diet or on high calcium or high cereal diet; often several in litter; may be depressed and anorexic	Focal hyperkeratotic plaques and crusts on head, trunk, and extremities; thickening and fissuring of footpads and planum nasale; lymphadenopathy common	Therapeutic trial with balanced diet and zinc; biopsy
Syndrome III	Associated with feeding some generic dog foods; onset of signs 2 to 4 weeks after feeding food without supplementation; may be lethargic and depressed; variable pruritus	Heavy crusting and scaling on distal extremities, face, pressure points, and trunk; variable erythema, alopecia, hyperpigmentation and lichenification	Same as above
Vitamin A–responsive dermatosis	Cocker spaniel has highest incidence; Labrador retriever and cairn terrier also affected; rancid skin odor	Follicular plugging and hyperkeratotic plaques; ventral and lateral trunk distribution; variable alopecia, scaling and papules; dry, dull haircoat	Therapeutic trial with vitamin A
Periappendageal dermatitis (sebaceous adenitis)	Highest incidence in standard poodles; also reported in samoyeds, Irish setters, golden retrievers, Labrador retriever, and collie; age of onset 1–5 years	Symmetric scaling and alopecia beginning on dorsum; secondary pyoderma common	Biopsy

DIAGNOSTIC KEY 9 (continued)

Keratinization Disorders (Seborrhea)

Etiologic Classification	*History*	*Clinical Signs*	*Screening/Definitive Tests*
Footpad hyperkeratosis	Secondary to many different primary diseases	Footpads are thickened, cracked, and scaly; other signs vary with primary etiology	Skin scraping; blood profile; fungal culture; biopsy; cats—feline serology
Lichenoid-psoriasiform dermatosis	Springer spaniels affected; age of onset <3 years; poor response to symptomatic treatment	Erythematous lichenoid papules and plaques; pinnae and ventral abdomen; may become generalized	Biopsy
Follicular dysplasia/dystrophy			
Color-mutant alopecia	Breed predilection for blue Doberman pinscher, dachshund, Great Dane, whippet, Italian greyhound, standard poodle and fawn Irish setter; sparse haircoat and slowly progressive alopecia at <1 year of age; poor response to symptomatic therapy	Generalized thin haircoat with patches of alopecia; papules and scale; often superficial folliculitis	Direct examination of hair shaft; biopsy
Black hair follicular dysplasia	Observed in mongrel, papillon, dachshund; black and white color; hair fails to grow on black patches	Alopecia on black skin; scaling	Biopsy
Acne	Dogs: Great Dane, Boxer, Doberman pinscher, English bulldog, bull terrier at highest risk; variable pruritus if secondary infection; age of onset—3–12 months; often spontaneous recovery	Papulopustular reaction; common to progress to nodules and furuncles; chin and lips	Biopsy
Schnauzer comedo syndrome	Miniature schnauzer predisposed; recurrent or persistent dorsal eruptive dermatitis; may have concurrent hypothyroidism	Soft, waxy comedones or crusted papules on dorsum of trunk and neck	Thyroid function tests; biopsy
Keratoses	Asymptomatic unless inadvertently traumatized	Gross appearance varies from plaques to proliferation hornlike growths; often hyperpigmented and greasy	Biopsy
Callus	Predisposed by repeated trauma on pressure points	Hyperkeratotic plaques; may be pustules, furnuncles, draining tracts; elbows; hocks, sternum	Biopsy

DIAGNOSTIC KEY 10

Canine Cutaneous Neoplastic and Cystic Disease

Etiologic Classification	*History*	*Clinical Signs*	*Screening/Definitive Tests*
Tumors of epithelial origin			
Epidermoid, sebaceous, and epidermal inclusion cysts	No discomfort or inflammation unless ruptured; slow increase or static in size	Fluctuant or firm nodule of varying size in dermis or subcutis; gray to brownish cheesy contents in lumen (sebaceous); hair in lumen (inclusion)	Aspiration biopsy; excision biopsy
Tumors of epithelial origin			
Perianal gland adenoma	Breeds at risk: dachshund, cocker spaniel, English bulldog, Samoyed, Afghan, beagle; male 8–12 years; rare in females; often pruritic	Solitary or multiple erythematous nodules located perianally and occasionally on prepuce; may be ulcerated	Aspiration biopsy; excision biopsy
Squamous cell carcinoma	Breeds at risk: Scottish terrier, Pekingese, boxer, poodle, Norwegian elkhound, dalmation, bull terrier, black Labrador retriever, black standard poodle; predisposed or exacerbated by sunlight on white skin; poor response to antibiotics and steroids	Erosion and ulceration of lips and nose; local invasion; may be diffuse ulceration of digit, pad, ventral abdomen, and eyelids	Incision biopsy; excision biopsy; radiographs of bone under lesion
Sebaceous gland tumor			
Nodular hyperplasia Adenoma Epithelioma	Breeds at risk: cocker spaniel, poodle, Kerry blue terrier, Boston terrier, beagle, dachshund, Norwegian elkhound, basset hound; slow growing, often static for years; usually no discomfort or inflammation	Firm, solitary or multiple 0.2- to 2-cm discrete dome or pedunculated nodules that are hairless, often multilobulated	Excision biopsy
Adenocarcinoma	Rapidly growing; locally invasive and metastatic; often local inflammation	Large, raised ulcerated mass lacking discrete borders	Excision biopsy
Papilloma (wart)	Breeds at risk: cocker spaniel, Kerry blue terrier; common in young dogs; usually multiple; occasionally dysphagic; spontaneous remission in 6–8 weeks	Initially small, whitish-raised mass on oral mucosa and lips; later rough, cauliflower-like surface; occasional small solitary or multiple nodules on medial thigh, face, or eyelid	Excision biopsy
Basal cell tumor	Breeds at risk: cocker spaniel, poodle; slow growth; age of onset >6 years; solitary	Firm, circumscribed, hairless discrete tumor; usually pink, glistening surface on lips, eyelids, pinnae, trunk, or legs	Excision biopsy
Trichoepithelioma	Breed at risk: cocker spaniel; locally invasive subcutaneous dorsal nodule	1- to 10-cm firm subcutaneous tumor on trunk; may be ulcerated	Excision biopsy
Intracutaneous cornifying epithelioma (keratoacanthoma)	Breeds at risk: generalized—German shepherd, Old English sheepdog, collie; multicentric—Norwegian elkhound, keeshond; young males <5 years	Dermal or subcutaneous nodules 0.5–4 cm with a pore opening to surface; keratin plug in pore; back, neck, thorax, and shoulder	Excision biopsy
Pilomatrixoma	Breeds at risk: Kerry blue terrier, poodle; solitary growth; average age of onset—6 years	Firm, circumscribed, alopecic, elevated; frequently ulcerated; variable size; calcification common	Excision biopsy
Tumors of mesenchymal origin			
Lipoma	Breeds at risk: dachshund, cocker spaniel, Weimaraner, Labrador retriever; slowly growing asymptomatic subcutaneous mass	Well-circumscribed oval or round subcutaneous mass of varying size; consistency is soft to firm	Aspiration biopsy; excision biopsy

DIAGNOSTIC KEY 10 (continued)

Canine Cutaneous Neoplastic and Cystic Disease

Etiologic Classification	*History*	*Clinical Signs*	*Screening/Definitive Tests*
Liposarcoma	Breeds at risk: dachshund, Brittany spaniel; male; >10 years; locally invasive; rarely metastatic	Poorly circumscribed, firm, subcutaneous mass of varying size; usually ventral abdomen or thorax	Excision biopsy
Mastocytoma (mast cell tumor)	Breeds at risk: boxer, Boston terrier, English bulldog, bull terrier, fox terrier, dachshund, Staffordshire terrier, Labrador retriever, Weimaraner; age of onset >6 years; single or multiple	Firm, solitary or multiple dermal or subcutaneous tumors of varying size; may be ulcerated; may have systemic signs with peripheral lymphadenopathy	Aspiration biopsy; excision biopsy; hemogram; buffy coat smear
Hemangiopericytoma spindle cell tumor, dermatofibroma	Breeds at risk: boxer, German shepherd, cocker spaniel, fox terrier, springer spaniel; onset at average age 10 years; slow growth	Firm, raised, smooth or lobulated mass on extremities, often with indistinct borders; ulceration and infection common	Incision biopsy; excision biopsy
Cutaneous histiocytoma	Breeds at risk: boxer, dachshund, cocker spaniel, Great Dane, Shetland sheepdog; age of onset <3 years; rapid growth; may spontaneously regress in 2–3 months	Solitary 0.3- to 5-cm dome or "button" shaped, firm, well-circumscribed, erythematous mass; occasionally ulcerated; rarely multiple	Excision biopsy
Hemangioma	Breed at risk: Boxer; most common in middle-aged dogs; range of 6 months to 15 years; ulcerated lesion that bleeds easily; solitary or multiple	0.5- to 3-cm ovoid, soft, spongy, discrete, dark red tumor of dermis or subcutis; often ulcerated; extremities, neck, and face	Aspiration biopsy; excision biopsy
Hemangiosarcoma	Breeds at risk: boxer, German shepherd, Bernese mountain dog; rapid growth; appears as subcutaneous hemorrhage; metastatic	Large, firm, poorly circumscribed tumor; inflammation in surrounding tissue	Hemogram; biochemical profile; radiographs; excision biopsy
Fibroma	Breeds at risk: boxer, fox terrier, dachshund; female predilection; aged dog; slow growing	Firm or soft, discrete raised tumors of variable size and shape; occasionally pedunculated; may have alopecic surface	Excision biopsy
Fibrosarcoma	Breed at risk: cocker spaniel; rapid course; locally invasive and metastatic	Firm, irregular shaped, poorly circumscribed tumor; often ulcerated; edema and secondary infection common	Hemogram; biochemical profile; radiographs; excision biopsy
Cutaneous lymphosarcoma	Breeds at risk: boxer, basset hound, St. Bernard, cocker spaniel, beagle, German shepherd, golden retriever, Scottish terrier; older dog of either sex; poor response to antibiotics and steroids; usually generalized; course of weeks to years; variable pruritus	Variable clinical signs and distribution; nodules, crusts, scales, erythema, ulceration, and alopecia	
Tumors of melanin-producing cells (melanoma)	Breeds at risk: Scottish terrier, cocker spaniel, Airedale, chow chow, springer spaniel, boxer, Irish setter, Irish terrier, Chihuahua, Doberman pinscher, Boston terrier; tumors of feet and mouth usually malignant; solitary skin tumors usually slow growing and benign; onset >7 years	Benign: discrete, alopecic, pedunculated dark masses; 1–4 cm in diameter; lip, eyelid, and occasional trunk distribution Malignant: poorly demarcated, variably pigmented, flattened or rounded tumors in the mouth or on the feet	Excision biopsy

DIAGNOSTIC KEY 11

Feline Cutaneous Neoplastic and Cystic Disease

Etiologic Classification	*History*	*Clinical Signs*	*Screening/Definitive Tests*
Tumors of epithelial origin			
Squamous cell carcinoma	High incidence in areas of intense sunlight; white cats predisposed; middle to older age; poor response to steroids and megestrol acetate	Usually solitary; firm, locally invasive; ulcerative with irregular borders on pinnae, lips, nose, or eyelid	Incision biopsy; excision biopsy
Basal cell tumor	Slow growing; >9 years average age of onset; usually small and solitary	Firm, well-circumscribed, round- or dome-shaped; often pigmented and ulcerated; occasionally has large central cyst	Excision biopsy
Trichoepithelioma	Slow growing; small and solitary	Small, firm, elevated growth; may be ulcerated	Excision biopsy
Sebaceous gland tumor			
Nodular hyperplasia, adenoma	Older cat; usually asymptomatic	Solitary; <0.5 cm in diameter; smooth or rough surface	Excision biopsy
Adenocarcinoma	Rare; older cat; locally invasive and metastatic; rapid growth	Solitary; firm, ulcerated mass lacking discrete borders; lymphadenopathy; lung lesions	Excision biopsy; radiographs
Papilloma (wart)	Older cat; predilection for face and limbs	Solitary; firm, discrete border; pedunculated; <0.6 cm in diameter; cauliflower-like surface	Excision biopsy
Tumors of mesenchymal origin			
Fibroma	Aged cat; usually solitary	Firm or soft; elevated; discrete border; variable size	Excision biopsy
Fibrosarcoma	Solitary tumors of aged cats; multiple tumors in kittens <4 months of age; locally invasive and metastatic	Aged cat: solitary, irregular or nodular growth of variable size; frequently ulcerated; limbs and trunk	
		Kitten: multiple tumors on trunk; often evidence of metastasis to lymph nodes and lung	Excision biopsy; radiographs
Mast cell tumor (mastocytoma)	Higher incidence in older males; majority are malignant; partial response to steroids and megestrol acetate	Variable clinical signs: firm, raised, dermal masses 0.5 to 5 cm in diameter; usually well-demarcated borders; some are soft and have nondiscrete borders; color pink, yellow or white; ulceration common; papules and plaques seen less frequently; splenomegaly and hepatomegaly common	Aspiration biopsy; excision biopsy
Hemangioma	Adult to aged cat; usually solitary	Discrete, 0.5 to 2 cm in diameter, round, bluish-red dermal or subcutaneous mass; friable	Excision biopsy
Lipoma	Adult to aged cat, slow growing	Well-circumscribed, subcutaneous mass of variable size and shape	Aspiration biopsy; excision biopsy
Tumors of melanin-producing cells (melanoma)	Uncommon; usually solitary; majority are malignant with metastasis at time of initial examination	Discrete, brown to black dome-shaped or pedunculated growth; variable size	Excision biopsy

DIAGNOSTIC KEY 12

Miscellaneous Diseases

Etiologic Classification	*History*	*Clinical Signs*	*Screening/Definitive Tests*
Physical/chemical disorders			
Irritant contact dermatitis	Sudden onset of pruritus at any age; clinical signs associated with recent exposure to potentially irritant physical or chemical agent	Acute erythema and edema; severe or chronic lesions with crusting, ulcerations, excoriation, and alopecia; may be scaling, hyperpigmentation, or scarring	Isolation and provocative exposure; skin scrapings; fungal culture; biopsy
Solar dermatitis (actinic dermatitis)			
Canine nasal solar dermatitis	Progressive lesions aggravated by sunlight; partial to complete response to steroids	Erythema, ulceration, crust, and scale at junction of haired and nonhaired skin of muzzle and planum nasale; hypopigmentation of planum nasale and nares	Biopsy; skin scrapings; fungal culture
Feline solar dermatitis	White cats with prolonged exposure to sunlight predisposed; chronic and progressive over years; variable pruritus	Initial: erythema of tips and margins of pinnae; alopecia, scales, crusts with chronicity; ear margins may curl Neoplastic stage: persistant ulceration; local invasion	Biopsy
Congenital and hereditary diseases			
Cutaneous asthenia (Ehlers-Danlos syndrome)	Breed predilection for springer spaniel and boxer dogs, Himalayan cats; multiple lacerations without trauma; skin tears easily, sags, and stretches excessively	Marked hyperextensibility of the skin; multiple lacerations; subcutaneous hematomas at site of skin lacerations	Biopsy
Color-mutant alopecia (dogs)	See Diagnostic Key 9		
Ectodermal defect	See Diagnostic Key 9		
Black hair follicular dysplasia	See Diagnostic Key 9		
Ichthyosis	See Diagnostic Key 9		
Diseases of unknown or multiple causes			
Acanthosis nigricans (dog)	Slowly progressive hyperpigmentation of axillae; variable pruritus; rancid odor; dachshund predisposed	Bilateral symmetric brown patch in axillae; then large gray to black acanthotic and lichenified patches, often seborrheic dermatitis; advanced lesions may involve forelegs, ventral thorax, and posterior abdomen	Biopsy
Canine acral lick dermatitis	Constant licking of localized area(s) of extremities; tendency for recurrence at same or new site following treatment	Alopecic, eroded or ulcerated plaques on extremities; variable size; periostitis may be present in chronic lesions	Biopsy, radiographs
Panniculitis	Acute onset; intermittent fever and anorexia; poor response to antibiotics; good response to steroids; age of onset in dogs often <6 months; occurs in older dogs; age of onset in cats 5–9 years	Multiple dermal nodules; variable size; usually firm but may be fluctuant; trunk and neck distribution; rupture with oily, brown exudate; secondary infection after rupture	Direct smear; deep biopsy; therapeutic trial with corticosteroids
Disease of anal sacs	Common in dogs, rare in cats; perianal scooting, biting, or licking; often diarrhea 1–3 weeks prior to signs; abnormal anal sac secretions or impaction; concomitant dermatoses observed	Abnormal anal sac secretions vary from greenish-yellow; exudate red, brown or black; opaque; dry and pasty; minimal odor to fetid; abscesses; perianal swelling and ulceration with tumors	Bacterial culture; direct smear; biopsy

DIAGNOSTIC KEY 13

Feline Dermatoses

Etiologic Classification	*History*	*Clinical Signs*	*Screening/Definitive Tests*
Eosinophilic granuloma complex			
Indolent ulcer (eosinophilic ulcer, rodent ulcer)	Nonpruritic; all ages; higher incidence in females; responsive to steroids and megestrol acetate; occasionally resolve without treatment	Well-delineated with ulcerated, necrotic center; variable size; mostly lip lesions; oral and trunk lesions seen	Feline serology; diet test; intradermal test; therapeutic trial of steroids
Eosinophilic plaque	Highly pruritic; age of onset 2–4 years	Well-circumscribed, raised, erythematous, exudative lesions; variable size; mostly on abdomen and groin; peripheral eosinophilia common	Complete blood count; diet testing; intradermal skin testing; therapeutic trial with steroids and parasiticides
Linear granuloma	Young cat; average age 1 year; higher incidence in females; often asymptomatic; spontaneous remission seen; steroid responsive	Well-circumscribed raised, erythematous to yellow; linear, papular or nodular; most common on caudal rear legs	Biopsy; diet testing; intradermal skin testing
Miliary dermatitis	Pruritus; may have hyperesthesia; personality changes; always associated with some primary cause (fleas and dermatophytes most often)	Multifocal papules or small crusts on dorsum; external parasites or flea excrement may be seen	Skin scrapes; Wood's lamp; fungal culture; fecal examination; complete blood count; diet testing; intradermal skin testing; therapeutic trial with parasiticides
Feline endocrine alopecia	Nonpruritic progressive alopecia; mostly neutered males and occasionally neutered females; middle-aged cats	Bilateral symmetric alopecia of perineum, ventral abdomen, thorax and forelimbs; no inflammation; easy epilation of hair	Hair examination; therapeutic trial with hormone replacement
Neurodermatitis (psychogenic alopecia)	Predilection for Burmese, Siamese, Himalayan, and Abyssinian; usually some change in life style preceding clinical signs; often poor response to steroids	Dermatitic form: solitary, discrete, excoriated, erosive, or ulcerated lesion; variable size; usually on an extremity, abdomen or flank Alopecic form: solitary or multifocal; partial alopecia with broken hairs; no inflammation	Skin scrapings; fungal culture; therapeutic trial with phenobarbital; intradermal skin testing
Feline leukemia virus infection	Systemic disease concurrent with skin problems secondary to immunosuppression	Cutaneous signs: chronic abscesses; susceptibility to other infections such as pyoderma and paronychia; cutaneous horns on footpads	Serology
Feline immunodeficiency virus infection	Systemic disease concurrent with skin problems secondary to immunosuppression	Cutaneous lesions: chronic abscesses, pyoderma, generalized parasitic infections (demodicosis, notoedric mange)	Serology
Poxvirus infection	Progressive, generalized dermatitis; no age, breed, or sex predilection; may have concurrent respiratory signs; usually spontaneous recovery in 1–2 months	Crusted papules, plaques, and nodules with erosive to ulcerative center and indurated borders; lips, face, feet, and dorsal trunk	Biopsy; serology; virus isolation

DIAGNOSTIC KEY 13 (continued)

Feline Dermatoses

Etiologic Classification	*History*	*Clinical Signs*	*Screening/Definitive Tests*
Hypereosinophilic syndrome	Rare, pruritic, eruptive dermatitis associated with tissue and peripheral eosinophilia	Maculopapular eruptions; crusts and scales	Biopsy; complete blood count; fecal examination
Plasma cell pododermatitis	Nonpainful swelling of multiple footpads; concurrent hypergammaglobulinemia	Soft, swollen footpads; usually central metatarsal or metacarpal pads; occasional ulceration; occasionally plasma cell stomatitis is observed	Aspiration biopsy; incisional biopsy
Xanthomatosis	Rarely seen concurrently with primary lipid metabolism disorders and more commonly secondary to factors that alter cholesterol or triglyceride metabolism (diabetes mellitus, progestagens)	Papules, plaques, ulcers, subcutaneous nodules; head and bony prominences	Biopsy; biochemical screen

Chapter 3

DERMATOTHERAPEUTICS

Lowell Ackerman, DVM
Gene H. Nesbitt, DVM, MS

The veterinarian can choose from a large number of topical and systemic drugs when treating canine and feline dermatologic diseases. Each class of drugs has its own indications for use in treating particular problems. To determine the appropriate therapy, the clinician must first recognize and characterize the lesions and try to categorize their cause. For example, is the lesion moist or dry, scaly or exudative, and deep or superficial? The veterinarian must also know the characteristics of the specific drugs so that the desired therapeutic effect on the lesion can be matched with the drug most likely to produce that effect.

Most skin conditions require routine monitoring by the veterinarian or pet owner to assess the success or failure of the treatment regimen. Many therapeutic failures are caused by poor or inadequate communication between the pet owner and veterinarian. Another common cause of ineffective therapy is failure to pursue a systematic approach to definitive diagnosis, which results in administering medications that are not the best choice. Inadequate or excessive doses as well as discontinuation of medications before total resolution of the problem also can result in treatment failure.

Dermatologic drugs can be divided into two groups, topicals and systemics. The purpose of this chapter is to review these drugs with respect to classification, general modes of action, and indications for use.

TABLE 3-1

Common Forms of Topical Dermatologic Agents

Form	*Actions/Characteristics*	*Indication*	*Disadvantages*
Wet dressings	Cleans, maintains drainage, soothes; keratolytic, antiinflammatory, antimicrobial, analgesic, antipruritic	Acute moist dermatoses with edema, erythema, pustules, vesicles, exudate, ulcers, and pain Subacute dermatoses with erythema, minor exudation, and ulceration	Requires frequent or prolonged application; penetrates poorly; often drying to skin
Gels, creams, ointments	Protects, soothes, softens, penetrates; antipruritic; vehicle for specific agents	Chronic nonpainful dermatoses with dry scale, lichenification, acanthosis	Occlusive, greasy, messy
Powders	Cools, soothes, protects, reduces friction; absorbent; vehicle for residual agents	Intertriginous lesions	Nonpenetrating; tends to form a dry, occlusive covering that must be removed before each new application; cannot use on open lesions
Lotions	Cools, soothes, dries, protects, allows some drainage; astringent; antiinflammatory; antipruritic	Acute moist dermatoses	Poor penetration; somewhat occlusive; may be drying and irritating; leaves deposit; not indicated on chronic lesions
Rinses (dips)	Vehicle for residual agent	Parasitic dermatoses; seborrheic dermatoses (emollient bath oils)	Parasitic rinse; odiferous; may be irritating Emollient rinse; oil film on hair if too concentrated

TOPICAL DERMATOLOGIC DRUGS

Topical dermatologic agents are available in many forms (Table 3-1). They are also classified according to their mode of action based on active components. There are usually many specific formulations in each class (Table 3-2).

Topical Corticosteroids

Topical corticosteroids are commonly used in general practice either individually or as a component of a multidrug formulation. It is important to note that percutaneous absorption of topical corticosteroids does occur and Cushing's disease secondary to the topical application of corticosteroids has been reported. It is important, therefore, to be aware of the actions and indications of topical corticosteroids (Table 3-3). When corticosteroids are incorporated into multidrug formulations (Table 3-4), the corticosteroid dose should be the limiting factor to the duration of treatment.

Topical Antibacterials

Topical antibacterials (Table 3-2) are useful for superficial pyodermas and localized bacterial eruptions. The most common antibiotics used in this fashion are cuprimyxin, bacitracin, polymyxin B, thiostrepton, spectinomycin, and furacin.

Antiseptics also are commonly used in veterinary practice. Chlorhexidine acts as a broad-spectrum antibacterial and antifungal agent with rapid microbial "kill," good residual activity, and little potential for sensitization. Povidone-iodine solutions are commonly used to flush wounds. Dilute solutions (0.1–1%) are more effective than full-strength solutions (10%). Because its bactericidal activity lasts only for 4 to 6 hours, povidone-iodine must be used several times daily for best results. Hydrogen peroxide (3%) is commonly used to irrigate wounds but is damaging to tissues. It has some sporicidal effects and should be reserved for use in wounds with suspected clostridial contamination.

Topical Antifungals

Topical antifungals (Table 3-2) are commonly used individually and in combination with antibacterials and corticosteroids. Such products as clotrimazole (Lotrimin® —Schering; Lotrisone® —Schering; Mycelex® —Miles), miconazole (Conofite® —Pitman-Moore), tioconazole (Vagistat® —SmithKline), naftidine hydrochloride

TABLE 3-2

Classes of Topical Dermatologic Agents

Class	*Drugs or Agents*	*Action/Characteristics*	*Specific Indications*
Antipruritic	Menthol 0.12–1%; camphor 0.12–5%; hot or cold water	Substitutes itch sensation with heat or cold	Pruritus/temporary relief
	Ointments, creams, petrolatum	Protects skin from external influences	Focal pruritic lesions
	Local anesthetics (dibucaine 0.5%)	Anesthetizes peripheral sensory nerves	Focal pruritic lesions
	Glucocorticosteroids; hydrocortisone 1–2.5%; prednisolone 0.5%; methylprednisolone 0.25%; desoximetasone 0.25%; triamcinolone acetonide 0.1%; betamethasone 0.1%; fluocinonide 0.05%.	Antiinflammatory	Focal pruritic, erythematous, or excoriated lesions
Keratolytic	Salicylic acid 5–40%; coal tar 1–10%; resorcinol 2–30%; sulfur 2–10%; benzoyl peroxide hydrous 0.05%	Helps remove stratum corneum or reduces thickness by hydration, softening, and peeling	Seborrheic lesions; bacterial dermatitis
Keratoplastic	Salicylic acid 1–2%; coal tar 1–5%; sulfur 2–10%	Helps normalize keratinization by unknown mechanism	Seborrheic lesions; bacterial dermatitis
Antiseborrheic	Sulfur 2–5%; coal tar 1–5%; benzoyl peroxide hydrous 2.5–5%	Reduces inflammation, and pruritus by keratolytic or keratoplastic actions	Seborrheic lesions; bacterial dermatitis
Antiparasitic	Sulfur 1.0–5%	Kills adults, larvae, or ova by direct contact or ingestion	Mites, lice, chiggers
	Pyrethrums 0.05–0.4%	Acts as contact poison resulting in release of acetylcholine	Lice, flies, mosquitos, fleas
	Rotenone 2–10%	Glutamic acid inhibitor	Mites, fleas, lice, chiggers
	Lindane	Destabilizes neuronal membranes	Fleas, lice, mosquitos
	Organophosphates malathion 0.5% carbamates 5–8%	Cholinesterase inhibitor	Flies, lice, mosquitos, fleas, ticks
	Amitraz	Unknown (may act on CNS)	Demodectic mange, sarcoptic mange
Antimicrobial	Povidone-iodine	Bactericidal, fungicidal, and sporicidal; liberates hydrochlorus acid	Bacterial dermatitis; dermatophytosis
	Cuprimyxin 0.5%; chlorhexidine	Bactericidal and fungicidal	Bacterial dermatitis; dermatophytosis
	Sulfur 1–10%	Bacteriostatic and antifungal	Bacterial dermatitis; dermatophytosis
	Benzoyl peroxide hydrous 2.5–5%	Antibacterial and antiseborrheic	Bacterial dermatitis; dermatophytosis; acne
	Neomycin sulfate, bacitracin, polymyxin B, nitrofurazone, thiostrepton	Antibacterial	Bacterial dermatitis
Antifungal	Miconazole nitrate 2%; clotrimazole 1%; haloprogin 1%; thiabendazole; ketaconazole	Fungicidal; acts on cytoplasmic membrane of fungus	Dermatophytosis; yeast infections
	Tolnaftate 1%	Fungistatic	*Microsporum gypseum* only
	Nystatin	Anticandidal; causes cells to lose potassium ions	Candidiasis

TABLE 3-2 (continued)

Classes of Topical Dermatologic Agents

Class	*Drugs or Agents*	*Action/Characteristics*	*Specific Indications*
Emollient oil rinses	Bath oil	Protects, soothes; vehicle for other drugs; artificial sebum	Seborrhea sicca; dry skin
Astringent	Aluminum acetate; tannic acid 5%	Precipitates protein; decreases cell permeability	Moist, weeping lesions

TABLE 3-3

Topical Glucocorticosteroids

Drug: Generic Name (Commercial Name—Manufacturer)	*Action*	*Indications*	*Dosage/ Administration*	*Comment*
Hydrocortisone 1–2% cream, ointment	Antipruritic; antiinflammatory; superficial effect	Focal excoriation; erythema	tid–qid initially; then sid–bid	Not practical for large areas
Prednisolone 0.5% cream (Meti-Derm® —Schering-Plough Animal Health)	Same as above	Same as above	Same as above	Same as above
Triamcinolone acetonide 0.5%, cream (Vetalog® —Solvay Animal Health)	Same as above	Same as above	bid–tid initially; then sid–bid	Same as above
Desoximethasone 0.25% cream (Topicort® —Hoechst)	Antipruritic; antiinflammatory; marked penetration	Same as above	Same as above	Marked antiinflammatory effect; not practical for large areas
Betamethasone 17-valerate 0.1% cream, ointment (Valisone® —Schering-Plough Animal Health)	Same as above	Same as above	Same as above	Same as above
Fluocinonide 0.05% cream (Lidex® —Syntex)	Same as above	Same as above	Same as above	Same as above

(Naftin® —Herbert), haloprogin (Halotex® — Westwood), cuprimyxin, and ketoconazole (Nizoral® —Janssen) are effective against dermatophytes as well as *Candida* and *Malassezia* (*Pityrosporum*) yeasts. Products such as tolnaftate may have some efficacy against *Microsporum gypseum* but are considered inferior antifungals for use on animals.

Antiseptics such as chlorhexidine and tamed iodides also have antifungal activity. Lime sulfur and captan, two products used to treat fungi on plants, also are commonly used on animals. Both are used in a 2 to 3% solution once to twice weekly. Gloves should be worn because captan can cause contact sensitivities and lime sulfur is odoriferous and can stain hands as well as light haircoats.

Parasiticides

Topical parasiticides usually consist of one or more of pyrethrins, pyrethroids, carbamates, organophosphates, and organochlorines. Many have systemic effects despite their topical application. Parasiticides can be applied as sprays, shampoos, collars, dips, and powders; in the en-

TABLE 3-4

Topical Combined Glucocorticoids and Antibiotics

Drug: Generic Name (Commercial Name—Manufacturer)	*Action*	*Indications*	*Dosage/ Administration*	*Comment*
Nystatin, neomycin sulfate, thiostrepton, triamcinolone acetonide; cream, ointment (Panolog® —Solvay Animal Health)	Antipruritic; antiinflammatory; antibacterial; anticandidal	Focal excoriation; erythema; otitis externa	bid–tid	No efficacy for dermatophytes
Neomycin sulfate, fluocinolone acetonide; cream (Neo-synalar® —Syntex Animal Health)	Antipruritic; antiinflammatory; antibacterial	Focal excoriation; erythema	bid–tid	
Gentamicin sulfate, betamethasone valerate (Topagen® —Hoechst)	Same as above	Same as above	bid–tid	
Thiabendazole, dexamethasone, neomycin sulfate; solution (Tresaderm® —MSD AGVET)	Antipruritic; antiinflammatory; antibacterial; antifungal	Focal excoriation; erythema; otitis externa	bid–tid	

vironment, they can be applied as liquid sprays, powders, or foggers. A comprehensive listing of topical, systemic, and environmental parasiticides is presented in Table 3-5.

Shampoos

Most shampoos are used to remove scale, bacteria, and debris from the surface of the skin. Most antiseborrheic shampoos contain such ingredients as sulfur, salicylic acid, selenium disulfide, tars, and benzoyl peroxide. Sulfur, salicylic acid, and selenium disulfide are considered weak antiseborrheic agents, tars are intermediate, and benzoyl peroxides are the most potent of the antiseborrheic agents. The mildest product capable of doing the job should always be selected. Other products, such as chlorhexidine, iodine derivatives, triclosan, hexachloraphene, and benzoyl peroxides, have marked antibacterial action. To be effective, medicated shampoos must contact the surface of the skin for a sufficient amount of time, usually 10 to 15 minutes. Application of an oil rinse or humectant immediately after bathing will prolong and maximize the hydrating activity of water. Some shampoos are listed in Table 3-6.

Sulfur is keratolytic, keratoplastic, antibacterial, antifungal, antiparasitic, and antipruritic. It is not a good degreasing agent and can be drying at higher concentrations.

Salicylic acid is keratolytic and keratoplastic and has mild antipruritic and antibacterial action. Combining salicylic acid with sulfur enhances keratolytic action.

Selenium disulfide is keratolytic, keratoplastic, and has degreasing activity. It can be drying and potentially irritating to sensitive skin.

Tars are keratolytic, keratoplastic, antipruritic, and degreasing. Tars can vary greatly in their efficacy and potential side effects. Tar products are not recommended for use on cats. Drying and irritation increase with the ultimate concentration of the product. Tars also can result in staining of the haircoat, contact sensitivity, and photosensitization.

Benzoyl peroxide is keratolytic, antibacterial, antipruritic, and is a good degreasing and follicular flushing agent. Side effects include a drying effect and the potential for irritancy.

Hypoallergenic shampoos are not strictly nonallergenic, but are mild shampoos that lack many of the potentially irritating properties of medicated shampoos. In addition, they often include such moisturizing agents as sodium lactate, glycerin, essential fatty acids, lactic acid, urea, and aloe vera. Shampoos containing perfumes, astringents, and medication may be poorly tolerated by individuals with sensitive skin.

Moisturizers are designed to rehydrate the skin in dry, scaly conditions or after shampooing with drying agents, such as benzoyl peroxide. Moisturizers can be applied directly to the coat or applied as a final rinse after bathing. Common emollients include oils (such as olive, coconut, cottonseed, corn), fats (lanolin), humectants (carboxylic acid, lactic acid), and hydrocarbons (paraffin, petrolatum, mineral oil).

This listing is arranged according to product classes defined as follows:

- Class 1: aerosol spray and mist products for use on pets
- Class 2: nonaerosol spray and mist products for use on pets
- Class 3: shampoo products
- Class 4: collars
- Class 5: dip or sponge-on products
- Class 6: dust and powder products
- Class 7: any topical liquid preparation that is not a dip, sponge-on, spray, mist, or shampoo
- Class 8: cream rinse preparations
- Class 9: foggers for environmental use
- Class 10: liquid sprays for environmental use
- Class 11: tablet or liquid oral preparations

TABLE 3-5

Classification of Flea Control Products by Type of Product[a]

(Reprinted from *Veterinary Technician*, 11(4):232–243, 1990)

Company	Product Name[b]	Class[c]	Principal Active Ingredients	Action[d]	Species[e]	Frequency of Administration	Precautions[f]	Miscellaneous Comments
Aerosol Spray								
Coopers Animal Health (A Pitman-Moore Company)	Flair®	1	Pyrethrins, carbaryl	1, 3	D, C	Weekly or as needed	See product label	Also repels lice, fleas, mosquitoes, and gnats
EVSCO Pharmaceuticals	SECT-A-CHLOR™	1	Chlorpyrifos	1	D	As needed	See product label	
	SECT-A-SPRAY®	1	Pyrethrins, piperonyl butoxide	1	D, C	As needed	See product label	
KenVet Animal Care Group, Veratec	Pyreth-a-ban™	1	Pyrethrins, rotenone	1, 2, 3	D	Repeat as needed	Do *not* use on nursing puppies	Kills and repels fleas, ticks, lice, flies, gnats, chiggers
Schering Animal Health	Duration® 60	1	Chlorpyrifos	1	D	30–60 days for fleas, 14 days for ticks	See product label; cholinesterase inhibitor	Do *not* use on cats; do *not* use on puppies younger than 16 wks of age
Vet-Kem	Pet Spray	1	o-isopropoxyphenyl methylcarbamate	1	D, C	See product label	See product label	Pleasant smell; excellent coverage; long-lasting killing power
Veterinary Products Laboratories	VIP™ Flea Spray	1	d-limonene	1	D, C	As needed, every 2 days	Avoid contact with eyes, skin, clothing	Do *not* use more than once every 2 days
Virbac Laboratories	Parid™ Plus Pressurized Spray	1	Pyrethrins, 0.06%; carbaryl, 2.5%	1, 3	D, C	Weekly	Cholinesterase inhibitor	Contains no fluorocarbons; pressurized with CO_2
	Parid™ Pressurized Spray	1	Carbaryl, 2.5%	1, 3	D, C	Weekly	Cholinesterase inhibitor	Contains no fluorocarbons
VMx Pet Products	VM_x™ Flea & Tick Repellent	1	Fenvalerate, DEET	1, 3	D, C	Once weekly to once every 3 wks	See product label	Kills and repels ticks carrying Lyme disease
Nonaerosol Spray								
Adams Laboratories (A SmithKline Beecham Company)	Adams™ Flea & Tick 14-Day Residual Mist	2	Pyrethrins	1, 3	D, C	As needed	See product label; avoid treatment of nursing puppies, kittens	Use as often as necessary on dogs, cats, nonnursing puppies and kittens; do not oversaturate
	Adams™ Flea & Tick Mist	2	Pyrethrins with synergists and repellent	1, 3	D, C, H	As needed	See product label; avoid treatment of nursing puppies, kittens	

Company	Product Name[b]	Class[c]	Principal Active Ingredients	Action[d]	Species[e]	Frequency of Administration	Precautions[f]	Miscellaneous Comments
	Adams™ Flea & Tick Spray for Dogs with Dursban	2	Chlorpyrifos, pyrethrins	1	D	As needed	Dogs only; do *not* use on cats	
Bio-Ceutic Animal Health	14-Day Flea & Tick Spray	2	Pyrethrins, permethrin	1, 2	D, C	14 days for fleas, 7 days for ticks	See product label	
	Buzz Off™	2	Pyrethrin, methoxyclor	1, 2, 3	H	3–4 times a week	See product label	
	Buzz Off™ II	2	Permethrin	1, 2, 3	H	As needed	See product label	Water base
	Permectrin™ II Horse & Stable Spray	2	Permethrin	1, 2	H	See product label	See product label	Use as needed but not more than once every two weeks; also can be used as a premise spray
	Permectrin™ Pet, Yard & Kennel Spray	2	Permethrin	1, 2	D, C	See product label	See product label	Apply as needed but not more than once every two weeks; also can be used as a premise spray
Coopers Animal Health (A Pitman-Moore Company)	Expar® Insecticide/Repellent	2	Permethrin	1, 3	D, H	Do *not* use on cats		Controls and repels gnats, mosquitoes, biting flies, houseflies, cockroaches, silverfish, and spiders; can also be used as a premise spray
	Mistaway® Extra	2	Pyrethrins, piperonyl butoxide	1, 3	D, C, H	As needed	See product label	Controls lice; repels gnats, mosquitoes, biting flies
DVM	DuraKyl™ Pet Spray	2	Resmethrin	1, 3	D, C	Weekly	See product label	
	SynerKyl™ Pet Spray	2	Pyrethrins, permethrin	1, 3	D, C	As needed	Do *not* use on nursing puppies or kittens under 3 months of age	Kills fleas, ticks, lice; coat and skin conditioner; 16-oz plastic bottle
EVSCO Pharmaceuticals	LIQUI-BAN™	2	Chlorpyrifos, xylene range aromatic solvent	1	D	As needed	See product label	
Fort Dodge Laboratories	Nolvacide® Mist II with Nolvasan®	2	Pyrethrins, permethrin	1	D, C	Every 14 days or as needed	See product label; do *not* use on nursing kittens or puppies	Available as 16-oz pump spray or in gallon quantities
HAVER, Mobay Animal Health	PARA™ Mist	2	Pyrethrins	1	D, C	Daily if needed	See product label	Alcohol base
	PARA™ Mist W.B.	2	Pyrethrins	1	D, C	Daily if needed	See product label	Water base
KenVet Animal Care Group, Veratec	Kenlyte K-14 Canine Residual Flea and Tick Spray™	2	Pyrethrins, permethrin	1, 2	D	Repeat as needed	Do *not* use on nursing puppies	Kills fleas for up to 14 days and ticks for up to 7 days
	Kenlyte F-14 Feline Residual Flea and Tick Spray™	2	Pyrethrins, permethrin	1, 2	C	Repeat as needed	Do *not* use on nursing kittens	Kills fleas for up to 14 days and ticks for up to 7 days
SmithKline Beecham Animal Health	MYCODEX® '14' Spray	2	Permethrin, 0.25%; pyrethrins, 0.10%	1	D	As needed	See product label	Controls fleas up to 14 days; aqueous vehicle, no alcohol; mist
	MYCODEX® Aqua-Spray	2	Pyrethrins, 0.20%	1	D, C	As needed	See product label	Aqueous base, no alcohol

[a]Product labels should be reviewed carefully before any product is used. In all cases, keep insecticide products out of the reach of children and pets. Inclusion of a product in this guide does not represent endorsement by the publisher.
[b]Proprietary names are listed.
[c]Class key: 1 = spray/mist—aerosol; 2 = spray/mist—nonaerosol; 3 = shampoo; 4 = collar; 5 = dip/sponge-on; 6 = dust/powder; 7 = topical liquid preparation (other than dips, sponge-ons, sprays, mists, shampoos); 8 = cream rinse; 9 = foggers (environmental use); 10 = liquid sprays (environmental use); 11 = oral administration (i.e., tablets, liquid).
[d]Action key: 1 = adulticidal; 2 = larvacidal; 3 = repellent.
[e]Species key: D = dog; C = cat; H = horse. If no species is indicated, the product is for environmental use.
[f]Any product specified as a cholinesterase inhibitor should *not* be used in conjunction with other pesticides.

This listing is arranged according to product classes defined as follows:

- Class 1: aerosol spray and mist products for use on pets
- Class 2: nonaerosol spray and mist products for use on pets
- Class 3: shampoo products
- Class 4: collars
- Class 5: dip or sponge-on products
- Class 6: dust and powder products
- Class 7: any topical liquid preparation that is not a dip, sponge-on, spray, mist, or shampoo
- Class 8: cream rinse preparations
- Class 9: foggers for environmental use
- Class 10: liquid sprays for environmental use
- Class 11: tablet or liquid oral preparations

Company	Product Name[b]	Class[c]	Principal Active Ingredients	Action[d]	Species[e]	Frequency of Administration	Precautions[f]	Miscellaneous Comments
	MYCODEX® Mist Plus	2	Carbaryl, 2.5%; pyrethrins, 0.06%; piperonyl butoxide, 0.60%	1	D, C	As needed	See product label	Do *not* apply more than once a week
TechAmerica	Dermatological Mist	2	Pyrethrins	1	D, C	See product label	See product label	Contains aloe vera; safe for use on puppies and kittens
	Feline & Puppy Mist	2	Pyrethrins	1	D, C	See product label	See product label	Ideal for cats, kittens, puppies; convenient fingertip sprayer
	Flea Kill Mist	2	Pyrethrins	1, 3	D, C	See product label	See product label	Fast-acting; convenient trigger sprayer
3M/Animal Care	Sectrol® Pet and Household Flea Spray	2	Microencapsulated pyrethrin	1	D, C	As needed	See product label	Kills fleas on pets for 8 days; also a premise spray; odorless
	Sectrol® Two-Way Pet Spray	2	Pyrethrins, microencapsulated pyrethrin	1	D, C	Repeat as needed	See product label	Kills fleas on pets for 8 days; excellent knockdown; pleasant scent; kills ticks, including deer ticks
Vet-Kem	Ovitrol™ Plus Flea Spray	2	Pyrethrins, methoprene	1, 2	D, C, H	See product label	See product label	Kills fleas and flea eggs on animal before they fall into the environment; breaks the flea life cycle
	Vet-Kem® Flea & Tick Pump Spray	2	Pyrethrins, piperonyl butoxide	1	D, C	See product label	See product label	Kills fleas, ticks, lice; alcohol or water base
Vet Mate Labs	VET MATE™ 14 Day Flea & Tick Spray	2	Organic pyrethrins; permethrin	1, 3	D, C	As needed	See product label	Kill fleas up to 14 days and ticks up to 9 days; pleasantly scented water base
	VET MATE™ Flea & Tick Mist	2	Dual synergized organic pyrethrins	1, 3	D, C, H	As needed	See product label	Pleasantly scented with aloe and conditioners
	VET MATE™ Equine Fly Repellent Mist	2	Dual synergized organic pyrethrins	1, 3	D, C, H	As needed	See product label	Controls and kills on contact fleas, ticks, lice, stable flies, horseflies, deerflies, gnats, and mosquitoes
	VET MATE™ Equine Fly Spray for Sensitive Skin	2	Organic pyrethrins	1	D, C, H	As needed	See product label	Controls fleas, ticks, deerflies, stable flies, horseflies, gnats, and mosquitoes
	VET MATE™ Flea Spray for Sensitive Skin	2	Organic pyrethrins	1	D, C, H	As needed	See product label	Kills fleas and ticks; water base with aloe

Company	Product Name[b]	Class[c]	Principal Active Ingredients	Action[d]	Species[e]	Frequency of Administration	Precautions[f]	Miscellaneous Comments
	VET MATE™ Barn & Stable Spray	2	Permethrin	1, 3	D, H	As needed	See product label	Can be used as a premise spray in hospitals, feed rooms, dairies, horse barns, and poultry houses or directly on dogs and livestock via automatic foggers and spraying systems
	VET MATE™ Permethrin + Additive	2	Organic pyrethrins	1	D, C	As needed	See product label	Concentrate can be mixed with water for low-cost spray or dip or can be mixed with VET MATE™ Flea & Tick Shampoo for low-cost shampoo
Veterinary Products Laboratories	VIP™ Dermatological Flea & Tick Spray	2	Pyrethrins	1	D, C	As needed	See product label	Contains special skin and coat conditioners (coconut and aloe vera); noncholinesterase inhibitor
	VIP™ Flea Mist	2	Pyrethrins	1	D, C	As needed	Avoid contact with eyes, skin, clothing; harmful if swallowed	Pleasant citrus scent
	VIP™ Ovi-Cide™ Plus Pet Spray	2	Linalool, d-limonene	1, 2	D, C	As needed	See product label	Kills adult fleas, eggs, larvae, pupae
	VIP™ Pet Spray	2	d-limonene, linalool	1, 2	D, C	As needed, every 2 days	Avoid contact with eyes, skin, clothing	Kills all 4 stages of flea life cycle; pleasant citrus scent; do *not* use more than once every 2 days
Virbac Laboratories	DuoCide® Long Acting Spray	2	Pyrethrins, permethrin	1, 3	D, C	Twice weekly	See product label	In an Aqua-soothe™ water base vehicle; woodlands fresh fragrance
	D-F-T	2	Carbaryl, 2.5%	1, 3	D	Weekly	Cholinesterase inhibitor	
	D-F-T Plus	2	Pyrethrins, 0.06%; carbaryl, 2.5%	1, 3	D	Weekly	Cholinesterase inhibitor	
	Supra-Quick Mist™	2	Pyrethrins, 0.10%	1, 3	D, C	Daily or as needed	See product label	Will not irritate skin with dermatologic problems
	Ultra-Sect Mist™	2	Pyrethrins, 0.15%	1, 3	D, C	Daily or as needed	See product label	"Tamed alcohol" base has low odor; reduces sting to sensitive skin
Shampoo								
Adams Laboratories (A SmithKline Beecham Company)	Adams™ Flea & Tick Shampoo	3	Pyrethrins	1	D, C	Every 7-10 days	See product label	
Bio-Ceutic Animal Health	Sectilin™ Flea & Tick Mousse	3	Pyrethrins	1, 2	D, C	As needed	See product label	
	Sectilin™ Shampoo	3	Pyrethrins, 0.06%; piperonyl butoxide, 0.12%	1, 2	D, C, H	As needed	See product label	Contains protein-base surfactant
Coopers Animal Health (A Pitman-Moore Company)	Expar® Shampoo	3	Permethrin	1	D, C	As needed	See product label	Also kills lice

[a]Product labels should be reviewed carefully before any product is used. In all cases, keep insecticide products out of the reach of children and pets. Inclusion of a product in this guide does not represent endorsement by the publisher.
[b]Proprietary names are listed.
[c]Class key: 1 = spray/mist—aerosol; 2 = spray/mist—nonaerosol; 3 = shampoo; 4 = collar; 5 = dip/sponge-on; 6 = dust/powder; 7 = topical liquid preparation (other than dips, sponge-ons, sprays, mists, shampoos); 8 = cream rinse; 9 = foggers (environmental use); 10 = liquid sprays (environmental use); 11 = oral administration (i.e., tablets, liquid).
[d]Action key: 1 = adulticidal; 2 = larvacidal; 3 = repellent.
[e]Species key: D = dog; C = cat; H = horse. If no species is indicated, the product is for environmental use.
[f]Any product specified as a cholinesterase inhibitor should *not* be used in conjunction with other pesticides.

This listing is arranged according to product classes defined as follows:

- Class 1: aerosol spray and mist products for use on pets
- Class 2: nonaerosol spray and mist products for use on pets
- Class 3: shampoo products
- Class 4: collars
- Class 5: dip or sponge-on products
- Class 6: dust and powder products
- Class 7: any topical liquid preparation that is not a dip, sponge-on, spray, mist, or shampoo
- Class 8: cream rinse preparations
- Class 9: foggers for environmental use
- Class 10: liquid sprays for environmental use
- Class 11: tablet or liquid oral preparations

Company	Product Name[b]	Class[c]	Principal Active Ingredients	Action[d]	Species[e]	Frequency of Administration	Precautions[f]	Miscellaneous Comments
	Thionium® Shampoo with Expar®	3	Permethrin	1	D, C	As needed	See product label	Controls lice
	Thionium® Shampoo with Lindane	3	Lindane	1	D	Weekly	Do *not* use on cats	Controls lice and sarcoptic mange
DVM	DuraKyl™ Shampoo	3	Resmethrin	1, 3	D, C	As needed	See product label	
	SynerKyl™ Shampoo	3	Pyrethrins, permethrin	1, 3	D, C	As needed	Do *not* use on nursing puppies or kittens under 3 months of age	Kills fleas, ticks, lice; skin and coat conditioner; 8-oz plastic bottle or gallon size
EVSCO Pharmaceuticals	Theradex/D-Flea™	3	Pyrethrins, piperonyl butoxide	1	D, C	1–2 times weekly	See product label	
Fort Dodge Laboratories	Nolvacide® Shampoo with Nolvasan®	3	Pyrethrins	1, 3	D, C	Repeat as needed	See product label	Available in 8-oz or gallon volumes
HAVER, Mobay Animal Health	FLEATOL™ Shampoo	3	Pyrethrins	1	D, C	As needed	See product label	
Pitman-Moore	KFL® Insecticide Shampoo	3	Pyrethrin, 0.5%	1	D, C	As needed	See product label	
SmithKline Beecham Animal Health	MYCODEX® Pet Shampoo with 3X Pyrethrins	3	Pyrethrins, 0.15%; piperonyl butoxide, 1.5%	1	D, C	As needed	See product label	
	MYCODEX® Pet Shampoo with Allethrin	3	Allethrin, 0.12%	1	D, C	Semiweekly or weekly	See product label	Frequency of use determined by severity of affliction
	MYCODEX® Pet Shampoo with Carbaryl	3	Carbaryl, 0.5%	1	D, C, H	As needed	See product label	
	MYCODEX® Pet Shampoo with Pyrethrins	3	Pyrethrins, 0.05%; piperonyl butoxide, 0.5%	1	D, C	As needed	See product label	
TechAmerica	Flea and Tick Shampoo Plus	3	Pyrethrins	1, 3	D, C	See product label	See product label	Concentrate (lasts longer); leaves coat clean and glossy
Vet-Kem	Vet-Kem® Flea & Tick Shampoo	3	Pyrethrins, piperonyl butoxide	1	D, C	See product label	See product label	Kills fleas, ticks, lice
	Vet-Kem® Flea & Tick Shampoo Plus	3	Pyrethrins, piperonyl butoxide	1	D, C	See product label	See product label	Contains 0.15% natural pyrethrins; kills fleas, ticks, lice
Vet Mate Labs	VET MATE™ Flea & Tick Shampoo	3	Dual synergized organic pyrethrins	1, 3	D, C	As needed	See product label	Contains aloe, whiteners, and brighteners

Company	Product Name[b]	Class[c]	Principal Active Ingredients	Action[d]	Species[e]	Frequency of Administration	Precautions[f]	Miscellaneous Comments
	VET MATE™ Pyrethrin + Additive	3	Organic pyrethrins	1	D, C	As needed	See product label	Concentrate can be mixed with VET MATE™ Flea & Tick Shampoo for low-cost shampoo product or mixed with water for low-cost dip or spray
	VET MATE™ Sulfur Tar Shampoo	3	Sulfur, coal tar, menthol	4	D	As needed	See product label	Aids in control of fleabite dermatitis
Veterinary Products Laboratories	VIP™ Concentrated Flea Shampoo	3	Linalool	1	D, C	As needed	May cause eye irritation; harmful if swallowed	Conditions and deodorizes coat; 1:3 dilution
	VIP™ Flea Control Shampoo	3	d-limonene	1	D, C	As needed	May cause eye irritation; harmful if swallowed	Pleasant citrus scent
	VIP™ Ovi-Cide™ Plus Citrus Scent Shampoo	3	Linalool	1, 2	D, C	As needed	See product label	Kills adult fleas, eggs, larvae, pupae; pleasant citrus scent; noncholinesterase inhibitor
Virbac Laboratories	DuoCide® Shampoo	3	d-trans® allethrin, sumithrin	1	D, C	As needed	See product label	
	Parid-X™ Shampoo	3	Pyrethrins, 0.075%	1	D, C	As needed	See product label	Concentrated (12 oz makes 1 gal)
	Pesticidal Shampoo	3	Pyrethrins, 0.05%	1	D, C	As needed	See product label	
Collar								
Schering-Plough Animal Health	Duration® 6	4	Chlorpyrifos	1	C	Change 11 mo for fleas, 6 mo for ticks	See product label	Do *not* use on sick or debilitated cats or kittens younger than 12 wk of age; maximum effectiveness within 2–3 days
	Duration® 11	4	Chlorpyrifos	1	D	Change 12 mo for fleas, 7 mo for ticks	See product label	Do *not* use on sick or debilitated dogs or puppies younger than 12 wk of age; maximum effectiveness within 2–3 days
	Escort® Flea & Tick Collar for Cats	4	Diazinon	1	C	Change 5 mo for fleas and ticks	See product label	Do *not* use on sick or convalescing animals or on kittens younger than 12 wk of age; maximum effectiveness within 3–4 days
	Escort® Flea & Tick Collar for Dogs	4	Diazinon	1	D	Change 5 mo for fleas and ticks	See product label	Do *not* use on sick or debilitated dogs or on puppies younger than 12 wk of age; maximum effectiveness within 3–4 days
	Escort® Plus Flea & Tick Collar for Cats	4	Diazinon	1	C	Change 5 mo for fleas and ticks	See product label	Do *not* use on sick or convalescing animals or on kittens younger than 12 wk of age; maximum effectiveness within 3–4 days
	Escort® Plus Flea & Tick Collar for Dogs	4	Diazinon, fatty acids	1	D	Change 5 mo for fleas and ticks	See product label	Do *not* use on sick or debilitated dogs or on puppies younger than 12 wk of age; maximum effectiveness within 3–4 days

[a]Product labels should be reviewed carefully before any product is used. In all cases, keep insecticide products out of the reach of children and pets. Inclusion of a product in this guide does not represent endorsement by the publisher.
[b]Proprietary names are listed.
[c]Class key: 1 = spray/mist—aerosol; 2 = spray/mist—nonaerosol; 3 = shampoo; 4 = collar; 5 = dip/sponge-on; 6 = dust/powder; 7 = topical liquid preparation (other than dips, sponge-ons, sprays, mists, shampoos); 8 = cream rinse; 9 = foggers (environmental use); 10 = liquid sprays (environmental use); 11 = oral administration (i.e., tablets, liquid).
[d]Action key: 1 = adulticidal; 2 = larvacidal; 3 = repellent.
[e]Species key: D = dog; C = cat; H = horse. If no species is indicated, the product is for environmental use.
[f]Any product specified as a cholinesterase inhibitor should *not* be used in conjunction with other pesticides.

This listing is arranged according to product classes defined as follows:

Class 1: aerosol spray and mist products for use on pets
Class 2: nonaerosol spray and mist products for use on pets
Class 3: shampoo products
Class 4: collars
Class 5: dip or sponge-on products
Class 6: dust and powder products
Class 7: any topical liquid preparation that is not a dip, sponge-on, spray, mist, or shampoo
Class 8: cream rinse preparations
Class 9: foggers for environmental use
Class 10: liquid sprays for environmental use
Class 11: tablet or liquid oral preparations

Company	Product Name[b]	Class[c]	Principal Active Ingredients	Action[d]	Species[e]	Frequency of Administration	Precautions[f]	Miscellaneous Comments
	Escort® Signal Flea & Tick Collar for Cats	4	Diazinon	1	C	Change 5 mo for fleas and ticks	See product label	Do *not* use on sick or convalescing animals or on kittens younger than 12 wk of age; maximum effectiveness within 3–4 days; includes reflective strip
	Escort® Signal Flea & Tick Collar for Dogs	4	Diazinon	1	D	Change 5 mo for fleas and ticks	See product label	Do *not* use on sick or debilitated dogs or on puppies younger than 12 wk of age; maximum effectiveness within 3–4 days; includes reflective strip
SmithKline Beecham Animal Health	Norden Flea & Tick Collar with Dursban for Dogs	4	Chlorpyrifos	1	D	Change 11 mo for fleas, 6 mo for ticks	See product label	Contains Dursban insecticide
	Norden Safety Stretch Flea & Tick Collar with Dursban for Cats	4	Chlorpyrifos	1	C	Change 11 mo for fleas, 6 mo for ticks	See product label	Contains Dursban insecticide
Solvay Animal Health	Dirodan® Flea & Tick Collar for Dogs	4	Dursban, 8%; chlorpyrifos	1	D	12 mo for fleas, 7 mo for ticks	See product label; cholinesterase inhibitor	Do *not* use on sick or debilitated dogs or on puppies younger than 12 wk of age; also helps prevent sarcoptic mange for 5 mo; 24-in. collar
	Dirodan® Saf-T-Stretch Flea & Tick Collars for Cats	4	Dursban, 3%; chlorpyrifos	1	C	11 mo for fleas, 6 mo for ticks	See product label; cholinesterase inhibitor	Do *not* use on sick or debilitated cats or on kittens younger than 12 wk of age; collar gives if caught on fixed object; 13-in. collar
Vet-Kem	Breakaway™ Flea & Tick Collar for Cats	4	o-isopropoxyphenyl methylcarbamate	1	C	Change every 5 mo	See product label	Unique breakaway feature
	Dursban Flea & Tick Collar for Dogs	4	Chlorpyrifos	1	D	Change 11 mo for fleas, 7 mo for ticks	See product label	Helps prevent sarcoptic mange for up to 5 mo
	Flea & Tick Collar for Dogs	4	o-isopropoxyphenyl methylcarbamate	1	D	Change every 5 mo	See product label	Kills fleas and ticks for up to 5 mo
	Paramite® Insecticidal Collar for Dogs	4	Phosmet	1	D	Change every 7 mo	See product label	Kills fleas and ticks for up to 7 mo
	Tick & Flea Collar for Cats	4	o-isopropoxyphenyl methylcarbamate	1	C	Change every 5 mo	See product label	Kills fleas and ticks for up to 5 mo
Veterinary Products Laboratories	VPL Flea & Tick Collar	4	Propoxur	1	D, C	Change as needed	Avoid contact with eyes, skin, clothing	Metered release technology; heavy-duty metal release

Company	Product Name[b]	Class[c]	Principal Active Ingredients	Action[d]	Species[e]	Frequency of Administration	Precautions[f]	Miscellaneous Comments
Virbac Laboratories	DuoCide® Flea and Tick Collar for Cats	4	Chlorpyrifos, 3%	1	C	Up to 11 mo	See product label	Safety-stretch feature
	DuoCide® Flea and Tick Collar for Large Dogs	4	Chlorpyrifos, 8%	1	D	Up to 12 mo	See product label	
	DuoCide® Flea and Tick Collar for Small and Medium Dogs	4	Chlorpyrifos, 8%	1	D	Up to 12 mo	See product label	
Dip/Sponge-on								
Adams Laboratories (A SmithKline Beecham Company)	Adams™ Flea & Tick Dip	5	Malathion	1, 3	D	Repeat as needed	See product label	Use on dogs over 12 weeks old; do *not* use on cats
	Adams™ Flea & Tick Dip with Dursban	5	Chlorpyrifos	1, 3	D	28 days for fleas; 21 days for ticks	Dogs only; do *not* use on cats	
	Adams™ Pyrethrin Dip	5	Pyrethrins	1, 3	D, C, H	As needed	Do *not* use on puppies, kittens, foals less than 6 wk old	
Coopers Animal Health (A Pitman-Moore Company)	Expar® 3.2% EC	5	Permethrin	1, 3	D	Every 3 wk	Do *not* use on cats	Controls lice
DVM	DuraKyl™ Pet Dip	5	Pyrethrins, rotenone	1, 3	D, C	Weekly	See product label	
Fort Dodge Laboratories	Dermethrin™ Pet Dip	5	Permethrins	1	D, C	Every 2 wk	Do *not* use on sick, debilitated, or old animals; toxic to fish	Pleasant smelling
Pitman-Moore	Sprecto® -D Flea/Tick Dip	5	Permethrin, pyrethrins	1, 3	D, C	Four weeks	See product label	
TechAmerica	Flea and Tick Dip for Dogs	5	Chlorpyrifos	1	D	See product label	See product label	Kills fleas for 28 days; effective on ticks and mange mites
3M/Animal Care	Duratrol® Flea & Tick Dip for Dogs	5	Microencapsulated chlorpyrifos	1	D	Not more than every 21 days	See product label	Kills fleas on dogs for 28 days; no knockdown; kills ticks, including deer ticks
Vet-Kem	Paramite® Sponge-on or Dip	5	Phosmet	1	D	See product label	See product label	16-day control of fleas and brown dog ticks
	Vet-Kem® Pyrethrin Dip for Dogs & Cats	5	Pyrethrins	1	D, C	See product label	See product label	Kills fleas, ticks, lice, mites; 8-oz and 1-gal sizes
Vet Mate Labs	VET MATE™ Flea & Tick Dip	5	Malathion	1	D, C	Every 7-10 days	See product label	Kills fleas, ticks, mange mites; also can be used on lawns and in kennels
	VET MATE™ Pyrethrin Dip	5	Dual synergized organic pyrethrins	1	D, C	As needed	See product label	Kills fleas, ticks, mange mites
	VET MATE™ Pyrethrin + Additive	5	Organic pyrethrins	1	D, C	As needed	See product label	Concentrate can be mixed with water for low-cost dip or spray or mixed with VET MATE™ Flea & Tick Shampoo for low-cost shampoo

[a]Product labels should be reviewed carefully before any product is used. In all cases, keep insecticide products out of the reach of children and pets. Inclusion of a product in this guide does not represent endorsement by the publisher.

[b]Proprietary names are listed.

[c]Class key: 1 = spray/mist—aerosol; 2 = spray/mist—nonaerosol; 3 = shampoo; 4 = collar; 5 = dip/sponge-on; 6 = dust/powder; 7 = topical liquid preparation (other than dips, sponge-ons, sprays, mists, shampoos); 8 = cream rinse; 9 = foggers (environmental use); 10 = liquid sprays (environmental use); 11 = oral administration (i.e., tablets, liquid).

[d]Action key: 1 = adulticidal; 2 = larvacidal; 3 = repellent.

[e]Species key: D = dog; C = cat; H = horse. If no species is indicated, the product is for environmental use.

[f]Any product specified as a cholinesterase inhibitor should *not* be used in conjunction with other pesticides.

This listing is arranged according to product classes defined as follows:

- Class 1: aerosol spray and mist products for use on pets
- Class 2: nonaerosol spray and mist products for use on pets
- Class 3: shampoo products
- Class 4: collars
- Class 5: dip or sponge-on products
- Class 6: dust and powder products
- Class 7: any topical liquid preparation that is not a dip, sponge-on, spray, mist, or shampoo
- Class 8: cream rinse preparations
- Class 9: foggers for environmental use
- Class 10: liquid sprays for environmental use
- Class 11: tablet or liquid oral preparations

Company	Product Name[b]	Class[c]	Principal Active Ingredients	Action[d]	Species[e]	Frequency of Administration	Precautions[f]	Miscellaneous Comments
	VET MATE™ 21 Day Flea & Tick Dip	5	Permethrin	1, 3	D, C	As needed	See product label	User friendly for cats; kills fleas and ticks
Veterinary Products Laboratories	VIP™ Flea and Tick Dip for Dogs	5	Chlorpyrifos	1	D	Every 4 wk	Avoid contact with skin, eyes, clothing	Do *not* repeat treatment more than once every 4 weeks
	VIP™ Flea Dip	5	d-limonene	1	D, C	Every other day	Do *not* get into the eyes or on clothing or skin	Pleasant citrus scent; conditions and deodorizes coat; safe for use on cats
	VIP™ Pyrethrin Flea & Tick Dip	5	Pyrethrins	1	D, C	As needed	Harmful if swallowed; avoid contamination of feed & utensils	
Virbac Laboratories	Ban-Guard Dip	5	Dursban, 3.84%	1	D	Monthly	Cholinesterase inhibitor; do *not* use on cats	Controls sarcoptic mange mites
Dust/Powder								
Adams Laboratories (A SmithKline Beecham Company)	Adams™ Flea & Tick Dust II	6	Pyrethrins with synergist and carbaryl	1	D, C	As needed	See product label	Can use on cats, dogs, puppies, and kittens over 4 weeks old
Fort Dodge Laboratories	Carpet Control™	6	d-phenothrin, 0.46%; piperonyl butoxide, 1.63%	1, 2		As needed	Harmful if swallowed; avoid breathing dust or contact with eyes; see product label	Sprinkle on carpet, wait 30 minutes, then vacuum; if ticks are present, leave powder on surface for two weeks; also kills lice, ants, silverfish, roaches
Pitman-Moore	Diryl® Insecticidal Powder	6	Carbaryl, 0.05%; pyrethrins, 0.1%	1, 3	D, C	As needed	See product label	
SmithKline Beecham Animal Health	MYCODEX® Powder Plus	6	Carbaryl, 5%; pyrethrins, 0.1%	1	D, C	At least once weekly	See product label	
TechAmerica	Flea and Tick Dust Plus	6	Carbaryl	1, 3	D, C	See product label	See product label	Combines 3 effective insecticides; no offensive odor
Vet-Kem	Flea & Tick Powder	6	Carbaryl	1	D, C	See product label	See product label	Kills fleas & ticks; can be used on puppies and kittens older than 4 wk of age
	Paramite® Insecticidal Dust for Dogs	6	Phosmet	1	D	See product label	See product label	Aids in prevention of sarcoptic mange; 8-oz size
Vet Mate Labs	VET MATE™ Extra Strength Flea & Tick Powder	6	Organic pyrethrins, carbaryl	1, 3	D, C	As needed but not more than once a week	See product label	Controls fleas, lice, ticks; can be used on pet bedding and in vacuum cleaner bags
	VET MATE™ Flea & Tick Powder	6	Carbaryl, 5.0%	1, 3	D, C	As needed but not more than once a week	See product label	Nonscented triple-application sifter top

Company	Product Name[b]	Class[c]	Principal Active Ingredients	Action[d]	Species[e]	Frequency of Administration	Precautions[f]	Miscellaneous Comments
Veterinary Products Laboratories	VIP™ Flea & Tick Powder	6	Carbaryl, pyrethrins with amorphous silica gel	1	D, C	Once weekly	Do not breathe dust; avoid contact with skin	Quick knockdown with residual
Topical Liquid								
Fort Dodge Laboratories	Foam Control™	7	1% propoxur (gendran)	1	D, C	2 wk for fleas, 1 wk for ticks	See product label	A fast-breaking topical foam product (not a shampoo) that is applied along top line of animal's back; also kills lice
HAVER, Mobay Animal Health	PROSPOT® Solution	7	Fenthion	1	D	Every 2 wk	Cholinesterase inhibitor; do *not* use on puppies younger than 10 wk of age	Safe for heartworm-positive dogs; safe during all stages of pregnancy; 5 sizes for dogs weighing between 5 lb and 160 lb
3M/Animal Care	Sectrol® Two-Way Flea Foam	7	Pyrethrins, microencapsulated pyrethrins	1	D, C	As needed	See product label	Kills fleas on pets for 8 days; excellent knockdown; kills ticks, including deer ticks
Vet Mate Labs	VET MATE™ Fly Repellent Ointment	7	Dual synergized natural pyrethrins	1, 3	D, C, H	As needed	See product label	Provides maximum protection against flies, fleas, ticks, other insects; controls ear mites
	VET MATE™ Repellent Roll-on	7	Dual synergized organic pyrethrins	1, 3	D, C, H	As needed	See product label	Provides excellent control of flies, fleas, ticks, gnats, mosquitoes, ear mites, other insects
Virbac Laboratories	Supra-Quick Roll-on™	7	Pyrethrins, 0.10%	1, 3	D, C	Daily or as needed	See product label	Roll-on application; does not frighten pets
Cream Rinse								
Coopers Animal Health (A Pitman-Moore Company)	Expar® Cream Rinse	8	Permethrin	1, 3	D, C	Every 2–3 wk	See product label	Controls lice
Fogger								
Adams Laboratories (A SmithKline Beecham Company)	Adams™ Room Fogger with Dursban	9	Chlorpyrifos, pyrethrins	1, 2		Every 30 days for adults, 42 days for larvae	See product label; harmful if swallowed	
Coopers Animal Health (A Pitman-Moore Company)	Impass™ Fogger	9	Fenoxycarb, S-bioallethrin	1, 2, 4		Every 6 months	Do *not* apply to pets	Kills all stages of fleas, including eggs; residual activity stable in ultraviolet light
KenVet Animal Care Group, Veratec	Inacide-5®	9	Pyrethrins	1, 2		Repeat as needed	Do *not* apply to pets	For use in kennels, catteries, agricultural operations
Pitman-Moore	Professional Home Treatment Kit	9	2 Sprecto-CF (4 oz); 1 Sprecto-CF (8 oz); 1 Sprecto-CCR	1, 2		Every 4 wk	See product label	

[a]Product labels should be reviewed carefully before any product is used. In all cases, keep insecticide products out of the reach of children and pets. Inclusion of a product in this guide does not represent endorsement by the publisher.
[b]Proprietary names are listed.
[c]Class key: 1 = spray/mist—aerosol; 2 = spray/mist—nonaerosol; 3 = shampoo; 4 = collar; 5 = dip/sponge-on; 6 = dust/powder; 7 = topical liquid preparation (other than dips, sponge-ons, sprays, mists, shampoos); 8 = cream rinse; 9 = foggers (environmental use); 10 = liquid sprays (environmental use); 11 = oral administration (i.e., tablets, liquid).
[d]Action key: 1 = adulticidal; 2 = larvacidal; 3 = repellent.
[e]Species key: D = dog; C = cat; H = horse. If no species is indicated, the product is for environmental use.
[f]Any product specified as a cholinesterase inhibitor should *not* be used in conjunction with other pesticides.

This listing is arranged according to product classes defined as follows:

- Class 1: aerosol spray and mist products for use on pets
- Class 2: nonaerosol spray and mist products for use on pets
- Class 3: shampoo products
- Class 4: collars
- Class 5: dip or sponge-on products
- Class 6: dust and powder products
- Class 7: any topical liquid preparation that is not a dip, sponge-on, spray, mist, or shampoo
- Class 8: cream rinse preparations
- Class 9: foggers for environmental use
- Class 10: liquid sprays for environmental use
- Class 11: tablet or liquid oral preparations

Company	Product Name[b]	Class[c]	Principal Active Ingredients	Action[d]	Species[e]	Frequency of Administration	Precautions[f]	Miscellaneous Comments
	Sprecto® -CV Foggers	9	Permethrin, tetramethrin	1, 2		Every 4 wk	See product label	
SmithKline Beecham Animal Health	MYCODEX® Chlori-Fog	9	Chlorpyrifos, 1%; pyrethrins, 0.05%	1		See product label	See product label	Covers up to 3000 cu ft of unobstructed space
TechAmerica	EctoGuard Fogger	9	Fenoxycarb, pyrethrins, permethrin	1, 2		See product label	See product label	New; stops flea development in all 4 life cycle stages
Vet-Kem	Siphotrol® Plus Fogger	9	Methoprene, permethrin	1, 2		See product label	See product label	Kills preadult fleas for 30 wk
	Vet-Fog®	9	Permethrin	1		See product label	See product label	Kills fleas, ticks, roaches, flying moths, spiders, ants
Veterinary Product Laboratories	VIP™ Fogger	9	Fenvalerate	1, 2		See product label	See product label	Kills fleas, roaches, ants, spiders, flying moths, mosquitoes, flies, crickets; 4-oz size covers 4000 cu ft
Liquid Spray								
Adams Laboratories (A SmithKline Beecham Company)	Adams™ Anti-Crawl®	10	Pyrethrins with synergists and propoxur	1, 2		Repeat as needed	Do *not* apply to animals; harmful if swallowed	
	Adams™ Home & Kennel Spray with Dursban	10	Chlorpyrifos	1, 2		Every 2–3 wk	See product label; do *not* apply to animals	
	Adams™ Lawn & Kennel Spray Kit with Dursban	10	Chlorpyrifos	1, 2		Every 2–3 wk	Do *not* apply to animals	
	Adams™ Lawn & Kennel Spray Concentrate with Dursban	10	Chlorpyrifos	1, 2		Every 2–3 wk	Do *not* apply to animals	
	Adams™ Surface Spray	10	Allethrin, chlorpyrifos	1, 2		As needed	Do *not* apply to animals; do *not* apply to finished wood surfaces	
Bio-Ceutic Animal Health	Permectrin™ II Horse & Stable Spray	10	Permethrin	1, 2	H	See product label	See product label	Use as needed but not more than once every two weeks
	Permectrin™ Pet, Yard & Kennel Spray	10	Permethrin	1, 2	D, C	See product label	See product label	Use as needed but not more than once every two weeks
	Yard & Kennel Spray	10	Chlorpyrifos	1, 2		As needed	See product label	Hose-end spray

Company	Product Name[b]	Class[c]	Principal Active Ingredients	Action[d]	Species[e]	Frequency of Administration	Precautions[f]	Miscellaneous Comments
Coopers Animal Health	Expar® Home & Carpet Spray	10	Permethrin	1, 3		Every 10 wk	See product label; do *not* use on cats	Available as spray; for use on dogs and premises; also controls cockroaches, silverfish, spiders
KenVet Animal Care Group, Veratec	Chlorpyriban™	10	Chlorpyrifos, 12.6%	1, 2		Repeat as needed	Do *not* apply to pets	Sustained activity to 4 wk depending on environmental conditions
Pitman-Moore	Sprecto® Complete Carpet & Room Spray	10	Chlorpyrifos, d-trans allethrin	1, 2		As needed	See product label	
SmithKline Beecham Animal Health	MYCODEX® Lawn Spray Concentrate	10	Cyano, 1.72%	1		As needed every 7–14 days	See product label	Hose-end sprayer
	MYCODEX® Room & Carpet Accu-Spray	10	Chlorpyrifos, 0.5%; pyrethrins, 0.025%; piperonyl butoxide, 0.05%	1		As needed	See product label	Trigger-action aerosol liquid product
TechAmerica	EctoGuard House and Carpet Spray	10	Fenoxycarbon, permethrin	1, 2		See product label	See product label	New; stops flea development in all 4 life cycle stages
3M/Animal Care	Duratrol® Household Flea Spray	10	Microencapsulated chlorpyrifos	1, 2		As needed	See product label	Kills adult fleas for 90 days & flea larvae for 90 days; odorless, nonstaining; available with pump-up sprayer
	Duratrol® Yard and Kennel Spray	10	Microencapsulated chlorpyrifos	1, 2		As needed	See product label	Kills fleas outdoors for 30 days; comes with hose sprayer; also kills deer ticks
	Sectrol® Pet and Household Flea Spray	10	Microencapsulated pyrethrin	1		As needed	See product label	Also a pet spray for direct application to dogs or cats; kills fleas indoors for 30 days; odorless
Vet-Kem	Siphotrol Plus® II House Treatment	10	Methoprene, chlorpyrifos, pyrethrin	1, 2		See product label	See product label	Kills fleas, ticks, roaches; kills preadult fleas for 30 wk; 32-oz and 64-oz sizes; also available in kit that contains pump-up sprayer
	Vet-Kem® Siphotrol Premise Spray	10	Methoprene, pyrethrins	1, 2		See product label	See product label	Kills fleas; kills preadult fleas for 30 wk; can be used on dogs or premises
	Vet-Kem® Yard & Kennel Spray	10	Chlorpyrifos	1		See product label	See product label	Kills fleas & ticks in yards, kennels, and doghouses; 16-oz size; hose-end sprayer or refill
Vet Mate Labs	VET MATE™ Barn & Stable Spray	10	Permethrin	1, 3		As needed	See product label	Can be used as a premise spray in hospitals, feed rooms, dairies, horse barns, and poultry houses or directly on dogs and livestock via automatic foggers and spraying systems
Veterinary Products Laboratories	VIP™ Concentrated Yard Spray	10	Fenvalerate	1		7–14 days	Do not get into eyes or on skin or clothing	A noncholinesterase inhibitor

[a]Product labels should be reviewed carefully before any product is used. In all cases, keep insecticide products out of the reach of children and pets. Inclusion of a product in this guide does not represent endorsement by the publisher.
[b]Proprietary names are listed.
[c]Class key: 1 = spray/mist—aerosol; 2 = spray/mist—nonaerosol; 3 = shampoo; 4 = collar; 5 = dip/sponge-on; 6 = dust/powder; 7 = topical liquid preparation (other than dips, sponge-ons, sprays, mists, shampoos); 8 = cream rinse; 9 = foggers (environmental use); 10 = liquid sprays (environmental use); 11 = oral administration (i.e., tablets, liquid).
[d]Action key: 1 = adulticidal; 2 = larvacidal; 3 = repellent.
[e]Species key: D = dog; C = cat; H = horse. If no species is indicated, the product is for environmental use.
[f]Any product specified as a cholinesterase inhibitor should *not* be used in conjunction with other pesticides.

This listing is arranged according to product classes defined as follows:

Class 1: aerosol spray and mist products for use on pets
Class 2: nonaerosol spray and mist products for use on pets
Class 3: shampoo products
Class 4: collars
Class 5: dip or sponge-on products
Class 6: dust and powder products
Class 7: any topical liquid preparation that is not a dip, sponge-on, spray, mist, or shampoo
Class 8: cream rinse preparations
Class 9: foggers for environmental use
Class 10: liquid sprays for environmental use
Class 11: tablet or liquid oral preparations

Company	Product Name[b]	Class[c]	Principal Active Ingredients	Action[d]	Species[e]	Frequency of Administration	Precautions[f]	Miscellaneous Comments
	VIP™ Formula 4 System and Concentrate	10	Linalool	1, 2		As needed	Do not get into eyes or on skin or clothing	Kills all 4 stages of flea life cycle
	VIP™ Indoor Premise Spray	10	Chlorpyrifos, pyrethrins	1		As needed	Avoid contact with skin, eyes, clothing	
	VPL Lawn Spray Concentrate	10	Fenvalerate	1		7–14 days	Do not get into eyes or on skin or clothing	A noncholinesterase inhibitor; 8-oz size covers 3000 sq ft
Oral								
HAVER, Mobay Animal Health	PROBAN® Tablets & Liquid	11	Cythioate	1	D	Twice weekly or every third day	Cholinesterase inhibitor; do *not* use for greyhounds or pregnant dogs	Safe for heartworm-positive dogs and adults or puppies of all ages

[a]Product labels should be reviewed carefully before any product is used. In all cases, keep insecticide products out of the reach of children and pets. Inclusion of a product in this guide does not represent endorsement by the publisher.
[b]Proprietary names are listed.
[c]Class key: 1 = spray/mist—aerosol; 2 = spray/mist—nonaerosol; 3 = shampoo; 4 = collar; 5 = dip/sponge-on; 6 = dust/powder; 7 = topical liquid preparation (other than dips, sponge-ons, sprays, mists, shampoos); 8 = cream rinse; 9 = foggers (environmental use); 10 = liquid sprays (environmental use); 11 = oral administration (i.e., tablets, liquid).
[d]Action key: 1 = adulticidal; 2 = larvacidal; 3 = repellent.
[e]Species key: D = dog; C = cat; H = horse. If no species is indicated, the product is for environmental use.
[f]Any product specified as a cholinesterase inhibitor should *not* be used in conjunction with other pesticides.

TABLE 3-6

Medicated Shampoos

Ingredients	*Pros*	*Cons*	*Examples*
Sulfur	Safe; keratolytic; keratoplastic; antipruritic; antifungal; antibacterial	Nondegreasing; malodorus; may stain coat; may dry skin	Sebolux® (Allerderm) Sebalyt® (DVM) Sultex® (Dermavet) MicroPearls® (IGI) Sebbafon® (Winthrop)
Selenium disulfide	Keratolytic; mildly degreasing	Weak antiseborrheic	Seleen® (Ceva) Selenium (Vet Derm)
Salicylic acid	Mildly antibacterial; astringent; mildly antipruritic	Weak antiseborrheic	Medi-Clean® (Lambert Kay) Cerbinol® (Pitman-Moore) Soothing Medicated (Vet Derm)
Tar	Keratolytic; keratoplastic; degreasing; antipruritic	Poorly standardized; can stain coats; contact sensitivity; irritating; possibly carcinogenic	Allerseb I® (Allerderm) Lytar® (DVM) Pragmatar® (SmithKline Beecham) Clear Tar (Vet Prescription) Mycodex® Tar and Sulfur (SmithKline Beecham)
Benzoyl peroxide	Keratolytic; keratoplastic; antibacterial; mildly antipruritic; degreasing	Very drying; stains coat; may irritate skin; possibly carcinogenic; bleaches fabrics	Pyoben® (Allerderm) Oxydex® (DVM) Vet-Derm® (Vet Derm) Sulf Oxydex® (DVM) Benoxyderm® (Coopers)

SYSTEMIC DERMATOLOGIC DRUGS

Corticosteroids

Corticosteroids are the most used and often abused class of systemic dermatologic drugs. When treating dermatologic disease, familiarity with the actions (Table 3-7), length of adrenal suppression (Table 3-8), treatment protocols (Table 3-9), and side effects (Table 3-10) of corticosteroids is necessary.

Antibiotics

The antibiotic of choice in treating dermatologic problems is often different from those commonly selected for systemic diseases (Table 3-11). The selection of the antibiotic of choice is based on drug history, clinical signs, and in vitro bacterial culture and antibiotic sensitivity testing. In general, ampicillin, penicillin, and the tetracyclines are not routinely recommended for treating either primary or secondary pyoderma because of their relatively lower clinical efficacy. Bacterial resistance to these antibiotics is commonly observed. Bactericidal antibiotics should be used to treat deep pyoderma and chronic or recurrent superficial pyodermas. Bacteriostatic antibiotics are used initially for superficial and intermediate pyodermas in cases in which no immune compromise is suspected.

Therapeutic dosages of an efficacious drug should continue to be administered for a minimum of 7 to 10 days following a complete clinical response. If there is a minimal clinical response in 5 to 7 days, the treatment protocol should be reevaluated.

Systemic Antifungal Drugs

Systemic antifungal drugs are limited in their indications (Table 3-12). Griseofulvin is limited to treating dermatophytosis while nystatin is indicated only for candidal infection. Sodium iodide is used in treating sporotrichosis. Amphotericin B, 5-fluorocytosine, and ketoconazole are used in the treatment of systemic mycoses.

Amphotericin B is a polyene macrolide that binds to ergosterol and must be administered intravenously; phlebitis is a common sequela to perivascular leakage. It is strongly protein bound and slowly excreted via biliary and renal routes. It is normally suspended in 10 to 120

TABLE 3-7

Systemic Glucocorticoids

Drug: Generic Name (Commercial Name—Manufacturer)	*Action*	*Indications*	*Dosage/Administration*	*Comment*
Short-acting Prednisone Prednisolone Methylprednisolone (Medrol® —Upjohn)	Antipruritic; antiinflammatory	Pruritus (acute or chronic)	Loading dose: 0.5–1 mg/kg sid–bid for 2–5 days PO Maintenance dose: 0.5–1 mg/kg q2d or as needed PO	Polyuria, polydipsia, polyphagia; iatrogenic hyperadrenocorticism may result from chronic daily administration
Long-acting Dexamethasone (Azium® —Schering-Plough Animal Health)	Same as above	Acute pruritus of expected short duration	0.25–2 mg sid PO or IM	Polyphagia; do not use in chronic pruritus requiring long-term steroids; potential for iatrogenic hyperadrenocorticism
Residual Triamcinolone acetonide (Vetalog® —Solvay Animal Health)	Same as above	Acute pruritus of expected short duration	Loading dose: 0.01–0.02 mg/kg sid PO Maintenance dose: 0.02–0.04 sid PO; 0.2 mg/kg IM; repeat in 7–10 days if needed	Same as above
Methylprednisolone acetate (Depo-Medrol® —Upjohn)	Same as above	Dogs: Acute pruritus of expected short duration Cats: Eosinophilic granuloma complex and nonspecific pruritus	Dogs: 1 mg/kg IM Cats: 20 mg q4–6wk SC	Do not repeat more than once in dogs: no side effects reported with repeated injections in cats

TABLE 3-8

Length of Action of Systemic Corticosteroids

Type	*Length of Adrenal Suppression*	*Drug*	*Relative Antiinflammatory Effects*[a]
Short-acting	<36 hours	Hydrocortisone	1
		Prednisone	4
		Prednisolone	4
		Methylprednisolone	5
		Triamcinolone	5
Long-acting	>60 hours	Dexamethasone	10–20
		Betamethasone	10–20
		Flumethasone	20 or more
Residual	2–4 weeks	Triamcinolone acetonide	NK[b]
		Methylprednisolone acetate	NK
		Betamethasone dipropionate	NK

[a]When compared with hydrocortisone on a mg to mg basis.
[b]Not known.

TABLE 3-9

Short-Acting Corticosteroid Dosage Guidelines for Oral Route

Corticosteroid Treatment	Size of Dog					
	Small (<9 kg)		*Medium (9 to 23 kg)*		*Large (>23 kg)*	
	Initial	*Maintenance*	*Initial*	*Maintenance*	*Initial*	*Maintenance*
Pruritus						
Minimal	5 mg q2d	taper[a]	5 mg q24h	5 mg q2d and taper[a]	10 mg q24h	10 mg q2d and taper[a]
Moderate	5 mg q12h or q24h	5–10 mg q2d and taper[a]	10 mg q2d and taper[a]	10 mg q2d and taper[a]	10–20 mg q12h or q24h	20 mg q24h and taper[a]
Marked	10 mg q12h or q24h	10–15 mg q2d taper[a]	10–20 mg q12h or q24h	20–30 mg q2d and taper[a]	25 mg q12h or q24h	25–50 mg q2d and taper[a]

[a]Try to decrease dosage 50% each week, either in frequency or quantity.

TABLE 3-10

Side Effects of Chronic Daily and Alternate-Day Short-Term Corticosteroid Therapy

Clinical Sign	Frequency of Treatment		Pathogenesis
	Daily	**Alternate-Day**	
	Relative Frequency of Occurrence[a]		
Polyuria/polydipsia	++++	±	Unknown
Alopecia	++	−	Atrophy of hair follicles, sebaceous glands, and epidermis
Thin skin	+	−	Atrophy of epidermis, collagen, and fibroelastic tissue
Hepatomegaly	++	−	Glycogen accumulation within hepatocytes
Distended abdomen	+	−	Muscle weakness, hepatomegaly, and intraperitoneal fat deposition
Calcinosis cutis	+	−	Altered dermal protein matrix with dystrophic binding of calcium
Hyperpigmentation	++	−	Unknown
Infection	+	−	Antiinflammatory and immunosuppressive effects
Anestrus/testicular atrophy	+	−	Probable inhibition of gonadotropin release

[a]If on continuous long-term therapy (months to years using prednisone, prednisolone, or methylprednisolone).

ml of 5% dextrose and given over a 5- to 15-minute period, three times weekly. All systemic mycoses are normally treated for four weeks beyond apparent cure or as indicated by serologic tests. Nephrotoxicity is a common side effect that might possibly be minimized by the intravenous loading of physiological saline prior to administration of the drug.

Ketoconazole is administered orally and is effective against blastomycosis, coccidioidomycosis, cryptococcosis, histoplasmosis, dermatophytosis, candidiasis, sporotrichosis, and aspergillosis. Ketoconazole should be administered with food and not concurrently with antacids, cimetidine, or anticholinergics. Anorexia and vomiting are the most common side effects.

TABLE 3-11

Systemic Antibiotics

Drug (Generic Name)	*Action*	*Type*	*Dosage/Administration*	*Comment*
Oxacillin	Bactericidal	Penicillin	15–20 mg/kg tid PO	β-lactamase resistant
Cloxacillin	Bactericidal	Penicillin	15 mg/kg tid PO	β-lactamase susceptible
Penicillin G	Bactericidal	Penicillin	20,000 U/kg qid PO	Cat bite abscess
Ampicillin	Bactericidal	Penicillin	22 mg/kg PO	Bacterial feline dermatoses
Amoxicillin	Bactericidal	Penicillin	12 mg/kg PO	Bacterial feline dermatoses
Nafcillin	Bactericidal	Penicillin	20 mg/kg bid PO	β-lactamase resistant
Amoxicillin/clavulanate	Bactericidal	Penicillin	12–14 mg/kg PO	β-lactamase resistant
Cefadroxil	Bactericidal	Cephalosporin	22 mg/kg bid PO	May be given tid
Cephalexin	Bactericidal	Cephalosporin	22 mg/kg tid or 30 mg/kg bid PO	High efficacy
Cephradine	Bactericidal	Cephalosporin	20–30 mg/kg bid PO	High efficacy
Trimethoprim-sulfa	Bactericidal	T-sulfa	30 mg/kg sid or bid PO	Potential to lead to keratoconjunctivitis sicca
Gentamicin	Bactericidal	Aminocyclitol	4 mg/kg bid SC	Only used in generalized resistant deep pyoderma or septicemia; ototoxic; nephrotoxic
Enrofloxacin	Bactericidal	Fluoroquinolone	5 mg/kg bid PO	Not for use in young animals
Lincomycin	Bacteriostatic	Lincosamide	20 mg/kg bid PO	Good first-line antibiotic
Clindamycin	Bacteriostatic	Lincosamide	5.5 mg/kg bid PO	Abscesses, wounds
Erythromycin	Bacteriostatic	Macrolide	15 mg/kg tid PO	Vomiting common
Chloramphenicol	Bacteriostatic	Chloramphenicol	50 mg/kg tid PO	Good first-line antibiotic

TABLE 3-12

Systemic Antifungal Agents

Agent	*Action*	*Dosage/Route*	*Comments*
Griseofulvin (microsize)	Fungistatic	50–150 mg/kg PO	Feed with fat meal; teratogenic; bone marrow suppression
Griseofulvin (ultramicrosize)	Fungistatic	35–65 mg/kg sid PO	No fat meal required
Sodium iodide 20%	Sporicidal	20–40 mg/kg tid	Sporotrichosis; vomiting; depression
Flucytosine	Fungicidal	60 mg/kg tid PO	Candidiasis; cryptococcosis; rapid resistant and mutations; used in combination with other drugs
Amphotericin B	Fungistatic	Dogs: 0.25–0.5 mg/kg in dextrose 3× weekly IV Cats: 0.15 mg/kg in dextrose 3× weekly IV	Systemic mycoses; used in combination with amphoketaconazole or flucytosine; nephrotoxic; anemia; phlebitis, hypokalemia
Ketoconazole	Fungistatic	2.5–15 mg/kg bid PO	Systemic mycoses, candidiasis, dermatophytosis; inappetence; hepatotoxic

TABLE 3-13

Chemotherapeutic Agents

Agent	*Action*	*Administration*	*Comments*
Prednisolone Prednisone	Immunosuppressive	Taper if possible	Polydipsia, polyuria, polyphagia; increased susceptibility for infection; delayed wound healing
Cyclophosphamide	Alkylating agent; immunosuppressive	50 mg/m^2; 1.5 mg/kg 3–4 days per week	Leukopenia; hemorrhagic cystitis
Chlorambucil	Alkylating agent; immunosuppressive	0.2 mg/kg sid	Usually no adverse effects
Azathioprine	Antimetabolite	2.2 mg/kg sid or q2d PO	Leukopenia; thrombocytopenia; vomiting; use with caution in cats
Vincristine	Vinca alkaloid	0.5 mg/m^2 weekly or alternate weeks	Anemia; leukopenia; stomatitis
Methotrexate	Antimetabolite	2.5–15 mg/m^2 sid IV, IM, PO	Anemia; gastrointestinal disturbances
Aurothioglucose (chrysotherapy)	Immunosuppressive	Test dose: 1–5 mg IM; later Maintenance dose: 1 mg/kg weekly IM	Thrombocytopenia; stomatitis; dermatitis; nephritis
Gold sodium thiomalate (chrysotherapy)	Immunosuppressive	Same as above	Same as above
Dapsone (Avlosulfon)	Enzyme interference	1.1–1.5 mg/kg bid–qid; taper to q2d	Thrombocytopenia; anemia
Cyclosporine	Cyclic polypeptide	10–30 mg/kg sid	Vomiting; dermatitis
Vitamin E	Antioxidant	200–400 IU bid PO	

Chemotherapeutic Agents

Chemotherapeutic agents are principally used in dermatology in the treatment of immune-mediated disorders and occasionally neoplasia. The most common treatments used include corticosteroids, cyclophosphamide, azathioprine, chlorambucil, and dapsone (Table 3-13). Chrysotherapy (gold salt therapy), cyclosporine, and vitamin E also have potential application in the management of immune-mediated disorders. Chrysotherapy is indicated for the treatment of pemphigus, pemphigoid, and lymphocytic-plasmacytic dermatitides. Because its side effects may resemble the clinical manifestations of lupus erythematosus, it is considered contraindicated in the treatment of that disorder.

Hormones

Hormones are used in dermatology not only as replacement therapy but for their antiinflammatory action as well (Table 3-14). Fortunately, the progestagens, with their marked side effects, are used much less frequently now than in the past.

Retinoids

Retinoids are synthetic derivatives of vitamin A and depending on their formulation have a profound effect on keratinization and sebaceous gland function. Etretinate (Tegison® —Roche) has a more profound effect on disorders of keratinization, while isotretinoin (Accutane® —Roche) has a more marked effect on sebaceous

TABLE 3-14

Hormonal Medications

Drug (Generic Name)	*Action*	*Indications*	*Dosage/Administration*	*Comments*
Thyroid				
Thyroxine	T_4 replacement	Canine hypothyroidism as initial therapy	0.2 mg/kg q12h–q24h PO	Polydipsia and nervousness if excessive dosage
Triiodothyronine	T_3 replacement	Canine hypothyroidism if poor response to thyroxine	4.4 μg/kg q8h PO	Depresses serum T_4 value; seldom indicated
Combination thyroxine and triiodothyronine	T_3 and T_4 replacement	Same as above	Calculate dosage on basis of thyroxine content (0.2 mg/kg q12h)	Seldom indicated
Androgens Methyltestosterone Fluoxymesterone	Testosterone replacement; increases sebum production	Sertoli cell tumor—postsurgery; hypoandrogenism; seborrhea sicca	0.5 mg/kg daily PO	
Testosterone propionate	Testosterone replacement	Sertoli cell tumor—postsurgery; hypoandrogenism; feline endocrine alopecia (male)	2.2 mg/kg IM; repeat q2wk for dogs and q6wk for cats	
Progestins Progesterone (repository)	Progesterone replacement	Feline endocrine alopecia	2.2–20 mg/kg IM; repeat in 6 weeks if poor regrowth of hair	
Megestrol acetate	Progesterone replacement; antiinflammatory effect	Feline endocrine alopecia; eosinophilic granuloma complex	2.5–5 mg/cat q2d until regrowth of hair; then maintenance dose 2.5–5 mg q3d–q7d PO	Not approved for cats in United States; polyuria, polydipsia, polyphagia; mammary gland hyperplasia; personality change; diabetes mellitus
Estrogen Diethylstilbestrol	Estrogen replacement; decrease sebum production	Ovarian imbalance Type II; seborrhea oleosa in spayed female	0.02 mg/kg daily × 2 weeks PO; then q2d as needed	Monitor bone marrow if long-term usage; thromboembolism
Growth hormone	Growth hormone replacement	Growth hormone replacement	5 units q2d SC × 10 doses	Presently not commercially available in United States

gland disorders. Neither product is licensed for use in dogs or cats and side effects are commonplace. Liver function tests, blood counts, and cholesterol levels should be monitored in patients receiving these drugs. An empirical dosage for etretinate is 0.5 mg/kg/day and for isotretinoin, 1.0 mg/kg/day.

Antihistamines

Antihistamines have been downplayed in the past but have become more popular in the last few years. In most pruritic conditions, antihistamines must be given at relatively high doses that frequently result in some degree of sedation (Table 3-15). It is generally expected that approximately 25 to 35% of pruritic dogs will benefit from the administration of antihistamines.

Fatty Acid Supplements

The omega-3 fatty acids, including eicosapentaenoic acid, docosapentaenoic acid, and docosahexaenoic acid, are derivatives of alpha-linolenic acid and are most plentifully supplied in fish oils. The omega-6 fatty acids, of which gamma-linolenic acid is most important, are deriv-

TABLE 3-15

Antihistamines

Class	*Generic*	*Trade Name*	*Administration*
Phenothiazine	Promethazine	Phenergan® (Wyeth)	0.2–1.0 mg/kg tid
	Trimeprazine	Temaril® (SmithKline Beecham)	1–2 mg/kg bid
Ethanolamine	Diphenhydramine	Benadryl® (Parke-Davis)	1–2 mg/kg bid–tid
	Clemastine	Tavist® (Ancalab)	0.5–1.0 mg/kg bid
Alkylamine	Chlorpheniramine	Chlor-Trimeton® (Schering-Plough)	0.5–2 mg/kg bid–tid
Ethylenediamine	Pyrilamine	Triaminic® (Ancalab)	1–2 mg/kg bid–tid
Piperazine	Hydroxyzine	Atarax® (Pfizer)	2.2 mg/kg tid
Piperidine	Terfenadine	Seldane® (Merrell Dow)	5 mg/kg bid

TABLE 3-16

Immune Stimulants

Drug	*Dosage/Administration*		
Staphage lysate™ (Delmont Laboratories)	Day 1: 0.2 ml SC Day 2: 0.4 ml SC Day 3: 0.6 ml SC Day 4: 0.8 ml SC Day 5: 1.0 ml SC Day 12: 1.5 ml SC Weekly: 1.5 ml SC or 0.5 ml SC q3–4d		
Staphoid A-B® (Cooper) or Lysigin® (Bioceutic)	Day 1: 0.1 ml ID; 0.15 ml SC Day 2: 0.1 ml ID; 0.40 ml SC Day 3: 0.1 ml ID; 0.65 ml SC Day 4: 0.1 ml ID; 0.90 ml SC Day 5: 0.1 ml ID; 1.15 ml SC Day 12: 0.1 ml ID; 1.40 ml SC Day 19: 0.1 ml ID; 1.65 ml SC Day 26: 0.1 ml ID; 1.90 ml SC Monthly: 0.1 ml ID; 1.90 ml SC		
Levamisole	2.2 mg/kg 3 times/wk		
	Weight	*Dose*	*Frequency*
ImmunoRegulin® (Immunovet)	<17 lb (<8 kg) 17–33 lb (8–15 kg) 34–88 lb (16–40 kg) >88 lb (>40 kg)	0.25 ml IV 0.50 ml IV 0.75 ml IV 1.00 ml IV	Injections are given twice weekly for 2 weeks; then weekly until good clinical response

atives of linoleic acid. The special fatty acids have been shown to be antiinflammatory by virtue of their ability to interfere with the lipoxygenase pathway of arachidonic acid metabolism. Their principal use has been in the management of allergic inhalant dermatitis in dogs. Some formulations that include these functional fatty acids are DermCaps® (DVM), EFA Z-Plus® (Allerderm), OFA Plus® (Nutrispecialties), and Efavet® (Vet-Kem).

Immune Stimulation

Immune stimulants have been used in veterinary dermatology for many years (Table 3-16) and are presumed to enhance the cell-mediated immune competence of animals although this has only tenuously been documented. The most commonly used stimulants include levamisole and bacterins derived from staphylococci, propionibacteria, or mycobacteria. Newer nutritional alternatives (for example, thymus gland extracts and dimethylglycine) are currently being evaluated.

SELECTED READINGS

Ackerman L: The use of nutritional supplementation in canine dermatological disorders. *Vet Focus* 2(2):39–42, 1990.

Codner EC: New treatments for external parasites in small animals. *Vet Focus* 2(2):55–56, 1990.

DeBoer DJ, Moriello KA, Thomas CB, et al: Evaluation of a commercial staphylococcal bacterin for management of idiopathic recurrent superficial pyoderma in dogs. *Am J Vet Res* 51:636–639, 1990.

Eichenbaum JD, Macy D, Severin GA, Paulsen ME: Effect in large dogs of ophthalmic prednisolone acetate on adrenal gland and hepatic function. *JAAHA* 24:705–709, 1988.

Ihrke PJ: Topical therapy: Uses, principles and vehicles. Dermatologic therapy (Part I). *Compend Contin Educ Pract Vet* 2:28–35, 1980.

Ihrke PJ: Topical therapy: Specific topical pharmacologic agents. Dermatologic therapy (Part II). *Compend Contin Educ Pract Vet* 2:156–164, 1980.

Lee AN, Swaim SF, McGuire JA, Hughes KS: Effects of chlorhexidine diacetate, povidone-iodine and polyhydroxydine on wound healing in dogs. *JAAHA* 24:77–84, 1988.

Meyer DJ, Moriello KA, Feder BM: Effect of otic medications containing glucocorticoids on liver function test results in healthy dogs. *JAVMA* 196:743-744, 1990.

Moriello KA, Fehrer-Sawyer SL, Meyer DJ, Feder B: Adrenocortical suppression associated with topical otic administration of glucocorticoids in dogs. *JAVMA* 193:329–331, 1988.

Scheidt VJ: The basic principles of shampoo therapy. *Vet Focus* 2(2):58–61, 1990.

Swaim SF, Lee AN: Topical wound medication: A review. *JAVMA* 190:1588–1593, 1987.

Swartout M: Antifungal therapeutic agents meet the challenge. *Vet Focus* 2(21):43–45, 1990.

Chapter 4

ALLERGIC DISEASES

Gene H. Nesbitt, DVM, MS
Lowell Ackerman, DVM

Allergic diseases have been well documented in dogs and are being recognized more frequently in cats. Hypersensitivity is defined as an immune response which results in tissue damage. Allergy and hypersensitivity are often used synonymously. Diagnostic Key 2 (see end of Chapter 2) lists the most pertinent historical and clinical findings and diagnostic tests used to help differentiate the common causes of canine and feline allergic diseases.

HYPERSENSITIVITY REACTIONS

Four types of hypersensitivity reactions have been described. *Type I*, or *anaphylactic*, reactions are a humoral hypersensitivity associated with the binding of immunoglobulin E (IgE) to the surface of a mast cell or basophil which results in the degranulation of the cells and subsequent release of pharmacologic mediators of inflammation. *Type II*, or *cytotoxic*, reactions are antibody dependent. An antibody binds to the antigen or complement on the cell surface or on the basement membrane of the skin which results in cell death by phagocytosis. *Type III*, *Arthus* or *immune-complex* reactions, are associated with the formation of antigen-antibody complexes (immune complexes), which either exist free in the circulation or are lodged in small blood vessels or basement membranes. *Type IV, cell-mediated, lymphokine-mediated,* or *delayed* reactions, are associated with sensitized lymphocytes that react with tissue-associated antigens, resulting in macrophages causing nonspecific cell damage or destruction either directly or by the release of lymphokines.

CANINE ATOPY (INHALANT ALLERGY)

Atopy or atopic disease is an inherited predisposition to the development of IgE antibodies to environmental allergens resulting in allergic disease.

Etiologic Factors

The most common causes of atopic dermatitis are inhaled allergens, including tree, weed, and grass pollens; molds; house dust or house dust mites; animal danders; and miscellaneous allergens, such as kapok and cottonseed. Intrinsic allergens, including estrogen and progesterone, have been implicated as causes of atopic disease. Several miscellaneous causes have been identified, including endoparasites, ectoparasites, and food. It is common to have multiple causes for the clinical signs, for example, flea saliva and inhalant allergens.

Pathogenesis

The pathogenesis of canine atopic disease involves a Type I hypersensitivity reaction to an antigen. This is an immediate reaction in which a skin-sensitizing antibody becomes fixed to tissue mast cells and circulating basophils. The coupling of the specific antigen and antibody results in the degranulation of the cells and the subsequent release of vasoactive amines, including histamine, slow-release substance of anaphylaxis (SRS-A), and many macromolecular mediators, such as lysosomal and polymorphonuclear leukocyte enzymes. Smooth muscle contraction, capillary dilatation, increased capillary permeability, and pruritus follow. The respiratory system is considered to be the most common route of entry of the allergen. An inherited susceptibility, probably involving suppressor T cells that do not function normally resulting in excess production of IgE, is thought to be the determining factor in the development of a hypersensitivity reaction. Recently, an immunoglobulin G (IgG) antibody called IgGd has been associated with canine atopic disease.

History

An accurate, thorough history is the most important part of a diagnostic workup for atopic disease. The history for canine atopy is characteristic. The average age of onset is 1 to 3 years with a range of 6 months to more than 6 years.

The breeds reported to be predisposed to atopic disease include wire-haired fox terrier, Scottish terrier, Sealyham terrier, dalmatian, West Highland white terrier, English setter, Lhasa apso, English bulldog, Boston terrier, cairn terrier, Irish setter, miniature schnauzer, pug, and golden retriever. A lower frequency of atopy than expected has been reported for the German shepherd, Doberman pinscher, dachshund, cocker spaniel, and poodle. Atopy has been observed in almost every breed.

Face rubbing, foot licking, and axillary pruritus are the most common allergic signs reported; however, pruritic signs are variable among atopic dogs. Many dogs, especially when young, have a seasonal pattern with severe signs in warm weather. These seasonal patterns vary depending on geographic location, growing season of pollen-producing plants, and environmental factors, such as humidity, wind, temperature, and degree of exposure to the allergen(s). Some dogs have fall and winter seasonal patterns, which often correlate with low humidity and forced air heating systems. As the dog ages, it is common to see an increase in severity and duration of allergic signs. Some atopic dogs have a year-round (nonseasonal) history of allergic disease from the onset of clinical signs, especially in climates with minimal seasonal changes.

A decrease in pruritus usually is reported when corticosteroids are administered daily or on alternate days at a dosage of 0.5 to 1.0 mg/kg. A change in environment also may result in temporary improvement or worsening of signs depending on exposure to the allergen(s). Because of the anamnestic response, an atopic dog may have an allergic reaction even with infrequent exposure to the allergen.

Clinical Manifestations

Dogs with atopic dermatitis have variable clinical manifestations. The lesions may be acute or chronic, localized or generalized, and are commonly found periorbitally and on the feet, ear pinnae, flank, perineum, ventral abdomen, and axillae (Plate I-1 and I-2). Most lesions are secondary to pruritus and usually are characterized by various secondary morphologic changes. Alopecia is variable. Signs of acute inflammatory reaction include erythema and edema of the skin and ears. Chronic inflammation is characterized by thickening of the skin, hyperpigmentation, and lichenification (Plate I-3). Common concurrent problems associated with atopic disease include salivary staining of the hair and superficial folliculitis. Some atopic dogs will have marked pruritus without gross lesions on the skin.

Definitive Diagnostic Tests

Allergy testing, both in vivo and in vitro, is performed so that the offending allergens can be identified, thus allowing for specific treatment with immunotherapy or occasionally avoidance. If symptomatic treatment is the only method of treatment to be used, allergy testing is not indicated because a tentative diagnosis can be made on the basis of history and clinical findings.

In vivo testing uses the intradermal injection of allergen resulting in the release of histamine at the injection site of positive reactions. The in vitro method quantitates the allergen-specific IgE serum levels.

Intradermal Allergy Testing

Intradermal (ID) allergy testing is the most widely accepted method of identifying the atopic dog. A positive ID reaction only indicates that the dog or cat has mast cell–bound IgE antibodies to the allergen injected. It does not necessarily mean that the dermatologic problem is caused by atopic disease. A history of exposure to the allergens must be confirmed.

The client must fully understand the procedures of allergy testing and hyposensitization before testing is initiated. A dissatisfied or misinformed client is the first step toward short- and long-term problems in managing an atopic dog or cat. It is important to consider the time of year when performing ID testing. An animal's intensity of reaction to the specific ID test may be directly correlated with the degree of exposure to the allergen(s). The best time to test for seasonal allergens generally is within 1 to 2 months after exposure, or postseasonally. Weaker or negative ID allergy test reactions may be expected if several months have elapsed after exposure to a seasonal allergen.

At the time of testing, the dog or cat must not be under the influence of immunosuppressive drugs. It often is difficult to determine the waiting time necessary after the last medication has been administered because of variable factors, including type of medication, route, dosage, and duration of treatment. A guideline for the waiting time after daily administration of oral short-acting glucocorticoids is a minimum of 2 weeks or until a marked increase in pruritus is observed. The longer the duration of treatment, the more prolonged the waiting time. After administration of injectable corticosteroids, the waiting time is unpredictable; a reasonable guideline is to wait at least 3 weeks after the expected duration of the effect of the drug or until the animal shows a marked increase in pruritus. Another guideline is to wait 1 week for every month a dog has been on daily or alternate-day oral corticosteroids. Wait at least 7 days after antihistamine administration and 1 day after the administration of a tranquilizer.

Intradermal allergy testing has proven to be an effective diagnostic test in experienced hands; however, there are reports of less than satisfactory results by clinicians or technicians who have not mastered the techniques because of infrequent testing or lack of familiarity with the many potential problems related to selection and handling of antigens. Lack of uniformity of injections or difficulty with grading and interpreting test results can also render the procedure ineffective. It is recommended that one veterinarian in a large group practice be designated to do all the ID allergy testing. If there is insufficient volume in the practice for the individual to develop the necessary skills, dogs should be referred for the diagnostic procedure.

Type and Concentration of Test Allergens. Only aqueous antigens are used for ID skin testing. Antigen concentration is defined in protein nitrogen units (PNU). When measuring, 1 mg of protein nitrogen is equivalent to 100,000 PNU. The final concentration of antigen routinely used is 1000 PNU. Another common measurement is weight per volume (w/v). Most testing concentrations are 1:1000 w/v. A 1:10 w/v is defined as 1 gram of raw material extracted in 10 ml of extracting or diluting fluid.

The actual concentration used for each allergen is dependent on the threshold concentration, which is defined as the maximum concentration at which a minimum number of nonallergic animals will develop skin test reactions. Most allergens are used at a concentration of 1000 PNU/ml. The exceptions include house dust and house dust mites, which are diluted to 250 PNU/ml, and *Rhizopus nigricans*, wool, silk, horse meat, and mixed feathers at 500 PNU/ml.

Selection of Testing Allergens. Allergens are generally grouped on the basis of the taxonomic classification of plants and organisms or are available as individual allergens. Each group contains variable percentages of the individual antigens (for example, 5 to 40%). In addition, several single antigens are routinely used, such as house dust and flea antigen.

The selection of allergens for testing is based on several factors, including the source of the allergens, the geographic location, the history (seasonal, perennial), and the maximum number of allergens to be used. Before selecting the allergens to be used in any given area, the most common problem allergens in the area for both humans and animals should be identified. The most common regional allergens are listed in Table 4-1.

The use of groups of antigens versus individual antigens for testing is controversial. There is limited to no cross-reactivity among some allergens within the same family. Most weeds are antigenically distinct. It is thought that the various animal fibers (epidermals) do have some cross-reactivity. Molds usually are grouped. Because the concentration of the testing antigen usually is standardized at 1000 PNU/ml or 1:1000 w/v, dilution

TABLE 4-1

Distribution of Major Allergens by Region[a]

Nonseasonal allergens common to all regions of the United States:
Molds: *Alternaria, Aspergillus, Fusarium, Helminthosporium, Cladosporium, Penicillium, Phoma, Rhizopus*
Epidermals: horse, cat, and dog epithelium; chicken, duck, and goose feathers; human dander; sheep wool
Miscellaneous: house dust, kapok, silk, orris root, pyrethrums, cottonseed

	Seasonal Pollens		
Region (States)[b]	*Grass Pollens*	*Weed Pollens*	*Tree Pollens*
Northwest (Oregon, Washington)	June, orchard, redtop, rye, timothy	Sagebrush, mugwort, Russian thistle, pigweed, English plantain	Cedar, elm, oak, walnut, sycamore, birch, box elder
California	Bermuda, johnson, june, rye, timothy, orchard, redtop	English plantain, sagebrush, pigweed	Oak, walnut, sycamore, cedar, birch, cypress, elm
Intermountain (Colorado, Idaho, Montana, Nevada, Utah, Wyoming)	June, rye, timothy, orchard, redtop	Cocklebur, kochia, pigweed, ragweed, Russian thistle, mugwort, lamb's quarters, sagebrush, English plantain	Birch, cedar, maple, oak, cottonwood
Southwest (Arizona, New Mexico, Texas)	Bermuda, johnson, rye, june, timothy	Cocklebur, English plantain, lamb's quarters, pigweed, Russian thistle, mugwort, sagebrush, ragweed	Ash, juniper, oak, cottonwood
North Central (Michigan, Minnesota, North Dakota, South Dakota)	June, orchard, redtop, rye, timothy	Pigweed, English plantain, ragweed, cocklebur, kochia, lamb's quarters	Cottonwood, elm, hickory, maple, oak, walnut, sycamore
Midwest (Illinois, Indiana, Iowa, Ohio)	June, orchard, redtop, rye, timothy	Kochia, lamb's quarters, pigweed, cocklebur, English plantain, ragweed, Russian thistle	Ash, cottonwood, elm, hickory, oak, sycamore, walnut
South Central (Arkansas, Kentucky, Louisiana, Mississippi, Oklahoma, Tennessee)	Bermuda, johnson, rye, orchard, june, timothy, redtop	Cocklebur, English plantain, marsh elder, pigweed, ragweed, Russian thistle	Ash, birch, cedar, elm, oak, pecan, walnut, sycamore, hickory
Northeast (Connecticut, Delaware, New Hampshire, New York, New Jersey, Pennsylvania, Maine, Massachusetts, Rhode Island, Vermont)	June, orchard, rye, timothy, meadow fescue, redtop, rye, sweet vernal	Lamb's quarters, ragweed, pigweed, English plantain, mugwort	Ash, birch, elm, maple, oak, pecan, sycamore
Southeast (Alabama, Florida, Georgia, Maryland, North Carolina, South Carolina, Virginia, West Virginia)	Bermuda, johnson, june, orchard, redtop, rye, timothy	Cocklebur, English plantain, lamb's quarters, pigweed, mugwort, ragweed	Ash, birch, cedar, elm, oak, pecan, walnut, sycamore

[a]Adapted from Weiss NS, Rubin JM: *Practical Points in Allergy*, ed 2. Garden City, NY, Medical Examination Publishing, 1980; and from data courtesy of Center Laboratories, Fort Washington, NY.
[b]There are differences in the specific plant populations among states in a given region and within individual states. This is not all-inclusive of important allergens in any given state.

is a factor to consider with grouped antigens. A tree mix with equal parts of 10 tree antigens at a concentration of 1000 PNU/ml of mixture will only contain 100 PNU/ml of each antigen. If one of the tree pollens was the only allergen of clinical importance, a false-negative reaction could occur because of an inadequate concentration of that antigen.

The number of allergens that can be tested at any given time is not standardized. The majority of screening testing kits use 10 to 15 grouped and individual allergens, but this generally is an inadequate number to arrive at the most definitive diagnosis of the specific causes of the atopic disease. Most definitive tests will include 30 to 50 different groups and individual allergens.

All allergens tend to become less stable, biodegrading more rapidly as they are diluted. Thus, allergens diluted for testing must be replaced every 2 to 4 weeks. If a commercial test kit is used, observe the dating closely and discard all outdated materials. The allergens also lose antigenicity on prolonged exposure to heat and thus must be kept refrigerated except when being used.

Each ID test has two controls. The positive control is histamine phosphate at a dilution of 1:100,000. The negative control is sterile buffered saline or sterile water.

Technique. Place the dog or cat in lateral recumbency. Most animals are tested without the use of any chemical restraint. Xylazine, ketamine, or gas anesthesia can be used without interfering with skin test results. Gently clip the lower lateral thoracic wall with a No. 40 blade, avoiding excessive heat or trauma to the skin. Mark the injection sites with a felt pen, leaving 3/4 to 1 inch (2.5 cm) between sites, and avoid areas that are irritated or otherwise look abnormal. To make the ID injections use a 1.0-ml tuberculin syringe and a 26-gauge, 3/8-inch needle with the bevel dorsal. The recommended volume of each allergen injected varies from 0.02 to 0.05 ml or a minimum bleb. The injection of an equal volume of allergen in each site is more important than volume itself. Unequal volume at the different sites makes interpretation difficult. It is equally important to place each injection at the same shallow depth in the dermis. All air bubbles in the syringe must be expelled before injection.

Grading of ID Reactions. Grading can be subjective or objective. Criteria for both methods are listed in Table 4-2. The test is read 15 minutes after injection (Plate I-4). Most tests are easier to read in a darkened room using indirect light (pen light). The grading of the reactions in cats usually is more difficult than for dogs because the wheal tends to be flatter and borders are less defined, which is probably a result of the thinner feline dermis and epidermis.

False-negative ID allergy test reactions can be caused by improper injection techniques, such as subcutaneous injections or injection of air instead of allergen; influence of immunosuppressive agents; and the use of outdated, impotent, or improperly prepared test antigens. The dilution effect of mixed antigens for ID allergy testing may result in false-negative reactions. A contaminated or irritant control (for example, glycerin) may result in a larger wheal being used for comparison. If there is a greater reaction than expected associated with the negative control, the test should be repeated using fresh buffered saline solution. The negative control wheal should measure no more than 4 mm in diameter 15 minutes after the injection of 0.05 ml of sterile buffered saline solution.

TABLE 4-2

Criteria for Grading Intradermal Skin Test Reactions

I. Subjective
  1. Compare size and color of wheal and steepness of wall.
  2. Compare positive and negative controls with allergen reaction.
  3. Grade individual reactions 0 through 4:
     a. Negative control = 0
     b. Positive control = 4
     c. 2 × size of negative control = 1
     d. 3 × size of negative control = 2
     e. 4 × size of negative control = 3
     f. Equal to size of positive control = 4
  4. Increased erythema and/or steep walls has positive influence on the grade.
  5. Known mild irritant reaction of allergen has negative influence on grade.

II. Objective
  1. Measure diameter of negative control
  2. Measure diameter of individual reactions.
  3. Grading:
     a. Negative reaction = < 3 mm larger than negative control.
     b. Positive reaction = > 3 mm larger than negative control.
        or
     c. Average the diameter of negative and positive controls. Any wheal greater than this average is a positive reaction.

False-positive ID allergy test reactions may be a result of contamination of diluted extracts, irritant reactions to the allergen or diluent used, excessive concentration or volume of test allergens, or cross-reactivity with related allergens.

Interpretation. Several factors are important to consider when interpreting ID allergy test results. It is imperative that positive ID reactions correlate with a history of exposure to the specific allergen. In general, there is a poor correlation between the grade of the positive reaction and the degree of hypersensitivity. Factors that influence the severity or grade of the ID reaction include the time of testing relative to exposure and the antigenicity of the testing extract.

In Vitro Allergy Testing

Two in vitro methods of testing are commercially available in the United States and Canada, the radioallergosorbent test (RAST) and the enzyme-linked immunosorbent assay (ELISA). Both tests are relative measures of the serum levels of allergen-specific IgE. Although there is a paucity of data based on controlled studies, there appears to be much variability in the specificity and reproducibility of these assays. The reproducibility of repeated assays on the same sample appears to be higher with the ELISA than with the RAST. There is much variation between ID allergy test reactions and in vitro reactions. Preliminary data suggest that both in vitro tests may result in a higher number of false-positive reactions than the ID allergy test. False-negative reactions can result from interference with immunosuppressive drugs. The RAST test is reported by the laboratory to be reliable while the dog is on immunosuppressive drugs, although preliminary data suggest that both the ELISA and RAST procedures are affected by corticosteroids.

In vitro testing has several advantages. The office testing is quick and painless for the dog, the investment in skin testing materials and time to perform the tests is eliminated, and the condition of the dog's skin does not affect the ability to perform the test.

In vitro testing also has some disadvantages. Presently, regionalized groups of allergens are used, which may not reflect specific allergen reactions or may lead to false-negative reactions because of the dilution effect. The in vitro tests are relatively expensive on a per allergen basis. Significant cross-reactivity appears to exist among some allergens and between species which can result in false-positive reactions. The time of testing in relation to exposure can affect the in vitro tests in the same way that ID test reactions are affected. If IgGd is found to be clinically significant, the specificity of in vitro tests that measure IgE may be decreased.

Based on the present state of the art of in vitro tests, we suggest that when possible, intradermal tests should be performed rather than in vitro tests. There appears to be minimal value in performing screening in vitro tests with a limited number of allergen groups because the history and clinical signs should be as suggestive of a diagnosis of atopy.

The in vitro tests are indicated if the ID tests are negative or correlate poorly with the history. If the condition of the skin is such that ID allergy testing is not possible, in vitro testing may be indicated.

It is imperative that all positive in vitro test reactions be correlated with the history of exposure and the occurrence of clinical signs *before* a hyposensitization program is recommended based on the in vitro tests.

Management

General considerations in managing atopic dogs include the avoidance of allergens whenever possible, using topical and/or systemic medications when needed, considering hyposensitization, and treating all concurrent problems.

The clinician and client should be aware of the "allergic threshold" concept. An allergic load may be tolerated by a dog without disease manifestations; however, a small increase in the load may push the dog over the threshold and initiate clinical signs (allergic breakthrough). Combined stresses of immunologic, genetic, climatic, and physiologic origins may precipitate the allergic disease. The allergic threshold is not fixed and can be raised or lowered by various factors that may affect the dog, including the general condition of the skin, the nutritional state, infection, external parasites, and the environment.

Medical Management

All manifestations of disease in atopic dogs must be treated simultaneously. Antiseborrheic and antibacterial shampoos help remove excessive scales and reduce surface bacterial flora. Daily water soaks for 15 minutes followed by an oil rinse are indicated for treating dry skin. Antibiotics are indicated if there is bacterial dermatitis.

Corticosteroids are routinely used to relieve focal or generalized pruritus. Topical corticosteroid ointments or creams (see Table 3-3) may help relieve pruritus or pain in a focal inflamed or excoriated area. These ointments and creams are not practical if lesions are generalized or the haircoat is thick or long.

Short-acting oral corticosteroids are preferred to mask pruritic signs and relieve acute inflammation because they can be discontinued when pruritus stops. A loading dose of prednisone or prednisolone followed by a step-down dosage schedule, preferably alternate-day in the morning, is recommended (see Table 3-9). Intermediate, long-acting, or residual injectable corticosteroids are not indicated for chronic nonseasonal pruritus but can be used for short, seasonal pruritus when one or two injections are all that is required for the entire year, or if oral administration is not possible (see Table 3-8). Oral corticosteroids should not be used concurrently with the injections.

Antihistamines are reported to be satisfactory antipruritics in approximately 25 to 35% of atopic dogs. Hydroxyzine (Atarax® — Pfizer) and clemastine (Tavist® — Ancalab) have provided the highest percentage of control (see Table 3-15).

The omega-3 and omega-6 fatty acids (eicosapentaenoic acid and gamma linolenic acid) have been shown to have some beneficial effect in approximately 20% of atopic dogs. Eicosapentaenoic acid, which has a structure similar to that of arachidonic acid, competes for the utilization of enzymes which results in the formation of fewer inflammatory mediators.

Because many mediators play a role in canine pruritus, it is logical to combine different drugs with effects on different mediators to achieve a maximum antipruritic effect. Antihistamines and omega-3/6 fatty acids are routinely used concurrently. Antihistamines used concurrently with short-acting corticosteroids may allow use of a lower corticosteroid dosage to control the pruritus.

Biologic Management

Hyposensitization (immunotherapy) is the biologic method used to treat atopic dogs. The standard theory of the immunologic mechanism has been that hyposensitization stimulates IgG antibodies. These antibodies have a selective affinity for specific allergens, and thus block the IgE antibody-antigen reaction and prevent the release of chemical mediators from the target mast cells. More recent investigations have shown that hyposensitization stimulates specialized T-lymphocyte suppressor cells and helper cells. Suppressor cells prevent IgE production and helper cells turn on B lymphocytes that produce IgG.

Hyposensitization should be considered when the allergic signs last for 4 months or more each year; or when a dog exhibits side effects from medical treatment, regardless of the duration of allergic signs; or is not controlled with medical treatment.

The client must understand all aspects of hyposensitization, including the procedure, short- and long-term costs, and prognosis. Most dogs require booster injections for life. The time required for response to immunotherapy is variable. Approximately 25% of those that respond will improve within the first 3 months, 50% in 3 to 6 months, and the remaining 25% between 6 and 12 months. Most dogs will respond within the first 9 months if they are going to respond. The prognosis for response is dependent on many variables, including the experience of the clinician with testing and interpreting ID reactions, concurrent problems, and owner attitudes and perceptions. The most common causes of hyposensitization failure include persistent flea infestation, secondary bacterial infection, concurrent allergies (such as food, contact), and occasionally newly acquired inhalant allergies.

Selection of Antigens. The selection of antigens to include in the treatment should be based on the correlation of positive ID reactions, history of exposure to the specific test-positive ID antigens, and the inability to avoid exposure. If there is a poor correlation between the positive ID reaction and the history of exposure, the allergen is not incorporated in the allergen extract. Likewise, if the allergen can be eliminated from the environment, it should be excluded from treatment.

The total number of allergens or the total PNU load that an allergic dog can tolerate is variable and subject to discussion among veterinary allergists. Some clinicians use a maximum of 10 different allergens, individual or grouped, while others include all allergens deemed clinically important regardless of the total number. Treatment protocols use individual or groups of antigens similar to those used for testing (see Table 4-1). If a limited number of dogs are being hyposensitized in a practice, it will be cost-effective to order individual treatment sets from the manufacturer; however, there usually is a minimum of 4 weeks or longer before specially ordered treatment sets are received. If there is sufficient practice volume, stocking the individual or grouped antigens is cost-effective. The stock concentrated antigens are subsequently diluted for both testing and treatment.

The two types of treatment antigens currently available are the aqueous and alum-precipitated types. The major considerations for selecting these antigens are given in Table 4-3. In the United States and Canada, aqueous antigens are the predominant type used because of availability and cost.

Treatment Schedules. The initial treatment protocols for aqueous antigens vary among clinicians. The standard protocol used by one of the authors (GN) is found in Table 4-4. The dosage schedule for alum-precipitated allergens is found in Table 4-5.

TABLE 4-3

Comparison of Aqueous and Alum-Precipitated Treatment Allergens

Criteria	*Aqueous*	*Alum-Precipitated*
Cost of vaccine per unit	Low	High
Assortment of antigens	Many	Limited
Average number of injections in initial series	15–20	6–9
Frequency of injections for initial series	Every 3–7 days	Every 7–21 days
Frequency of booster injections	1–4 weeks	1–3 months
Side effects	Increased pruritus if over tolerance	Increased pruritus if over tolerance; nodule at injection site
Stability of vaccine	Loses potency in weak dilutions	Stable for dating

TABLE 4-4

Hyposensitization Schedule for Aqueous Antigens[a]

Day	*Vial No. 1 (ml)*	*Vial No. 2 (ml)*	*Vial No. 3 (ml)*
1	0.1		
4	0.2		
7	0.4		
10	0.8		
13	1.0		
16		0.1	
19		0.2	
22		0.4	
25		0.8	
28		1.0	
31			0.1
34			0.2
37			0.4
40			0.8
43			1.0
50			1.0
57			1.0

Vial No. 1: 10 ml of 10:1 dilution of Vial No. 2 (100–200 PNU[b]/ml)

Vial No. 2: 10 ml of 10:1 dilution of Vial No. 3 (1000–2000 PNU/ml)

Vial No. 3: 10 ml of allergen mixture, that is, 1 ml of 10,000–20,000 PNU solution of each single or grouped allergen up to a maximum of 10; if there is less than 10 ml of allergen, the difference is made up with sterile saline or sterile diluting solution.

Boosters are given whenever the dog begins to show more pruritic signs. If there is a seasonal allergy, the injections may be maintained year-round with 1.0-ml doses of vial No. 3 administered every 4 to 8 weeks during the nonallergenic season. If the injections are discontinued for several months start with vial No. 2 (0.4 ml) when recommencing hyposensitization.

[a]Protocol used by the authors.
[b]PNU, protein nitrogen units.

TABLE 4-5

Hyposensitization Schedule for Alum-Precipitated Allergens

Week	*Amount of Single Antigen or Group[a] Used (PNU)[b]*
1	100
2	200
3	400
5	600
8	1500
12	2000
16	3000
20	6000
24	10000
Boosters as needed[c]	

[a]Mixture of related antigens, such as mixed molds.
[b]Protein nitrogen unit.
[c]Given when pruritus starts to increase.

The protocol for allergen boosters for each atopic dog is based on response to the initial hyposensitization and the anticipated pattern of occurrence of clinical signs. The general guideline is to give an injection whenever there is an increase in pruritus. There often is an advantage to giving periodic boosters during the nonallergic season to dogs with a seasonal allergic pattern. If a long interval exists between injections (2 months or longer), the booster may have to be reinitiated at a less than maximum dose to prevent exacerbation of pruritus. The first indication that an excessive amount of antigen was administered is a marked increase in pruritus within 24 hours after the injection. This response must be differentiated from a milder, transient increase in pruritus a few hours after the injection. A written treatment schedule and instruction sheet should accompany every treatment program.

Antihistamines, omega-3/6 fatty acids, and/or short-acting alternate-day glucocorticoids can be used concurrently with immunotherapy if needed.

Prognosis

The reported average response rates and their ranges are excellent, 36% (21–60); good, 30% (21–42); fair, 19% (14–24); and poor, 22% (14–35). The definition of response is variable, especially when the owner's expectations are considered. Most dogs with atopic dermatitis can be controlled with either immunotherapy or medical therapy alone or with a combination of both types of therapy.

Client Education Handout

Treatment of canine atopy requires a major commitment by the owner in terms of time and expense; thus, it is imperative that all aspects of diagnosis, treatment, and prognosis are understood. Multiple family members often are involved in the decision-making process although only one member has been involved in the consultation. Client education handouts that summarize the pertinent facts should be given to the client after the initial consultation (Table 4-6).

FELINE ATOPY

Ample evidence exists for the presence of airborne-related allergies in cats based on history, ID allergy tests, and response to immunotherapy.

TABLE 4-6

Client Education Handout—Atopic Dermatitis

Facts about Canine and Feline Atopic Dermatitis

1. Canine atopic dermatitis is an inherited predisposition to develop allergic symptoms following repeated exposure mostly to inhaled allergens.
2. Age of onset of allergic symptoms is usually between 1 and 3 years of age. Symptoms may be seasonal or year-round. They tend to become worse and have a longer season as the dog ages.
3. Due to the hereditary nature of the disease several breeds, such as golden retrievers, most terriers, Irish setters, and Old English sheep dogs, have a higher incidence.
4. Cats manifest the allergic reaction usually between 6 months and 2 years of age. Either seasonal or year-round symptoms are seen.
5. Common causes include pollens, (trees, weeds, grasses), molds, dust, wool, cat dander, and feathers.

Clinical Signs

The primary clinical signs are scratching, biting, or licking, most often under the arms, face, feet or lower abdomen in dogs. Head and neck scratching is most common in cats, although it can be generalized. Hair loss, redness, scaly skin, bad odor, and darkening of the skin are often associated with scratching.

Diagnosis

The best way to identify specific allergens is to skin test the dog. The dog *must not* be under the influence of cortisone (steroids). Waiting time following the oral administration of cortisone may vary from 2 to 4 weeks. There may be up to 2 months waiting time after some cortisone injections or long-term oral treatment.

Treatment

1. Hyposensitization (allergy vaccine):
   A. This involves giving allergy vaccine for the life-time of the dog.
   B. An initial series of injections, usually every 3 days for 6 weeks, is given under the skin.
   C. Periodic boosters are usually required every 1 to 4 weeks. If scratching is seasonal, the vaccine may not be given all year.
   D. Expected response time: 25% within 3 months; 50% in 3 to 6 months; 25% within 6 and 12 months.
   E. Expected response rate: 70% of dogs hyposensitized will be controlled satisfactorily with allergy vaccine.
   F. Cortisone or antihistamines may be given while hyposensitizing if needed to control itching.

2. Cortisone (steroids):

   Cortisone is the only drug that is consistently effective in masking the allergic symptoms. It is preferable to administer the cortisone orally on alternate days in the morning to minimize side effects. Common side effets of cortisone include increased water intake, frequency of urination, and appetite. Long-term cortisone usage may cause increased susceptibility to infection, hair loss, thin skin, liver damage, gastrointestinal problems, and muscle weakness.

3. Antihistamines:

   Antihistamines are given two or three times per day to a mild sedative dose. If there is poor control of scratching and biting with sedation, antihistamines are discontinued. If they control the symptoms satisfactorily, antihistamines are a safe alternative to cortisone.

4. Omega-3 and omega-6 fatty acids:

   Specific fatty acid supplements will result in improvement of symptoms in 20 to 30% of dogs. They are commonly used in conjunction with other forms of treatment, especially antihistamines and hyposensitization.

Etiologic Factors

Positive intradermal test reactions have been observed with most of the allergens, including grass and weed pollens, molds, house dust, animal danders, feathers, and kapok.

Pathogenesis

A hereditary predisposition has not been identified in the feline population. A feline reaginic antibody has been identified that has characteristics similar to IgE of other species although feline IgE has not been verified. Therefore, the designation "feline atopy" is based on similarities to canine atopy without verification of a hereditary basis or the presence of a specific IgE-mediated reaction.

History and Clinical Signs

There is a paucity of data concerning feline atopy. Most cats present with a history of pruritus and often excoriation. A seasonal history often is elicited, which may be correlated with a spring/summer onset, or a fall onset associated with the heat being activated indoors. The age of onset is variable, usually between 6 months and 2 years. No sex predilection has been reported. The pruritus should be responsive to corticosteroids, especially to methylprednisolone acetate (Depo-Medrol® — Upjohn).

The clinical signs are variable. The majority of cats are presented with signs of miliary dermatitis, alopecia with minimal or no inflammation, or indolent ulcer, eosinophilic plaque, or linear granuloma lesions suggestive of the eosinophilic granuloma complex (see Chapter 13).

The distribution of the pruritus may be localized to the head and neck region or may be generalized (Plate I-5). Some cats are presented with signs of feline asthma as the only clinical sign. A few will have some respiratory symptoms as well as dermatologic signs.

Diagnosis

Screening diagnostic tests help to rule out other differential diagnoses. Skin scrapings, fecal flotations, and fungal cultures are negative. Diet testing does not result in clinical improvement. Cutaneous biopsy findings are consistent with allergic dermatitis with dermal edema and increased numbers of mast cells and eosinophils. A nonspecific, subacute to chronic dermatitis or microscopic lesions consistent with the eosinophilic granuloma complex may be seen (see Chapter 13).

The definitive diagnostic test for feline atopy is the intradermal (ID) allergy test. The selection of antigens and testing technique is the same as that described previously for dogs. Because of the thin skin of cats, a new needle should be used for each injection to ensure an intradermal route. Ketamine HCl can be used in the case of a fractious cat, although most cats tolerate the ID testing without any chemical restraint.

Corticosteroids and megestrol acetate will interfere with allergy test reactions. The chronic administration of megestrol acetate has been shown to suppress the pituitary/adrenal axis for as long as 4 months.

The grading of feline ID reactions is more difficult than in dogs because the well-defined urticarial wheal is seldom observed. Most of the reactions are slightly raised, mildly erythemic areas with poorly defined borders. The positive reaction occurs very rapidly in cats and thus should be read several times starting immediately after completing the battery of ID injections. Most reactions have subsided within 15 minutes.

Management

Managing a cat with feline atopy is similar to the protocol followed for atopic dogs. Cats with dermatologic signs often have a poor response to the short-acting daily or alternate-day oral corticosteroids. The corticosteroid of choice is methylprednisolone acetate (Depo-Medrol) administered at a dosage of 5.5 mg/kg subcutaneously at 4-week or longer intervals. Few long-term side effects have been reported if it is not administered more often than monthly. Chronic megestrol acetate often is effective in controlling allergic signs, but is not recommended because of many side effects, including predisposition to mammary gland hyperplasia and neoplasia, diabetes mellitus, and iatrogenic Cushing's syndrome.

Cats with respiratory signs of asthma often respond well to the oral short-acting corticosteroids. Antihistamines also have been used to control the respiratory allergic signs. Chlorpheniramine maleate is reported to have a high degree of efficacy (73%) in the control of feline pruritic dermatoses.

Immunotherapy is recommended for cats with perennial atopy. Cats respond to hyposensitization protocols similar to those recommended for dogs (see Tables 4-4 and 4-5). A limited number of reports suggest a response rate of 65 to 75%. Some cats do not tolerate as high a concentration of allergen for maintenance and are maintained on Vial 2 rather than Vial 3 (see Table 4-4).

Prognosis

Most cases of confirmed feline atopy can be controlled with either medical therapy or immunotherapy. Some cats will develop new allergens over several years.

Client Handouts

A client handout explaining all aspects of feline atopy is extremely helpful. A general handout can be used for both canine and feline atopy (Table 4-6).

ALLERGIC CONTACT DERMATITIS

Contact dermatitis usually is classified into two etiologic categories: irritant and allergic. It often is difficult and unnecessary to differentiate between the two entities clinically although different pathomechanisms are involved. Allergic contact dermatitis is immune-mediated, while irritant contact dermatitis is caused by nonimmunologic factors of a physical or chemical nature. An irritant contact reaction may predispose to an allergic reaction after repeated exposure. The following discussion focuses on allergic contact dermatitis. Irritant contact dermatitis is discussed in Chapter 12, although differentiating characteristics of the two diseases are presented here.

Etiologic Factors

Many agents have been incriminated as causes of allergic contact dermatitis (Table 4-7). Wool, nylon, and

TABLE 4-7

Etiologic Factors of Allergic Contact Dermatitis in Dogs and Cats

Chemicals and ions	
	Chrome
	Nickel
	Iodine
	Formaldehyde
	Dyes
	Finishes (floor, fibers)
	Oleoresins
	Sterols
	Antioxidants
Materials and products	
	Wood
	Cotton
	Synthetic fibers
	Rubber
	Plastic
	Cleaning materials
	Polishes
	Leather
	Topical drugs (neomycin, parasiticides, bases)
	Flea collars
	Fertilizer
	Fish scale

other synthetic fibers generally are thought to cause an irritant rather than an allergic contact reaction. The dyes and finishes used in the manufacture of carpeting, blankets, and furniture may be the primary factors associated with allergic problems. The number of topical medications reported to cause allergic contact dermatitis is limited. In many cases it is not apparent whether the active drug or the vehicle is causing the contact problem. The reaction may be irritant or allergic, or a combination of both.

Incidence

The incidence of contact dermatitis in dogs and cats is not well documented, partially because it is difficult to differentiate between allergic and irritant etiologic factors. Pruritus in 1 to 5% of dogs presented to a dermatology referral practice has been reported to be of contact origin. The condition is rare in cats.

Pathogenesis

A delayed hypersensitivity (Type IV) reaction is the basis of allergic contact dermatitis. Contact allergens usually are substances of relatively low molecular weight. They are incomplete antigens or haptens, which attach to a structural epidermal protein to form a complete antigen. A subpopulation of lymphocytes develops that has been sensitized to the antigen and a migration of sensitized lymphocytes to the antigen site follows. Chemical mediators (lymphokines) are released, resulting in pruritus and inflammation.

Three clinical stages in the pathogenesis of allergic contact dermatitis have been identified. The *refractory phase* is characterized by no detectable evidence of skin change or immunologic activity. In the *incubation phase,* the contactant or antigen does not produce clinical evidence of a contact reaction; however, immunologic activity can be detected by in vitro methods. The third phase is that of *hypersensitivity* with clinical evidence of changes in the skin.

All contact reactions that are allergic require repeated exposure to the allergen. Thus, it is common for a substance to be a primary irritant on the first exposure and to cause an allergic response on subsequent exposure.

Several factors can predispose an animal to contact sensitivity, including trauma or irritation to the skin, which results in a break of continuity of the protective epidermal surface; continued or repeated wetting of the skin, which softens the keratin layer; use of wetting agents; the dose-time relationship of exposure to the contactant; the vulnerability of the skin; environmental factors, such as temperature and humidity; and prior exposure. The nutritional status of the animal with mineral and vitamin deficiencies may alter the responsiveness of the skin. The epidermal protein in ichthyosis and defatted skin is more susceptible to conjugation with an incomplete antigen. Endocrine imbalances and metabolic disturbances may cause variations in the integrity of the skin. Once an allergic reaction has been established, the severity of signs associated with subsequent exposure to the contactant may be enhanced by irritants, abrasives, and skin alkalinity.

History

The single most important factor in the evaluation of an animal with contact dermatitis is the history. The age of onset varies because the development of an allergic response requires repeated exposure to the contactant. An immediate reaction on first exposure is seen with an irritant contactant. The total length of the refractory and sensitizing periods is in excess of 2 years in 70% of the cases of allergic contact dermatitis, and is rarely less than 6 months. No specific breed susceptibility to allergic contact dermatitis has been verified.

Most dogs and cats with allergic contact dermatitis have nonseasonal pruritus, although some seasonal patterns may be identified with solid contactants such as fibers or oleoresins of plants. The distribution of lesions is regionalized and occurs on the ventral and lateral aspects of the body in most animals. When liquid contactants such as shampoos have been used, the distribution may be generalized. Pet owners frequently observe increased pruritus associated with a particular area of the environment, such as one room, one rug, or a dog run. Improvement of clinical signs and pruritus is often reported in association with a change in the environment, such as that produced by traveling or boarding. Usually only one animal in a multiple-animal household is affected. A history that reveals a sudden onset of pruritus and associated clinical signs correlated with recent exposure to potentially irritant chemicals is suggestive of an irritant rather than an allergic reaction.

Clinical Manifestations

A physical examination reveals variable signs that depend on many factors, such as severity of pruritus, location of lesions, and degree of secondary skin change. Acute allergic contact dermatitis usually is characterized by erythema and a moist edematous lesion (Plate I-6). The most common primary morphologic lesions are erythematous papules or macules, often lacking bilateral symmetry. Occasionally, wheals are observed. Dogs with chronic allergic contact dermatitis usually have secondary morphologic lesions including excessive scaling, hyperpigmentation, and occasionally lichenification accompanied by varying degrees of alopecia. Excoriation and crusts are observed in self-traumatized lesions. Lesions localized to the ventral and lateral aspects of the trunk are suggestive of a reaction to floor cleaners, bedding, grass resins, or other ground or floor contactants. A generalized distribution of lesions is suggestive of a reaction to shampoo or insecticide. If allergic reactions occur with specific medications, the area of involvement tends to be localized or regionalized to the areas of contact with the medication. In long-haired dogs and cats, the lesions may be localized to the least protected areas of the body.

Concurrent skin disorders are common in dogs with allergic contact dermatitis. Distribution of lesions may be generalized in these dogs. A secondary superficial pyoderma frequently is present.

Diagnosis

Diagnosis of allergic contact dermatitis is based on history, clinical signs, and screening and definitive diagnostic tests. The routine screening diagnostic tests and some definitive tests do not identify allergic contact dermatitis, but they do help to rule out other primary etiologic factors. These tests include skin scraping, fungal culture, bacterial culture, biopsy, intradermal allergy testing, and hypoallergenic diet testing. Results of hematologic and biochemical testing generally are normal. Cutaneous biopsy is not a specific test for either irritant or allergic contact dermatitis although some microscopic changes are consistent with a delayed hypersensitivity reaction.

Isolation followed by provocative exposure is the definitive diagnostic test for allergic contact dermatitis. The time that the dog or cat must be isolated from the suspected contactant is variable. Acute clinical signs resolve within 4 to 7 days in some animals, while 14 days of isolation are required for other animals. During the isolation period there should be a marked reduction of pruritus and acute inflammation.

Once the animal is clinically normal or stabilized in a less reactive state for 24 to 48 hours, maximum exposure to the suspected contactant should be allowed. Signs of an allergic reaction should return with 48 to 72 hours of reexposure if continuous contact is maintained. It is not unusual to see obvious exacerbation of signs within 24 hours. If more than one contactant is suspected, isolate the dog or cat from all contactants initially; then provocatively expose the animal to each one individually until all suspected contactants have been ruled out as the cause of the skin problem. If there is a reaction to one contactant, isolate the animal again until clinical signs resolve. Then provocatively expose the animal to the next suspected contactant. Hospitalizing or boarding the dog or cat is often a satisfactory alternative to isolation at home. If an animal shows improvement in a hospital environment, maximum provocative exposure to some allergens can be achieved by placing remnants of the material in the cage with the animal.

Patch testing is a definitive diagnostic test for allergic contact dermatitis, although it is seldom needed or used. An open patch test using chemical extracts of vehicles may be performed. The major problem is obtaining the extracts or vehicles of suspected contactants in a concentration that will produce an allergic reaction and be nonirritating. The reader is referred to lists of suggested concentrations and vehicles (Walton, 1977).

The closed patch test is not generally accepted as a practical diagnostic test for dogs or cats. It is reserved for situations in which treated fibers, such as rugs, are suspected but isolation is impossible and open patch testing for the various possible chemicals is not practical.

Management

Treatment alternatives for allergic contact dermatitis are limited. The best method is to avoid exposure to the contactant material or chemical. If complete avoidance is not possible, every effort should be made to minimize exposure, such as using a cover over the carpet to reduce direct contact. In many cases the life-style of the dog or cat must change in order to reduce to a minimum the contact time with the primary allergen. When it is not possible to avoid the offending material or chemical, a low dose alternate-day maintenance dose of corticosteroids (see Table 3-9) usually is required.

All concurrent dermatologic problems, such as pyoderma and external parasites, must be treated as well to achieve maximum control of clinical signs.

FOOD HYPERSENSITIVITY AND FOOD INTOLERANCE

Adverse reactions to foods (including food allergy or food hypersensitivity and food intolerance) are clinical entities that can affect several target areas, including the cutaneous, respiratory, gastrointestinal, neurologic, and hematologic systems, and can manifest in a variety of clinical signs. Adverse reactions may have an immunologic or nonimmunologic basis. Food intolerance is an abnormal physiologic response to an ingestant of an idiosyncratic, metabolic, pharmacologic, or toxic nature. Food idiosyncrasy is an abnormal response to an ingestant resembling hypersensitivity but not involving immune mechanisms. It is impossible to differentiate between these reactions on clinical evaluation.

Etiologic Factors

Most basic food components have the potential to cause an allergic reaction. These components include lipoproteins, glycoproteins, lipopolysaccharides, and carbohydrates. The antigenicity of an allergen is often altered by preingestion, cooking, or processing or by digestion, which either enhances or destroys its allergenic character. Artificial flavors, dyes, and preservatives can act as direct allergens or as haptens. Some specific foods reported to cause food allergies in dogs and/or cats include milk, wheat, raw and cooked beef, dog biscuits, eggs, chicken, cat food, rabbit food, pork, fish, horse meat, mutton, and cod liver oil.

Incidence

The true incidence of food hypersensitivity is not known; reported figures vary from 1% of all dermatologic cases to 23% of cases of nonseasonal allergic dermatitis. In one study, 23% of dogs with confirmed food allergies based on diet testing also had some other allergic condition.

Pathogenesis

Type I, III, and IV hypersensitivity reactions have been associated with food hypersensitivities. If the time of onset in relation to the ingestion of the allergen is immediate (occurring within minutes), soluble, whole food molecules are incriminated. If there is a delay of one to several hours after the ingestion of an allergen before clinical signs occur, insoluble molecules that require digestion are suspected. These degradation products are most likely to be the allergens. Hypersensitivity reactions to foods must be differentiated from food intolerance that results from enzymatic deficiencies, reduced gastric hydrochloric acid, reduced bile secretions, and mechanical factors.

History

Most animals with food hypersensitivities are presented for nonseasonal pruritus. The owners may observe some correlation with diet change and clinical signs. There are no breed or sex predilections.

Most food allergies are observed in adult dogs and cats. Over 70% of all animals with food allergies have had constant exposure to the specific antigen(s) for at least 2 years. Occasionally, there may be a recent history of a dietary change. The exception to the prolonged time of exposure is the young pruritic dog. A food hypersensitivity should always be considered in the dog under 6 months of age that is presented with a history of chronic pruritus and is negative for external parasites. Although a nonseasonal pruritus is most common, the animal that is fed a varied diet with intermittent exposure to the allergen may present with a seasonal or intermittent pattern of clinical signs.

Stress can lower the allergic threshold, and other concurrent allergies may predispose to exacerbation of clinical signs caused by food allergies. Occasional gastrointestinal signs (diarrhea, flatulence) may be a concurrent problem, occurring more frequently in dogs than in cats. Respiratory signs of sneezing and rhinitis have been reported.

The response to corticosteroids is variable. Many dogs and cats with food hypersensitivities are reported to be more refractory to antiinflammatory dosages of corticosteroids, while other animals respond well.

Clinical Signs

Canine

Clinical signs are variable. A dry, thin, or lusterless haircoat may be observed. Urticarial wheals or angioedema may be present (Plate I-7). The most common primary morphologic changes include papules and erythematous macules. There may be many secondary morphologic changes, including hyperpigmentation, hyperkeratosis, crusts, scale, and frequently focal or generalized excoriation. Erythema and alopecia are variable, depending on the degree of pruritus. In chronic food allergies, a secondary keratinization disorder (seborrhea) or pyoderma may be noted. The distribution of lesions is variable and indistinguishable from contact or atopic disease.

Gastrointestinal signs can vary from mild flatulence to acute, profuse watery or hemorrhagic diarrhea. Minimal general depression usually is associated with the gastrointestinal signs, which may help to differentiate food allergy from other systemic diseases. In chronic food allergies vomiting may be observed. The feces are often intermittently or chronically soft.

Respiratory signs include sudden onset of rhinitis and sneezing without concurrent evidence of conjunctivitis. These signs usually appear within a few minutes of ingestion of the food allergen and resolve within 1 to 2 hours without treatment.

Feline

Several different clinical signs have been associated with feline food allergies, including pruritic, ulcerative, or erosive dermatitis of the head (Plate I-8), neck, and axillae; pruritus without lesions; a miliary eczema-like eruption; and pruritic, urticaria-angioedema. Focal ulcerative or plaque lesions on the abdomen also have been observed. Excoriations, crusts, and variable alopecia and erythema are frequently seen.

Diagnosis

The diagnosis of food allergy is based on the history, clinical signs, and screening as well as definitive diagnostic tests. The routine diagnostic tests do not identify a food allergy, but they do rule out other primary etiologic factors. These screening tests include skin scrapings, fungal and bacterial cultures, biopsy, isolation and provocative exposure, and ID allergy testing. Results of hematologic and biochemical testing are generally within normal limits. Cutaneous biopsy is not specific for food allergy, but may be consistent with the diagnosis of allergic dermatitis. ID allergy testing for food allergens is not recommended in dogs and cats. Positive ID reactions would be consistent with an atopic dermatitis, but do not rule out a concurrent food allergy.

Diet Testing (Test Meal Investigation)

The basis of diet testing is to avoid ingestion of the offending allergen(s). Because many components of the normal diet may be the cause, it is recommended to limit the test diet to foods to which the dog or cat has not been previously exposed. In some instances this is not possible because of such factors as lack of knowledge of basic components of the normal diet, expense of feeding an elimination diet, and unwillingness of the owner to subject the dog or cat to a restricted diet. Concurrent dermatologic problems, such as pyoderma and fleas, should be controlled before starting the diet. If there is a concurrent active atopy, it may be difficult to evaluate the response to the elimination diet.

Dietary testing can be started by withholding all food for 2 days and then administering a saline cathartic before starting a test meal. Most diet testing for dogs is initiated by feeding lamb or mutton and rice or potatoes, proportioned 1:2 or 1:4, for 21 to 28 days. If there has been minimal previous exposure other acceptable protein sources include fish, rabbit, venison, turkey, or chicken. Most commercial diets contain both meat and poultry by-products, thus making chicken and beef unacceptable. It is recommended to substitute well water or water from municipal sources (which may contain algae or fungi) with distilled water.

Commercial hypoallergenic diets consisting of lamb and rice or egg and rice are available. The canned food, Prescription Diet® d/d® (Hill's Pet Products), is a mutton and rice diet that is reported to cause a flare of the pruritus or vomiting and/or diarrhea in 10 to 50% of the dogs that respond to a homemade restrictive diet. These problems have not been reported with the dry food, Nature's Recipe (a lamb and rice kibble) or with dry Prescription Diet d/d (an egg and rice kibble).

The hypoallergenic diet is fed at approximately the same quantity as the regular diet. Good client education and communication is an integral part of a successful diet testing program because strict compliance to the nonallergenic diet is essential. All other foods, snacks, chewables and treats must not be fed during the trial.

Similar options for the protein source are suitable for the cat's restrictive diet. Most cats will not eat much of the carbohydrates; thus, baby food with the specific restrictive protein is an acceptable elimination diet. Overcooked meat (same kind as the baby food) can be given as a chewable. Most cats will eat and tolerate canned Prescription Diet d/d.

At the end of the test period, individual components of the normal diet (such as beef or chicken) can be provocatively tested or one commercial component of the regular diet (such as kibble or canned food) can be reintroduced. If there is no exacerbation of clinical signs within 7 days, an additional component is added. These steps are repeated weekly until the dog or cat is back on the regular diet. If at any time clinical signs are provoked with the addition of one of the components, the restrictive diet or the diet immediately prior to the reaction should be started and continued until signs subside; then provocatively expose the animal to other foods based on an assessment of which is least likely to precipitate problems. The goal is to find a commercial diet that is tolerated or to build a balanced homemade diet.

Management

The only satisfactory method of treating a food allergy is complete and permanent removal of all the allergenic foods and substances that caused the reaction. If this is not possible, glucocorticoids can be administered, preferably on an alternate-day basis, to control the pruritus and self-trauma. In cats methylprednisolone acetate (Depo-Medrol) injections monthly have given good results (see Table 3-7).

Prognosis

The prognosis generally is good if the allergen(s) is identified and avoided; however, other food allergies may develop later.

Client Education Handout

Specific instructions must be followed to have a valid dietary elimination trial; thus, a client education handout should be given to the client (Table 4-8).

TABLE 4-8

Client Education Handout—Food Allergy

Facts about Canine and Feline Food Allergies

1. Food allergies are most commonly caused by an allergic reaction to one or more of the animal proteins: horse meat, beef, pork, chicken, milk, eggs, or fish. Preservatives, dyes, or other components of the food may cause allergic problems.

2. Symptoms may be seen at any age. A young animal or an older one that has been on the same diet for years may develop a food allergy.

3. It is not possible to differentiate a food allergy from other causes of allergies without diet testing.

4. Many animals with food allergies will not significantly improve by changing commercial diets. All commercial diets (canned, semi-moist, dry) will contain one or more common components.

5. Food allergies are found concurrently with other allergies.

Clinical Signs

Clinical signs include scratching, biting, or licking and occasionally digestive signs (loose stool, excessive gas).

Diet Testing Procedure

A. Feed only foods to which the dog or cat has had no previous exposure.
B. Suggested diets include:
   a. Lamb (1/3) and boiled white rice (2/3) or potatoes.
   b. Prescription Diet d/d (canned or dry)
   c. Fish, venison, or rabbit if no previous exposure.
   d. Lamb baby food for cats.
C. Feed the approximate quantity of test diet as the regular diet.
D. Feed the test diet for 21 to 28 days with NO OTHER FOOD, TREATS, OR SUPPLEMENTS. Observe for less severe symptoms. There may not be complete remission if other concurrent problems are present.
E. At the end of the test period, if animal improves
   a. The animal is reexposed to one basic component of the regular diet (one brand and flavor of commercial food or one protein).
   b. If symptoms do not become more severe within the 7 days, add a second component of the regular diet. This procedure is followed until a balanced diet is tolerated.
   c. If a problem is identified with the provocative testing, revert back to the last step in which no problem was observed. Remain at this step until symptoms have subsided and then add another component of the regular diet.

FLEABITE HYPERSENSITIVITY

Flea allergy dermatitis (fleabite hypersensitivity) is an immune-mediated reaction to the saliva of the flea.

Etiologic Factors

The common dog and cat flea, *Ctenocephalides felis*, and the human flea, *Pulex irritans*, are the most common fleas associated with flea allergy dermatitis. Other species that can cause flea allergy dermatitis include the sticktight flea, *Echidnophaga gallinacea*; the sand flea, *Tunga penetrans*; the rat flea, *Xenopsylla cheopis*; and the mouse flea, *Leptopsylla segnis*. *C. canis* is seldom observed in the dog and cat population. There is a lack of host specificity as well as a sharing of common antigens among most if not all flea species.

Incidence

Flea allergy dermatitis is the most common cause of allergy in most geographic areas of the United States and Canada and perhaps even the world. Areas of high elevation, above 5000 feet, generally have a low flea population.

Pathogenesis

Allergen-specific IgE and IgG have been identified in flea-allergic dogs. Dogs exposed to fleas early in life are less likely to develop clinical allergy than are those exposed at a later age. Both immediate and delayed hypersensitivity reactions occur in a random sequence, or more commonly they occur concomitantly. Dogs with continuous exposure to fleas appear to develop a tolerant state in which they are free of clinical signs associated with a flea infestation. If the flea exposure changes to intermittent, clinical flea allergy dermatitis will develop. A higher incidence of positive skin tests to flea antigen is seen in atopic dogs; thus, the atopic state may predispose dogs to the development and/or maintenance of flea allergy. Cutaneous basophil hypersensitivity has been shown to contribute to the clinical signs.

History

Pruritus is nearly always the primary complaint. There are no breed, sex, or haircoat-type predispositions. The majority of dogs with fleabite allergies that live in an area endemic for fleas develop clinical signs between 1 and 4 years of age. In areas with seasonal flea infestations, the age of onset of hypersensitivity reactions is variable, as it is partially dependent on the indoor flea population. There is more variability in age of onset in cats with flea allergy dermatitis.

Flea infestations usually are observed by the owners, preceding or concurrent with an increase of pruritus. In some cases, the owner has not observed fleas nor have any been seen on the dog or cat on previous examinations. Fleabite hypersensitivity commonly occurs simultaneously with other allergic disease, especially atopy in dogs. The clinical signs attributable to the fleabite may be severe, even though only a small number of fleas or only flea excrement is observed. Frequently, only one dog or cat in a multiple-animal household manifests signs of flea allergy dermatitis.

Clinical Signs

Canine

The lesions are most commonly distributed over the dorsal caudal back, tail, and perineum. They are found frequently on the flanks and caudal ventral abdomen, and less commonly in the axillae and on the cranial trunk. A few dogs manifest a generalized distribution, most commonly associated with atopic dermatitis. Fleas and/or flea excrement usually are present.

The primary morphologic lesions most frequently observed are erythematous papules on the ventral abdomen and occasionally in the axillae. Diffuse erythema of the dorsal cranial tail region (Plate I-9) is commonly accompanied by secondary morphologic signs including hyperkeratosis and occasionally lichenification. Alopecia is variable, from mild to marked, although the distribution may be localized or involve the entire posterior half of the trunk and perineum. Superficial folliculitis is associated with approximately 10% of flea-allergic dogs. Acute moist dermatitis and secondary keratinization disorders (seborrhea) are frequently seen.

Feline

The most common signs are those of miliary dermatitis with papules and crust distributed on the dorsal caudal trunk, dorsal neck and shoulders, perineum, and ventral abdomen (see Plate X-5). A generalized distribution occasionally is observed. Fleas and flea excrement usually are present. Other signs associated with the pruritus include excoriation, ulcers, and variable alopecia and erythema. Eosinophilic plaques and linear granulomas have been found to occur with feline flea allergy dermatitis (see Plates X-3 and X-4).

Diagnosis

History or observation of flea infestation correlated with a distribution of lesions regionalized to the dorsal caudal back, perineum, and caudal ventral abdomen and accompanied by intense pruritus is suggestive of canine flea allergy dermatitis. Lesions on the dorsal neck and back are frequently observed in cats.

Screening diagnostic tests are used mainly to rule out other causes of the clinical signs. Skin scrapings are negative for mites. A flea egg or larvae may occasionally be seen in the scraping. Skin biopsy findings are not specific for flea allergy dermatitis, although they are consistent with allergic dermatitis. Many tissue eosinophils are seen on microscopic examination.

The intradermal allergy test using a 1:1000 w/v flea antigen is a supportive test for flea allergy dermatitis. The test is performed as previously described for atopy and is read at 15 minutes. If it is negative, read the test again at 24 to 48 hours to evaluate a delayed reaction characterized by a small area of erythema and mild focal edema at the injection site.

The most widely used diagnostic test for flea allergy dermatitis is a therapeutic trial with parasiticides. A complete flea control program must be initiated and maintained, including fumigation of the indoor environment and continuous flea control on all animals in the household (see Table 3-5). A 100% clinical response to the flea control program is considered diagnostic for flea allergy dermatitis. If the response is less than complete, other concurrent problems, such as atopy, food allergy, and secondary pyoderma, must be considered (see Table 2-2).

Management

An effective control program for flea allergy dermatitis in dogs and cats must include three objectives: (1) to break the flea life cycle in the environment; (2) to minimize infestations of all animals in the environment; and (3) to control the allergic reaction to the fleabite.

Control of fleas in the indoor environment may necessitate thorough vacuuming of carpets and hard surfaces, removal of debris and old bedding, and spraying or fumigation of the entire premises. Spraying of the kennels and yard helps to reduce the outdoor exposure. To minimize animal infestation, the prophylactic treatment of all animals on a continuous basis is required. The use of powder and spray two or three times per week usually is effective on small, short-haired dogs and most cats. Flea collars or medallions can be used on cats and small dogs, but powder or spray may need to be used concurrently. An insecticidal dip every 7 to 10 days is often the most satisfactory method of continuous flea control for medium to large dogs and for long-haired dogs. A few insecticidal dips are approved for cats; these usually are effective but often are more difficult to use than powders. Insecticidal foams may be tolerated better by some cats. Systemic insecticides are not effective in the flea-allergic animal because they do not prevent fleabites and the deposition of the antigen in the tissue.

Problems can occur with any of these methods of flea control. Powders and sprays often are difficult to work through hair to the skin. Sprays and dips can evaporate rapidly in areas of high environmental temperatures, resulting in a shortened residual effect. There is potential for systemic side effects from the storage of insecticides in the body tissues if absorbed through the skin after application of sprays and dips; this tends to be more of a problem in cats than in dogs. Local dermatitis may be associated with flea collars.

One of the major problems with continuous insecticidal therapy is the development of resistance to the common insecticides among the endemic flea population. It often is necessary to change the insecticide periodically.

The control of the allergic reaction to the fleabite is most commonly achieved by using oral (see Table 3-9) or injectable corticosteroids (triamcinolone acetonide; see Table 3-7). Oral corticosteroids can be given for 1 to 2 weeks while good flea control is initiated (see Table 3-5). If there is adequate flea control and no concurrent problems, corticosteroids usually are not required for a prolonged time. Therefore, the long-acting residual corticosteroids usually are not indicated.

The use of flea antigen for hyposensitization is not effective in most animals. Flea hyposensitization can be used as a "last resort" in an animal that has historical and clinical manifestations of flea allergy dermatitis, other causes of clinical signs have been ruled out, and good flea control in the environment and on the animal(s) has not resulted in a good clinical response. The duration of effect of the flea antigen is relatively short. Weekly injections of 0.5 to 1.0 ml are given for 6 to 12 weeks.

Prognosis

If a diligent flea control program is maintained, the prognosis is good for many animals. In flea-endemic areas, however, 100% flea control often is impossible. Thus, the prognosis for good control is fair to guarded.

TICK BITE HYPERSENSITIVITY

Tick bite hypersensitivity is uncommonly recognized in dogs. It is suspected when the tick bite is associated with pruritus or a more severe skin reaction at the attachment site. Lesions associated with a tick bite hypersensitivity reaction are erythematous and granulomatous; occasionally, more proliferative and ulcerative lesions are seen. Cutaneous basophil hypersensitivity is thought to play a role in tick bite hypersensitivity.

EAR MITE HYPERSENSITIVITY

Otodectes cynotis has been associated with both a Type I and Type III hypersensitivity reaction in cats and these reactions are presumed to occur in dogs. The animal with a severe pruritus associated with the ear mite infestation is presumed to have ear mite hypersensitivity.

AUTOSENSITIZATION (ID) REACTIONS

Autosensitization or "id" reactions occur when a hypersensitivity develops after cutaneous sensitization that results in lesions at a distant site. Dermatophytes are a common source of antigens, but anal sac material also has been implicated to cause an id reaction. The antigens may become blood or lymphatic borne and in this way affect distal sites.

Affected animals often will have been exposed to dermatophytes or even have a clinical dermatophytic infection. Autosensitization reactions usually are quite pruritic. In humans, id reactions have a variable clinical appearance and can be vesiculobullous, papular, or erythema multiforme-like or present as cellulitis. History and inability to culture dermatophytes from active lesions, combined with positive intradermal trichophytin testing, is supportive of the diagnosis. Histopathology is not diagnostic but can be supportive. Treating the primary source of antigen is the major therapeutic goal. Topical or systemic corticosteroids and systemic sulfonamides have been reported helpful in controlling the distal lesions.

HORMONAL HYPERSENSITIVITY

Hormonal hypersensitivity is a rare, pruritic condition in which the dog develops a hypersensitivity reaction to its own endogenous sex hormones. The pathogenesis is unknown.

History and Clinical Signs

The condition is recognized most often in intact females, although intact males may also have a hormonal hypersensitivity. The most suggestive history is that of a recurring maculopapular pruritic eruption observed at the same stage of each estrus cycle. Initially, the pruritic signs subside, but both pruritus and gross skin changes become progressively worse with each recurrence. In males, the cyclic pattern is not observed, resulting in a progressive nonseasonal pruritus.

The distribution is localized initially to the lower back, perineum, and posteromedial thighs. Early signs are that of pruritus without gross lesions. Gross lesions are variable, with papules, alopecia, and hyperpigmentation observed. In chronic hormonal sensitivity, hyperpigmentation is marked and lichenification also is observed. Vulvar hyperplasia is common.

Diagnosis

The diagnosis of hormonal hypersensitivity is based on the cyclic history, the regional distribution of lesions with the progressive hyperpigmented dermatoses, and the response to neutering. Intradermal tests using aqueous progesterone, estrogen, or testosterone have been advocated, but have not had widespread acceptance.

Treatment

The treatment of choice is neutering. Hormonal injections using repository testosterone or human chorionic gonadotropin (HCG) have been suggested as an alternative to surgery (see Table 3-14).

Prognosis

The prognosis for remission of most clinical signs is good after surgery.

SELECTED READINGS

Ackerman L: Recognizing the signs and sources of canine inhalant allergies. *Vet Med* 83:770–778, 1988.

Ackerman L: Diagnosing inhalant allergies: Intradermal or in vitro testing? *Vet Med* 83:780–789, 1988.

Ackerman L: Medical and immunotherapeutic options for treating atopic dogs. *Vet Med* 83:790–797, 1988.

Ackerman L: Food hypersensitivity: A rare, but manageable disorder. *Vet Med* 83:1142–1148, 1988.

August JR: Dietary hypersensitivity in dogs: Cutaneous manifestations, diagnosis and management. *Compend Contin Educ Pract Vet* 7:469–477, 1985.

DeBoer DJ: Survey of intradermal skin testing practices in North America. *JAVMA* 195:1357–1363, 1989.

Gorman NT, Halliwell REW: Mechanisms of immunological injury in hypersensitivity reactions. In: Halliwell REW, Gorman NT (eds): *Veterinary Clinical Immunology*. Philadelphia, WB Saunders Co, 1989, pp 212–229.

Halliwell REW, Gorman NT: Atopic diseases. In: Halliwell REW, Gorman NT (eds): *Veterinary Clinical Immunology*. Philadelphia, WB Saunders Co, 1989, pp 232–234.

Halliwell REW, Gorman NT: Nonatopic allergic skin diseases. In: Halliwell REW, Gorman NT (eds): *Veterinary Clinical Immunology*. Philadelphia, WB Saunders Co, 1989, pp 253–281.

Jeffers JG, Shanley KJ, Meyer EK: Diagnostic testing of dogs for food hypersensitivity. *JAVMA* 198(2):245–250, 1991.

Kleinbeck ML, Hites MJ, Loker JL, et al: Enzyme-linked immunosorbent assay for measurement of allergen-specific IgE in canine serum. *Am J Vet Res* 50:1831–1839, 1989.

Kunkle GA: Contact dermatitis. *Vet Clin North Am [Small Anim Pract]* 18:1061–1068, 1988.

Kwochka KW, Bevier DE: Flea dermatitis. In: Nesbitt GH (ed): *Dermatology, Contemporary Issues in Small Animal Practice*, vol 8. New York, Churchill Livingstone, 1987, pp 21–27.

Miller WH, Scott DW: Efficacy of chlorpheniramine maleate for management of pruritus in cats. *JAVMA* 197:67–70, 1990.

Moriello KA: Oh, no! Not fleas again! *Vet Focus* 1:19–28, 1989.

Nesbitt GH: Feline dermatoses. In: Nesbitt GH (ed): *Dermatology, Contemporary Issues in Small Animal Practice,* vol 8. New York, Churchill Livingstone, 1987, pp 209–231.

Nesbitt GH, Kedan GS, Caciolo P: Canine atopy. Part I: Etiology and diagnosis. *Compend Contin Educ Pract Vet* 6:73–84, 1984.

Nesbitt GH, Kedan GS, Caciolo P: Canine atopy. Part II. Management. *Compend Contin Educ Pract Vet* 6:264–278, 1984.

White SD: Food hypersensitivity. *Vet Clin North Am [Small Anim Pract]* 18:1043–1048, 1988.

Willemse TA: Atopic dermatitis. In: Nesbitt GH (ed): *Dermatology, Contemporary Issues in Small Animal Practice*, vol 8. New York, Churchill Livingstone, 1987, pp 57–72.

Chapter 5

IMMUNE-MEDIATED SKIN DISEASES

Lowell Ackerman, DVM
Gene H. Nesbitt, DVM, MS

Immune-mediated skin diseases are those that result directly from an aberrant immune response. Autoimmune skin diseases are immune-mediated in nature, yet not all immune-mediated disorders are autoimmune. Diagnostic Key 3 (see end of Chapter 2) lists the most pertinent historical and clinical findings and diagnostic tests used to help differentiate the common causes of canine and feline immune-mediated skin diseases.

LUPUS ERYTHEMATOSUS

Pathogenesis

Lupus erythematosus is characterized by multiple circulating autoantibodies that participate in immune-mediated tissue injury directed against the animal's own system. Two forms of the condition have been recognized in animals and people: systemic lupus erythematosus and cutaneous (discoid) lupus erythematosus.

History and Clinical Signs

The most common clinical findings in dogs with systemic lupus erythematosus (SLE) are arthritis, fever unresponsive to antibiotics, kidney disease (glomerulonephritis) with protein loss in the urine, anemia, and skin disease. The diversity of clinical presentations and the fact that affected dogs may only have a few signs causes systemic SLE to mimic other syndromes (Plate II-1). The skin disorders seen with SLE also are diverse and can include scaling, red maculopapular eruptions, scarring, exfoliative dermatoses, pyoderma, lymphedema, rheumatoid-like nodules, hair loss, panniculitis, purpura, loss of pigment, and erosive-ulcerative lesions of the mucous membranes (mouth, nose, anus, vulva, penis, nail beds).

Cutaneous (discoid) lupus erythematosus (DLE) is generally regarded as a less harmful variant of SLE, wherein systemic involvement is absent and autoantibodies are rarely found. The most common presenting sign is red, scaling dermatitis of the face, often including the nose and nasal mucosa (Plate II-2). Loss of pigment from the nares often is noted.

Diagnosis

Specific diagnostic testing for SLE includes the antinuclear antibody test, the lupus erythematosus cell test, and biopsies for histopathologic and immunopathologic evaluation.

The antinuclear antibody (ANA) test, performed on serum, detects antibodies directed against cell nuclei and is a good screening test (up to 90% of dogs with SLE will have a positive titer with active disease), although false-positive results are common. The lupus erythematosus (LE) cell test is performed on clotted or heparinized blood and about 60% of affected dogs have LE cells. Animals with strictly cutaneous LE usually are negative when evaluated for ANA or LE cells. Positive ANA tests with a speckled pattern of fluorescence are more likely to be the result of an immune-mediated process.

Biopsies taken for histopathologic examination may show changes as variable as the clinical presentation but characteristic changes at the junction between the dermis and epidermis (interface dermatitis) are highly suggestive. A positive "lupus band" evident on immunopathologic evaluation is supportive but nonconfirmatory. Systemic and cutaneous forms of LE can not be differentiated on the basis of cutaneous biopsies for histopathology or immunopathology.

Treatment

The treatment of SLE must be individualized for each patient. In general, it is attempted with immunosuppressive doses of corticosteroids, with or without chemotherapy (for example, azathioprine, cyclophosphamide), or plasmapheresis (see Table 3-13).

The treatment of DLE differs from that of SLE in that immunosuppressive therapy usually is not warranted. Anti-inflammatory doses of corticosteroids (1.0–1.5 mg/kg daily then tapered to alternate-day therapy) together with vitamin E at 400 IU twice daily often are sufficient to control the condition. Limited exposure to sunlight or the use of sunscreens is an additional measure likely to benefit patients with DLE.

PEMPHIGUS

Pathogenesis

The term *pemphigus* is used to describe a complex of disorders characterized by autoantibody deposition within the epidermis that causes the separation of epidermal cells from one another such that spaces are created. Four variants of pemphigus currently are recognized in animals: pemphigus vulgaris, pemphigus foliaceus, pemphigus erythematosus, and pemphigus vegetans. There is mounting evidence to support the supposition that the lesions of pemphigus in people result from the binding of an autoantibody to an antigen (or antigens) in or near the epidermal cell membrane. Pemphigus in dogs and cats bears many similarities to its human counterpart and therefore the pathomechanisms are presumed to be similar.

History and Clinical Signs

Pemphigus vulgaris is an ulcerating disease primarily involving nonhaired mucous membranes (mouth, anus, conjunctiva, nasal mucosa, vagina, prepuce) and their junctions with the skin (Plate II-3) before becoming generalized. Oral lesions are found in the majority of cases. Mucous membrane lesions rarely occur as intact blisters because of the fragility of the blister roof. Secondary bacterial complications develop, and severely affected individuals can be anorectic, depressed, and febrile.

Pemphigus vegetans is the least common form of pemphigus and is currently believed to be a less harmful variant of pemphigus vulgaris in individuals with increased resistance to the disease. Groups of pustules evolve into eruptive papillomatous lesions and verrucous vegetative masses, often studded with pustules and erosions and exuding serum.

Pemphigus foliaceus is probably the most common variant in animals and is characterized by a scaling, crusting and/or pustular dermatitis that often originates on the head and ears before becoming generalized (Plate II-4). Mucosal and mucocutaneous involvement is not prominent, but the footpads are frequently involved and are hyperkeratotic. Intact vesicles can appear transiently, but rapidly become purulent and usually are sterile on culture. Secondary infection is less common. Animals usually do not become systemically ill.

Pemphigus erythematosus is indistinguishable from pemphigus foliaceus clinically but usually remains localized to the head and face. Occasionally the footpads are involved.

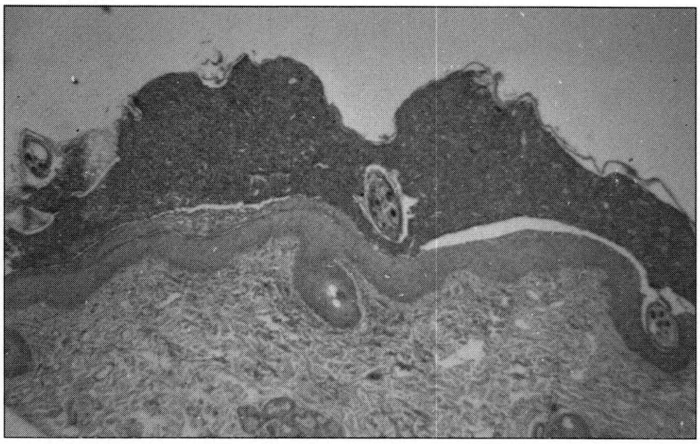

Figure 5-1. Subcorneal bulla/pustule seen in pemphigus foliaceus.

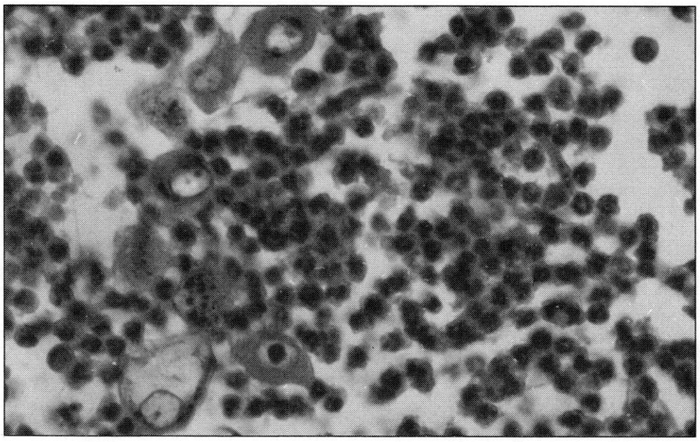

Figure 5-2. Cytology of acantholytic keratinocytes.

Diagnosis

Diagnosis of pemphigus relies on clinical examination and biopsies for histopathologic examination, with or without immunopathologic assay. The formation of blisters within the epidermis is classic but infrequently seen because of the thinness of the epidermis in animals (Fig. 5-1). Direct immunofluorescence testing (immunopathologic examination) of normal-appearing perilesional tissue may reveal autoantibodies in the intercellular spaces in about 65% of cases. Pemphigus erythematosus may occasionally present additionally with autoantibody deposition at the dermoepidermal junction. Important supportive findings on cytologic evaluation include the presence of numerous acantholytic cells and neutrophils in the blister/pustule (Fig. 5-2).

Nikolsky's sign is characteristic of pemphigus although it also may be seen in toxic epidermal necrolysis and sometimes in pemphigoid. A positive Nikolsky sign is obtained when finger pressure applied laterally to an erosion or to normal-appearing skin dislodges the epidermis from the dermis and creates a new erosion.

Treatment

Treatment of all forms of pemphigus is similar but differs in degree, depending on the particular variant involved, the individual susceptibility, and the initial response to therapy. Pemphigus vulgaris is the most aggressive form, followed by pemphigus foliaceus, with pemphigus erythematosus and pemphigus vegetans representing the least harmful variants. Immunosuppressive doses of prednisone remain the initial treatment of choice, but alternative or adjunctive treatments include azathioprine, cyclophosphamide, and gold salts (chrysotherapy) (see Table 3-13). Animals with nasal dermatitis and depigmentation will also benefit from the application of commercial sunscreens and being kept indoors during peak periods of sunshine as solar ultraviolet irradiation may exacerbate lesions.

PEMPHIGOID

Pathogenesis

Pemphigoid refers to a complex of blistering conditions characterized by autoantibody deposits at the junction between the epidermis and dermis, with blister formation immediately deep to the epidermis. Current evidence suggests that bullous pemphigoid in people is an autoimmune inflammatory disorder in which autoantibodies are directed against an antigen found in the lamina lucida of the basement membrane zone of squamous epithelium. Bullous pemphigoid has been well-documented while cicatricial pemphigoid has been suspected in animals.

History and Clinical Signs

The principal lesions of bullous pemphigoid are transient blisters, crusts, epidermal collarettes, and ulcerations (see Plate II-5). The mucous membranes, head, neck, axillae, ventral abdomen, and the footpads are commonly affected. There is an apparent breed predilection for collies, Shetland sheepdogs, and perhaps Doberman pinschers. Cicatricial, or mucous membrane pemphigoid, is a rare, chronic blistering disease primarily affecting the oral and ocular mucous membranes.

Diagnosis

Impression smears made from these blisters may reveal inflammatory cells but few or no detached epidermal cells (acantholytic keratinocytes) (Fig. 5-2). Diagnosis relies on characteristic histopathologic findings and supportive immunopathology. Bullous pemphigoid and cicatricial pemphigoid are indistinguishable on the basis of histopathology and immunopathology but can be differentiated by their clinical presentation.

Treatment

Treatment of pemphigoid is identical to that of pemphigus and includes immunosuppressive dosages of corticosteroids, adjuvant chemotherapy, and chrysotherapy (see Table 3-13). Cicatricial pemphigoid usually does not require such drastic therapy and may respond to topical corticosteroids or cyclosporine.

DRUG ERUPTION
Pathogenesis

Drug eruption, an immune-mediated reaction to medications, is any dermatologic manifestation that results from administering a drug orally, parenterally, topically, or as an inhalant. All four types of hypersensitivity reactions can be associated with immune-mediated drug eruption as well as irritant contact reactions. The low-molecular-weight drugs act as haptens, combining with plasma or epidermal proteins. There is often a lag period of 5 to 21 days before humoral antibodies are formed or tissue lymphocytes become sensitized. Cross-reactions between drugs can occur; affected animals have reacted to antibacterials, antifungals, antiparasitics, vaccines, topicals, hormones, tranquilizers, antineoplastic agents, and other drugs. More extreme manifestations of drug eruption may include erythema multiforme and toxic epidermal necrolysis. Table 5-1 lists the cutaneous reactions associated with specific drugs.

History

Careful questioning of owners will reveal that the animal currently is receiving some medication, either topical or systemic, or that medication has recently been discontinued. In immune-mediated drug eruption, a history of repeated exposure or prolonged therapy is obtained. Pruritus is variable. There may be a history of poor response to symptomatic treatment if the animal is still receiving the medication.

No sex or age predilection has been reported for drug eruptions. Adverse reactions to sulfa drugs have been documented in Doberman pinschers and serious reactions, sometimes fatal, have been reported in collies after administration of ivermectin at parasiticidal doses.

Clinical Signs

Drug eruption is characterized by a history of cutaneous eruptions that might be maculopapular, erosive/ulcerative, vesiculopustular, or exfoliative, after the administration of a specific drug (Plate II-6). The clinical lesions and distribution are variable and mimic many other bullous and nonbullous skin diseases. The distribution of a drug eruption often includes the head and dorsal spine if a systemic reaction has occurred. A local reaction occurs when there is an allergic reaction to a topical drug or to a fixed drug eruption. Other clinical signs reported in cats include miliary dermatitis, urticaria/angioedema, ulceration (Plate II-6), and variable alopecia.

Fixed drug eruptions are quite rare in dogs and present as uniformly well-circumscribed erythematous lesions starting with edema that may form bullae and ulcerate.

Diagnosis

The history is the most important clue in diagnosing drug eruption. A drug eruption is suspected when there is marked improvement of clinical signs within 7 to 14 days after discontinuing the drug and when there is no recurrence of clinical signs. Occasionally, clinical signs persist for several weeks. Drug eruptions vary in their histologic characteristics. A drug eruption can cause hydropic degeneration of basal cells, subepidermal vesicles, and epidermal necrosis. Provocative exposure to the suspected drug is not recommended to verify the probable cause of clinical signs because of the danger to the patient; exposure may occur inadvertently, however, when a specific medication is repeated.

Treatment

The treatment of choice for a drug eruption is discontinuing and avoiding further use of the suspect drug. Clinical signs are treated symptomatically. Corticosteroids are indicated on a short-term basis to decrease the immune-mediated reaction and problematic pruritus. Drugs of similar chemical structure to the suspected ones should be avoided because cross-reactivity can occur.

ERYTHEMA MULTIFORME
Pathogenesis

Erythema multiforme is an uncommon syndrome that presumably is immune-mediated. In most cases, it represents an adverse cutaneous reaction to drugs, infections, or internal disorders.

Clinical Signs

The eruption is usually symmetric and often involves the limbs and ventrum. Manifestations include macules, papules, urticarial plaques, vesicles/bullae, erosions, and ulcerations. Lesions often spread centrifugally, leaving a central clear area, commonly referred to as a "target" or "iris" lesion, but also can be serpiginous or arciform.

Diagnosis

Diagnosis is based on clinical presentation and consistent histopathologic findings. Immunopathology is seldom beneficial.

Treatment

Most cases in dogs have been secondary to staphylococcal folliculitis or reactions to drugs. If the causative insult can be addressed, the condition can be expected to regress spontaneously.

TABLE 5-1

Cutaneous Drug Reactions in Dogs and Cats

Class/Drug	*Species*	*Route*[a]	*Clinical Signs or Lesions*
Analgesic			
Phenylbutazone	cat	NA	Alopecia
Anticonvulsant			
Primidone	dog	PO	Alopecia
Antimicrobials			
Amoxicillin	dog	NA	Skin rash
Ampicillin	dog/cat	Inj	Fixed reaction, wheals, alopecia, pruritus, injection site inflammation, toxic epidermal necrolysis
Cephalexin	dog	NA	Epidermal necrosis, ulceration, alopecia, erosion, crusting
Chloramphenicol	dog	PO	Epidermal necrosis, ulceration
Gentamicin	dog/cat	Inj	Pruritus, alopecia, erythema, edema, injection site inflammation
Griseofulvin	dog	PO	Eczematous
Hetacillin	cat	PO	Alopecia, pruritus
Miconazole	cat	Top	Erythema, alopecia
Neomycin	dog/cat	Top	Contact dermatitis
Neomycin/triamcinolone/thiostrepton	dog	Top	Eczematous
Penicillin	dog/cat	NA	Epidermal necrosis, eczematous, urticaria, angioedema
Procaine and benzathine penicillin G	dog/cat	Inj	Sterile abscess
Povidone-iodine	dog/cat	Top	Exfoliative
Streptomycin	dog	NA	Cutaneous eruption
Sulfasoxizole	cat	PO	Eczematous
Tetracycline	dog/cat	PO	Urticaria, angioedema
Trimethoprim/sulfamethoxazole	dog/cat	NA	Facial edema, purpura, thrombocytopenia, papules
Triple sulfa	dog	PO	Eczematous, alopecia, erosion, crusts
Tylosine	cat	Inj	Irritation at injection site
Antiparasitic			
Amitraz	dog	Top	Pruritus, papules
Bunamidine	cat	PO	Oral lesion
Chlorinated hydrocarbon/pyrethrum, mineral oil	cat	Top	Otitis externa
Diclorvos	cat	Top	Contact dermatitis, alopecia, ulceration
Diethylcarbamazine	dog	PO	Pruritus, eczema
Organophosphate/organochlorine	dog/cat	Top	Erythroderma
Thiabendazole	cat	PO	Pemphigus vulgaris-like lesion
Cardiac/Respiratory			
Phenylhydantoin	dog	PO	Vesicobullous
Quinidine	dog	PO	Exfoliative
Chemotherapeutic			
Azathioprine	dog	PO	Alopecia, pyoderma
Bleomycin	dog		Ulceration at pressure points, onychomadesis
Chlorambucil		PO	Alopecia, hyperpigmentation
Cyclosporine			Hirsutism, papillomatosis, lymphoplasmacytoid dermatosis
Doxorubicin	dog		Erythema, alopecia, hyperpigmentation
5-Fluorocytosine	dog	PO	Eczematous
Hydroxyurea			Alopecia
Tranquilizer/Anesthetic			
Acepromazine	dog	PO	Scales, erythema, alopecia
Tetracaine	dog	Top	Cutaneous eruption
Xylazine	dog	Inj	Urticaria/hives
Vaccine/serum			
Feline leukemia antiserum	cat	SC	Toxic epidermal necrolysis
Panleukopenia vaccine	cat	Inj	Angioedema

TABLE 5-1 (continued)

Cutaneous Drug Reactions in Dogs and Cats

Class/Drug	*Species*	*Route*[a]	*Clinical Signs or Lesions*
Miscellaneous			
Aminopropazine	dog	Inj	Injection site necrosis
Benzoyl peroxide shampoo and gel	dog	Top	Erythroderma
Coal tar shampoo	dog	Top	Eczematous
Copper naphthenate	dog	Top	Skin burn
Glucocorticoids	dog	PO/Inj	Alopecia
Isotretinoin	dog	PO	Mucocutaneous erythema and crusting
Megestrol acetate	cat	PO	Alopecia
Methoxypyridazine	dog	PO	Alopecia
Propylthiouracil	cat	PO	Facial edema/pruritus
Sodium arsenite 44%	dog	NA	Necrosis, edema, ulceration
Sulfurated lime	dog	Top	Skin burn, edema, exfoliative
Synthetic estrogen	dog	NA	Cutaneous eruption
Thiacetarsamide	dog	NA	Alopecia, dermatitis
Thyroid extract	dog	PO	Cutaneous eruption

[a]NA = no data available; PO = per os; Inj = injection; TOP = topical; SC = subcutaneous.

TOXIC EPIDERMAL NECROLYSIS

Pathogenesis

Toxic epidermal necrolysis is a life-threatening disease involving the mucosal and skin surfaces. It most commonly results from a response to an underlying infection, drug reaction, or metabolic disorder. It forms one extreme of a spectrum that ranges from drug eruption, through erythema multiforme, to toxic epidermal necrolysis.

History and Clinical Signs

Toxic epidermal necrolysis is characterized by large, painful, ulcerative areas on any part of the body (Plate II-7). There may be a mucocutaneous component and a positive Nikolsky sign may be evident. In dogs, the disease is always associated with some predisposing disease, such as a staphylococcal infection, drug administration, or systemic neoplasia.

Diagnosis

Toxic epidermal necrolysis can be diagnosed by biopsy; necrosis of the entire thickness of the epidermis and the formation of subepidermal vesicles will be evident.

Treatment

Treatment is initiated with a higher loading dose followed by low-dose corticosteroids. Supportive topical therapy with astringents and systemic antibiotics usually is indicated. The primary disease must also be treated concurrently if the condition is to resolve.

CUTANEOUS VASCULITIS

Pathogenesis

Cutaneous vasculitis is a collection of disorders in which the underlying problem includes destructive and inflammatory changes in the blood vessels. Cutaneous vasculitis can occur secondary to a number of processes, including infections (bacterial, mycoplasmal, rickettsial, viral, fungal), drug reactions, eruptions caused by foods and food additives, immune-mediated disorders (systemic lupus erythematosus, scleroderma, dermatomyositis, rheumatoid arthritis), exposure to cold, trauma, reactions to injections (vaccinations), chronic diseases (diabetes mellitus, chronic respiratory disease, cancer), and arthropod bites, or for no apparent cause.

Clinical Signs

Vasculitic lesions are most frequent on the dependent parts of the body, feet and ears. The most common lesion visualized and felt is an elevated bruise, a so-called "palpable purpura." An erosive-ulcerative process is inevitable at some stage of the disease. In later stages when the blood vessels have been thoroughly compromised, the tissue may die, leaving a depressed area.

Diagnosis

Diagnosis is based on histopathologic and immunopathologic evaluation but many tests may be warranted to unearth the underlying cause (for example, antinuclear antibody, rheumatoid factor, hypoallergenic food trial, bacterial or fungal culture, titers).

Treatment

Treatment should be directed at the underlying cause if it is known. If no cause has been determined, therapy is often initiated with antiinflammatory or immunosuppressive doses of corticosteroids or dapsone.

JUVENILE CELLULITIS (PUPPY STRANGLES)

Pathogenesis

Juvenile cellulitis, or puppy strangles, is presumed to be an immune-mediated disease based on histopathologic features and response to immunosuppressive forms of therapy. Dachshunds, golden retrievers, Labrador retrievers, and pointers are most commonly affected.

Clinical Signs

In juvenile cellulitis the face and head are commonly swollen and inflamed (Plate II-8). The lesions are nodular, indurated, and there is frequently a concurrent submandibular lymphadenomegaly. Draining tracts often are present and scarring is a common sequel.

Diagnosis

Biopsies reveal an underlying cellulitis. Bacterial cultures sometimes reveal organisms, although they do not appear to be of primary significance.

Treatment

Treatment with a bactericidal antibiotic (see Table 3-11) and immunosuppressive doses of corticosteroids is required for about 2 weeks. The condition usually responds completely, with little chance of recurrence.

STERILE PYOGRANULOMA

Pathogenesis

Sterile pyogranuloma is a nonbacterial cause of pododermatitis in dogs and is presumed to be immune-mediated based on histopathologic presentation and response to corticosteroid therapy. Great Danes, St. Bernards, Newfoundlands, dachshunds, shar peis, pit bull terriers, and English bulldogs appear to be predisposed.

Clinical Signs

The condition appears as firm red nodular lesions between the toes which frequently ulcerate and drain (Plate II-9). The presentation is indistinguishable from any of the other types of pododermatitis.

Diagnosis

The diagnosis is based on histopathologic findings. Bacterial culture and sensitivity tests invariably are negative or reflect only contaminant growth.

Treatment

Therapy consists of either resection or treatment with antiinflammatory doses of corticosteroids (see Table 3-9).

UVEODERMATOLOGIC (VOGT-KOYANAGI-HARADA-LIKE) SYNDROME

Pathogenesis

The cause of uveodermatologic (Vogt-Koyanagi-Harada-like) syndrome is currently unknown, but it may represent an autoimmune attack against melanocytes.

History and Clinical Signs

The condition is characterized by a serious eye disorder (granulomatous panuveitis) and concurrent loss of pigment from the nose, lips, eyelids, and occasionally the entire body. Most affected individuals are young adults. Acute blindness can result if the inflammatory process is not arrested.

Diagnosis

The diagnosis of uveodermatologic syndrome relies on biopsies of affected tissues for histopathologic evaluation. There is a pronounced inflammatory reaction at the dermoepidermal junction. The histopathologic presentation of skin lesions bears little if any resemblance to the condition seen in people.

Treatment

The mainstay of therapy is topical and/or systemic corticosteroids. Once blindness has occurred the return of sight is unlikely, but early therapeutic intervention usually is successful. Repigmentation may be complete, partial, or unsubstantial.

ALOPECIA AREATA

Pathogenesis

Alopecia areata refers to a focal area of hair loss which usually is not accompanied by any significant inflammatory reaction. The exact pathogenesis in people is unknown, but there is some circumstantial evidence that autoimmunity is involved.

History and Clinical Signs

The clinical presentation of alopecia areata is that of a focal-to-multifocal, noninflammatory area of hair loss. There is no age, sex, or site predilection.

Diagnosis

The diagnosis of alopecia areata is confirmed by the characteristic biopsy findings. In later stages, the condition may be reported as an endocrine type of pattern on histopathology.

Therapy

Therapy for alopecia areata in animals can include conscientious neglect or intralesional corticosteroids. The condition is really cosmetic in nature and poses no health concern to the animal.

SCLERODERMA

Pathogenesis

Scleroderma is a rare connective tissue disease that can occur as a localized phenomenon (morphea) in dogs. Some evidence indicates that autoimmunity might play a role in the condition in humans.

History and Clinical Signs

In the few cases of scleroderma reported in animals, the clinical presentation is one of a localized hairless area of skin, which appears thickened on palpation.

Diagnosis

A diagnosis of scleroderma is confirmed by biopsy for histopathology that reveals sclerosis of the dermis and subcutis. On biopsy alone it is impossible to distinguish between the localized and systemic forms.

Treatment

Treatment often is attempted with corticosteroids in either systemic or topical regimens. The overall behavior of the localized form is often relatively benign and therefore overtreatment is to be avoided.

SJÖGREN'S SYNDROME

Pathogenesis

Sjögren's syndrome is a sicca complex characterized by dry eyes (keratoconjunctivitis sicca) and a dry mouth (xerostomia), often coupled with an autoimmune connective tissue disease.

History and Clinical Signs

Animals with Sjögren's syndrome usually are presented for ophthalmic disease but concurrent dermatologic manifestations (such as keratinization disorders, erythroderma, hypothyroidism) may be evident.

Diagnosis

Sjögren's syndrome should be considered in dogs with keratoconjunctivitis sicca, suggestive biopsies of the lacrimal glands, and not uncommonly, a positive ANA or rheumatoid factor.

Treatment

Treatment may be attempted with topical (see Table 3-3) or systemic (see Table 3-9) corticosteroids and, more recently, with a topical cyclosporine preparation.

DERMATITIS HERPETIFORMIS

Pathogenesis

Dermatitis herpetiformis in humans is a chronic, extremely pruritic dermatitis associated with a gluten sensitivity, elevation of IgA circulating gluten antigenemia, significant elevation of IgA circulating immune complexes, and irregular granular deposits of immunoglobulin A (IgA) in the papillary dermis. The pathogenesis is unknown but it has been suggested that immune complexes of gluten and antigluten may play a role.

Clinical Signs

Dermatitis herpetiformis has only rarely been suspected in dogs. Those patients have shown a papulocrustous, pruritic eruption involving principally the trunk, head, ears, and feet. Biopsies were supportive but not confirmatory.

Diagnosis

To properly confirm a diagnosis, an animal should have appropriate clinical signs, characteristic histopathologic lesions, a positive direct immunofluorescence test for IgA in granular deposits in the dermal papillae, and a favorable response to dapsone.

Treatment

The treatment of choice for dermatitis herpetiformis in people, and presumably in dogs as well, is dapsone and a gluten-limited diet.

SUBCORNEAL PUSTULAR DERMATOSIS

Pathogenesis

Subcorneal pustular dermatosis is a rare, presumably immune-mediated skin disease. Although there is no apparent age or sex predilection, miniature schnauzers appear to be predisposed.

History and Clinical Signs

The classical history is that of pustular dermatitis that does not respond to antibiotics or corticosteroids. The majority of bacterial cultures of the lesions are sterile. The age of onset varies, but the disease commonly occurs when the animal is 3 to 4 years old. Pruritus, frequently a primary complaint of the owner, is of variable intensity. The disease often waxes and wanes despite therapy with antibiotics and corticosteroids.

Generalized truncal lesions are the most common signs, but the head and medial thighs may also be involved. The lesions begin as erythematous macules, progressing to papules or pustules within 36 to 48 hours; these lesions subsequently rupture and form crusts. The healing stages include annular scaling with an erythemic border followed by a hyperpigmented alopecic lesion that persists for 8 to 10 weeks.

Diagnosis

The history and clinical signs suggest subcorneal pustular dermatosis. Cutaneous biopsy reveals subcorneal pustules with minimal dermal inflammation. A therapeutic trial with dapsone is also supportive.

Treatment

The treatment of choice for subcorneal pustular dermatosis is dapsone. The side effects of this drug in dogs include anemia, leukopenia, hepatic toxicosis, keratoconjunctivitis sicca, and thrombocytopenia.

STERILE EOSINOPHILIC PUSTULOSIS

Pathogenesis

Sterile eosinophilic pustulosis is a rare pustular disease with no apparent age, breed, or sex predilection. It is presumed to be immune-mediated based on its histopathologic presentation and response to corticosteroid therapy.

Clinical Signs

Primary skin lesions include papules and pustules and pruritus is moderate to severe. Scaling, crusting, hair loss, and hyperpigmentation are common sequelae.

Diagnosis

Diagnosis consists of biopsies and ruling out other potential causes of follicular and nonfollicular pustules.

Treatment

Treatment consists of antiinflammatory doses of corticosteroids daily or on alternate days on a long-term basis. Relapses are common when therapy is discontinued.

SELECTED READINGS

Ackerman LJ: Pemphigus and pemphigoid in the dog and cat. Part I. Pemphigus. *Compend Contin Educ Pract Vet* 7:89–97, 1985.

Ackerman LJ: Pemphigus and pemphigoid in the dog and cat. Part II. Pemphigoid. *Compend Contin Educ Pract Vet* 7:281–286, 1985.

Ackerman LJ: Dermatitis herpetiformis—Does it exist? *JAVMA* 185:633–635, 1984.

Ackerman LJ: Canine nodular panniculitis. *Compend Contin Educ Pract Vet* 6:818–824, 1984.

Ackerman LJ: *Practical Canine Dermatology*. Goleta, CA, American Veterinary Publications, 1989, 369 pp.

Ackerman LJ: *Practical Feline Dermatology*. Goleta, CA, American Veterinary Publications, 1989, 264 pp.

Cottrell BD, Barnett HC: Harada's disease in the Japanese Akita. *J Small Anim Pract* 28:517–521, 1987.

Daniel GB, Patterson JS: Toxic epidermal necrolysis: A case report. *JAAHA* 21:631–635, 1985.

Drazner FH: Systemic lupus erythematosus in the dog. *Compend Contin Educ Pract Vet* 2:243–254, 1980.

Giger U, Werner LL, Miilichamp NJ, Gorman NT: Sulfadiazine-induced allergy in six Doberman pinschers. *JAVMA* 186:479–484, 1985.

Grindem CB, Johnson KH: Systemic lupus erythematosus: Literature review and report of 42 new canine cases. *JAAHA* 19:489–503, 1983.

Kalaher KM, Scott DW: Subcorneal pustular dermatosis in dogs and in human beings: Comparative aspects. *J Am Acad Dermatol* 22:1023–1028, 1990.

Kaswan HL, Martin CL, Dawe DL: Rheumatoid factor determination in 50 dogs with keratoconjunctivitis sicca. *JAVMA* 183:1073–1075, 1983.

Kern TJ, Walton DK, Riis RC, et al: Uveitis associated with poliosis and vitiligo in six dogs. *JAVMA* 187:408–414, 1985.

McKeever PJ, Dahl MV: A disease in dogs resembling human subcorneal pustular dermatosis. *JAVMA* 170:704–707, 1977.

McMurdy MA: A case resembling erythema multiforme major (Stevens-Johnson syndrome) in a dog. *JAAHA* 26:297–300, 1990.

Medleau L, Chalmers S, Kirpensteijn, et al: Erythema multiforme and disseminated intravascular coagulation in a dog. *JAAHA* 26:643–646, 1990.

Medleau L, Shanley KJ, Rakich PM, Goldschmidt MH: Trimethoprim-sulfonamide–associated drug eruption in dogs. *JAAHA* 26:305–311, 1990.

Nesbitt GH: Cutaneous drug reactions in small animals. *Clin Dermatol* 4(1):190–192, 1986.

Randall MG, Hurvitz AI: Immune-mediated vasculitis in five dogs. *JAVMA* 183:207–211, 1983.

Scott DW: Localized scleroderma (morphea) in two dogs. *JAAHA* 22:207–211, 1986.

Scott DW: Sterile eosinophilic pustulosis in the dog. *JAAHA* 20:585–589, 1984.

Scott DW, Anderson WI: Panniculitis in dogs and cats: A retrospective analysis of 78 cases. *JAAHA* 24:551–559, 1988.

Scott DW, Miller WH Jr, Goldschmidt MH: Erythema multiforme in the dog. *JAAHA* 19:453–459, 1983.

Scott DW, Walton DK, Manning TO, et al: Canine lupus erythematosus. I. Systemic lupus erythematosus. *JAAHA* 19:461–479, 1983.

Scott DW, Walton DK, Manning TO, et al: Canine lupus erythematosus. II. Discoid lupus erythematosus. *JAAHA* 19:481–488, 1983.

Chapter 6

PARASITIC DISEASES

Gene H. Nesbitt, DVM, MS
Lowell Ackerman, DVM

Parasitic diseases represent one of the most common causes of dermatoses in dogs and cats. Diagnostic Key 4 (see end of Chapter 2) lists the most pertinent historical and clinical findings and diagnostic tests used to help differentiate the common causes of canine and feline parasitic diseases.

FLEA DERMATITIS

Flea dermatitis is a reaction of the skin to the physical presence of the flea or the mechanical trauma of the fleabite, which is not immune mediated. Although there is an academic distinction between the non–immune-mediated flea dermatitis and the immune-mediated fleabite hypersensitivity, the actual differentiation is often impossible as well as unnecessary. It has been suggested that any dog with clinical signs related to fleas has a hypersensitivity reaction. Flea allergy dermatitis is discussed in Chapter 4.

Etiologic Factors

The common cat flea, *Ctenocephalides felis*, is the primary parasite for both dogs and cats. *Pulex irritans* (human fleas) are found in large numbers of dogs in the southeastern United States. Other fleas reported to infest both dogs and cats include *Echidnophaga*

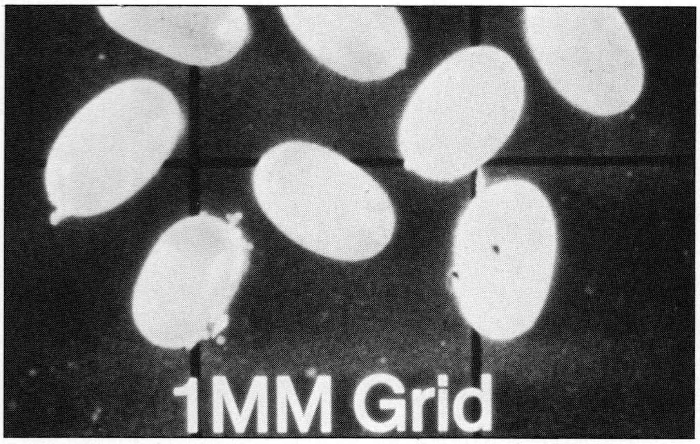

Figure 6-1. Flea eggs (Courtesy of VetKem).

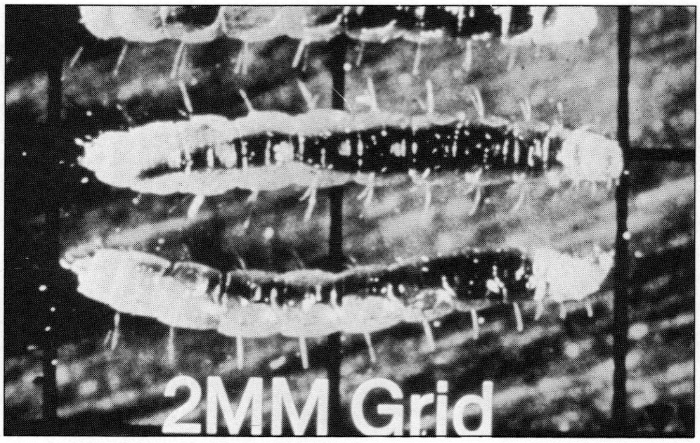

Figure 6-2. Flea larvae (Courtesy of VetKem).

gallinacea (chicken sticktight flea). Cats are infested by *Ceratophyllus* spp. (bird and hedgehog flea) and *Xenopsylla cheopis* (rat flea).

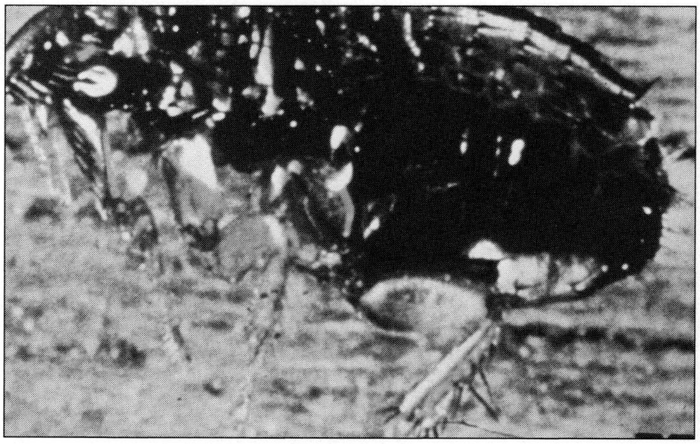

Figure 6-3. Adult flea (Courtesy of VetKem).

Incidence

Flea dermatitis is geographically dependent and is a major clinical dermatologic problem in areas with moderate temperatures, moderate to high humidity, and in areas where elevations are less than 5000 feet. In regions with a warm climate year-round, the flea problems are nonseasonal, whereas in regions with seasonal temperature and humidity extremes, flea infestation generally occurs only during the warmer months. A nonseasonal incidence of flea dermatitis will be observed in any climate, however, if there is an indoor infestation.

Pathogenesis

The flea saliva that is deposited in the skin contains histamine or histamine-like compounds. These chemicals initiate an inflammatory reaction at the bite site that is usually transient in duration. This is followed by an enzyme reaction in the skin which is mediated by the secretions of the flea. These enzymes dissolve parts of tissues and provide the flea access to the predilection site. A concurrent flea allergy dermatitis results if the dog or cat develops a hypersensitivity reaction to the enzymes which act as antigens (see Chapter 4).

Life Cycle

Knowledge of the flea life cycle is important for client education as well as for planning a protocol of treatment and control. The flea life cycle, including the egg, larva, pupa, and adult, can be completed within 3 weeks or can persist for 2 years. The eggs (Fig. 6-1) usually are laid in dust, cracks, or on damp ground. If they are laid on the host, they soon drop off. Approximately 3 to 18 eggs are laid at one time, with several hundred laid over a life span of 6 to 12 months. The incubation period varies greatly. With optimal conditions of 25°C (80°F) and 80% relative humidity the larvae can hatch in 2 to 4 days (Fig. 6-2). The larvae ingest organic material (such as fecal pellets) as well as the eggs of the tapeworm, *Dipylidium caninum*, and hide from light in such places as floor crevices and under carpets. They pass through three stages that can last from 9 to 200 days. A coccoon is spun during the third stage. The pupal stage can persist from 10 days to 1 year with low ambient temperature prolonging this stage. The adult flea (Fig. 6-3) must eventually feed on the host, but usually can survive 1 to 2 months separated from the host in the immediate environment. High humidity can prolong the survival time, while desiccation from low humidity can cause death of the adult in a few days.

History

There is no age, sex, or breed predilection for flea dermatitis. Pruritus and clinical signs vary from none to severe. The dog owner usually reports signs of biting over the dorsal caudal back and perineum with some alopecia and variable excoriation. Pruritus in cats is most common over the lumbar and dorsal neck areas. Fleas or flea excrement often are observed by the owner. Bathing and/or flea control (powders and sprays) usually give temporary relief. There is frequently a history of inadequate flea control, either on the animal or in the environment or both. Concurrent tapeworm infection is often reported.

Clinical Signs

The lesions of canine flea dermatitis commonly are distributed on the dorsal and caudal back, tail, and perineum (Plate III-1). Lesions also frequently occur on the flanks and caudal ventral abdomen (Plate III-2). In cats, the lumbosacral and dorsal neck area are most often associated with clinical signs (see Plate X-5). Flea excrement (dried blood), characterized by small, dark specks that look like dirt attached to the hair, often is observed with or without fleas. The specks streak out with a reddish color when placed on damp white paper.

The primary morphologic lesions most frequently observed in dogs are erythematous papules on the ventral abdomen (see Plate IV-3) and occasionally in the axillae. Diffuse erythema, scaling, hyperpigmentation, and hyperkeratosis are commonly seen on the caudal back, and perineal and tailhead regions. Alopecia varies from none to marked. The distribution may be localized or may be generalized. Severe flea dermatitis, accompanied by marked pruritus and excoriation, may have a generalized distribution. In dogs, superficial pyoderma may be observed concurrently, especially on the ventral abdomen.

In cats, miliary dermatitis, characterized by small adherent crusts on the dorsum (see Plate X-5), is common. Other lesions include focal excoriation and variable alopecia and inflammation.

Diagnosis

The history or observation of flea infestation (fleas or excrement) is the most important basis for a diagnosis of flea dermatitis. The distribution of clinical signs regionalized to the dorsum, perineum, and caudoventral abdomen are suggestive, especially if other possible causes for the clinical signs have been ruled out by skin scrapings, fungal cultures, diet testing, and intradermal allergy testing. The most definitive diagnostic test for flea dermatitis is a therapeutic trial with topical parasiticides for all animals, and the use of parasiticides in the environment (see Table 3-5). A 100% clinical response to the flea control program is considered diagnostic for flea dermatitis. If the response is less than complete, concurrent problems must be considered.

Management

The basic control program for flea dermatitis must include two objectives: breaking the flea life cycle in the environment, and minimizing infestation of all animals in the environment.

The control of fleas in the indoor environment or closed kennel can be accomplished by fumigation by a commercial exterminator; or with insect foggers, thoroughly vacuuming the carpets and immediately removing the vacuum cleaning bag from the premises, removing all debris and old bedding, and disinfecting hard surfaces using lindane, delnav, or bioresmethrin. It often is necessary to repeat these procedures several times at intervals of 2 to 4 weeks.

Methoprene is an insect growth regulator that prevents the fourth-instar larvae from completing metamorphosis into adults. The residual action of foggers containing methoprene is reported to be 75 days. Methoprene should be used in conjunction with a fast-acting insecticide that kills the adults. Methoprene may become unstable in ultraviolet light. A new product, fenoxycarb (Ecto-Gard® —Fermenta Animal Health) is reported to have all the characteristics of methoprene except it is stable in the presence of ultraviolet light.

Eliminating fleas in the outdoor environment is difficult. Periodic spraying of large areas of ground with lindane, chlordane, or malathion is helpful. If possible, animals should be kept away from outdoor areas favorable for flea propagation, such as grass and damp, overgrown areas. All debris and old bedding should be removed from areas that are frequented by the animal.

Minimizing the flea infestation on the animal involves continuous flea control on all animals in the environment (see Table 3-5). Treatment should include the use of flea powders or sprays twice weekly, flea collars or medallions, insecticidal dips repeated every 7 to 14 days, or systemic insecticides. No single universal control measure can be recommended. Flea sprays are less effective on long-haired dogs unless good penetration of the haircoat is achieved. The microencapsulated forms of sprays and foams provide a residual repellent effect on the hair. Flea powder on short-haired dogs and most cats is effective and safe. Powders are often difficult to apply adequately to long-haired animals because of the lack of penetration. Flea collars and medallions are not considered satisfactory in areas of moderate to heavy flea infestation or on the medium to large, long-haired dog. On small short-haired dogs or cats with minimal flea exposure, a flea collar often is satisfactory. Flea powder can be used concurrently with a collar to achieve better flea control in most animals without causing side effects. There have been few reported problems of flea collar dermatitis since the advent of the powder-impregnated collars; however, the owner should always be cautioned to look for signs of irritation for the first 2 weeks after a new collar is used.

Insecticidal dips often are the most satisfactory method of continuous flea control on the medium to large or long-haired dog. Most dips have a residual insecticidal effect for 7 to 14 days, but in hot climates evaporation may decrease the effective time. Dips are not practical for dogs that are frequently wet. When a dip is recommended to an owner, the veterinarian must give explicit instructions as to its use. The client may confuse the dip with an insecticidal shampoo and rinse it off. Frequently, the client is advised to bathe the dog or cat first and then apply the dip while the animal is still damp, letting it air-dry. Most insecticidal shampoos do not have a residual effect. Therefore, they should not be relied upon for continuous flea control. One insecticidal shampoo containing resmethrin, which can be used on both dogs and cats, is reported to have a 5- to 7-day residual effect (see Table 3-5).

Systemic organophosphate parasiticides, such as cythioate (Proban® —Haver) and fenthion (Pro-Spot® —Haver), can be used in dogs. Systemic insecticides are most effective when the dog is in a controlled indoor environment with no or very limited outside exposure. In this situation, the indoor environment can be kept relatively or completely free of flea infestation. The systemic insecticides should not be used as the definitive flea control if the dog is manifesting signs of flea allergy dermatitis because the flea is not killed until it penetrates the skin and contacts the agent in the blood. It can be used concurrently with topical parasiticides that are not anticholinesterase inhibitors, such as pyrethrins and pyrethroids.

A potential problem of insecticides administered orally, or sprays and dips applied topically, is systemic absorption and storage of the insecticide in the body, which can lead to chronic toxicity although this is seldom reported.

Development of resistance to insecticides is a major problem in endemic flea areas, with the most resistance observed to the carbamates. If there is a poor response to the routine control program, change types of insecticides, methods of application, or both.

All secondary or concurrent problems should be treated at the same time as the primary flea infestation. Often, flea control is sufficient to control pruritus; however, it is common to administer corticosteroids for 5 to 10 days while the flea control program is implemented to prevent continued self-trauma and to reduce inflammation. Antibiotics for a minimum of 10 to 14 days also are indicated when secondary superficial pyoderma is present.

SARCOPTIC MANGE

Sarcoptic mange, or canine scabies, is a commonly encountered parasitic disease of dogs caused by the mite *Sarcoptes scabiei* var. *canis*. It transiently infests humans, causing pruritic, papular dermatitis.

Pathogenesis

The transmission of sarcoptid mites can occur by direct or indirect contact with fomites or such objects as grooming instruments. The mites are more active and more likely to infest other animals at higher ambient temperatures. Other factors that favor mite infestation include a long, dirty haircoat and malnutrition. There is often a higher rate of recovery from mite infestation in younger dogs than older ones. It is postulated that the hypersensitivity reaction keeps the mite population lower, and at the same time is responsible for the generalized lesions in adult dogs.

The incubation period is variable, usually 4 to 6 weeks. Visible lesions can appear within 2 weeks. Pruritus associated with infestation may be caused by a combination of factors, including mechanical irritation by the mite, toxic materials produced by the mite, and secretion of allergenic substances to which the host becomes sensitized.

Life Cycle

The adult sarcoptic mite (Fig. 6-4A) lives for 3 to 4 weeks in the skin. Copulation occurs in the stratum corneum. The eggs (Fig. 6-4A) hatch within 3 to 10 days into six-legged mobile larvae. Eight-legged nymphs represent the third stage of life before becoming adult mites. The entire life cycle, which takes place on the host, is 17 to 21 days with a longer survival time when very humid.

History

Sarcoptic mange is characterized by marked pruritus and localized or generalized excoriation. There is no breed or sex predisposition. The distribution of lesions is often around the elbows and on the pinnal margins. Infestation can occur at any age, although the highest incidence is in the young dog. There often is a history of poor response to antiinflammatory doses (0.5 to 1 mg/kg/day) of short-acting corticosteroids. There may be a history of recent exposure to other pruritic dogs, boarding, or recent acquisition from a pet store. Human contagion is common, and the owner may report a pruritic, papular skin eruption that occurred at the same time as the dog's clinical signs.

Clinical Signs

Initially, the distribution of lesions is usually on the thin-haired areas, including ear margins and elbows

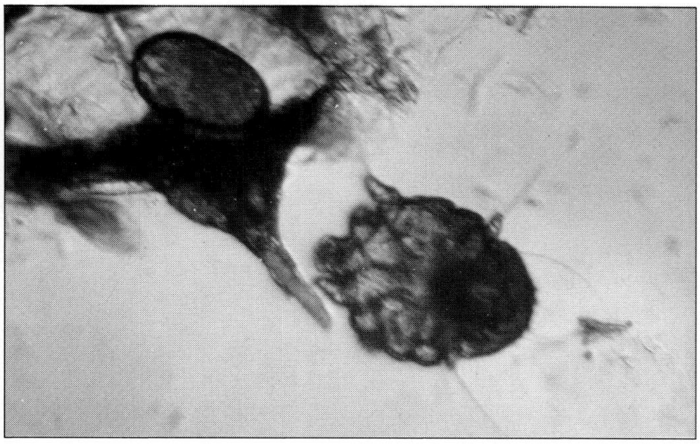

A

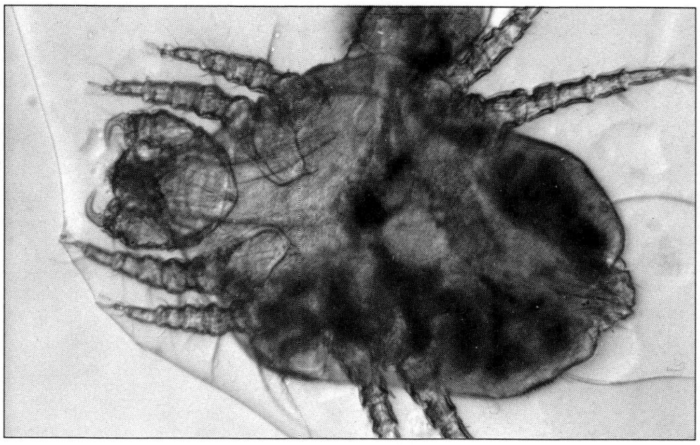

B

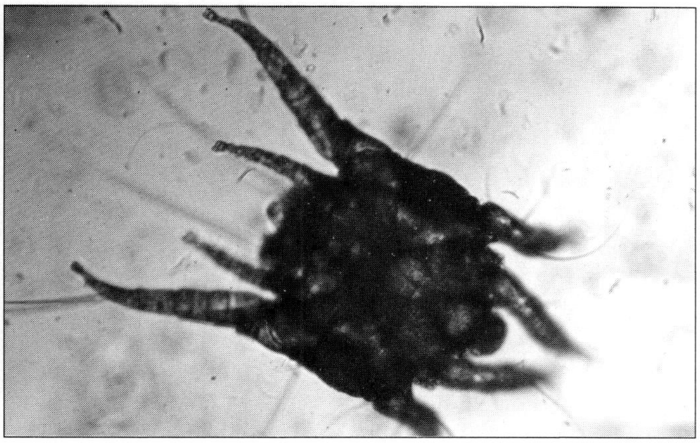

C

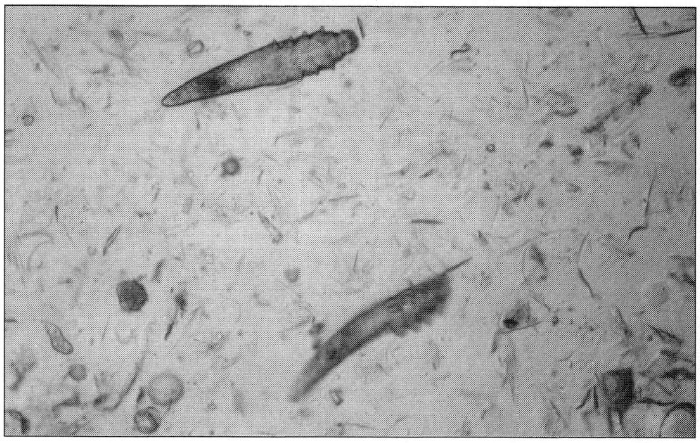

D

(Plate III-3). A predominantly ventral distribution or entire truncal distribution of lesions may be observed. Primary lesions include erythematous papules or pustules. The most common secondary and miscellaneous lesions are crusts, excoriation, erythema, and alopecia. Secondary superficial bacterial infection and secondary keratinization disorders (seborrheic dermatitis) are common. Although the clinical signs are suggestive, a definitive diagnosis of sarcoptic mange requires additional screening or definitive diagnostic tests.

Diagnosis

A history of an intense pruritus unresponsive to low-dose corticosteroids is suggestive as are crusts and excoriations on the ear margins and elbows. Concurrent pruritic papular dermatitis in members of the family is also supportive. A relatively high incidence of peripheral eosinophilia is reported. Mites are occasionally observed during routine fecal examination.

Skin scrapings are the most widely used screening and definitive diagnostic tests, and a positive scraping for adults, nymphs, larvae, or eggs (Fig. 6-4A) is diagnostic.

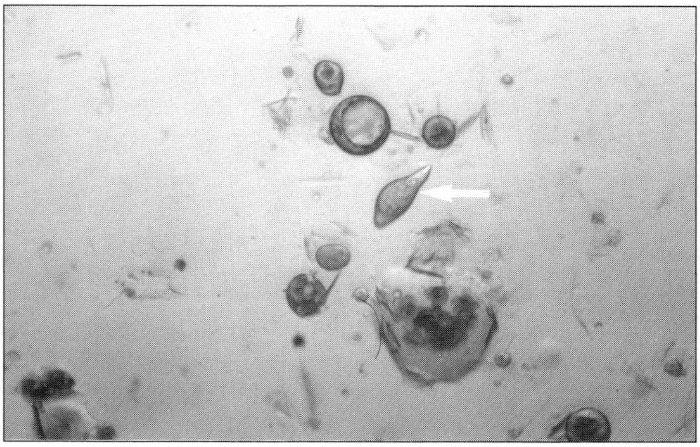

E

Figure 6-4. Ectoparasites. **A**, *Sarcoptes scabiei* adult and egg; **B**, *Cheyletiella yasguri* (courtesy of G.S. Kedan); **C**, *Otodectes cynotis*; **D**, *Demodex canis* adults; **E**, *Demodex canis* egg in scraping (arrow); **F**, trombiculid mite (courtesy of W.H. Miller, Jr., New York State College of Veterinary Medicine, Cornell University); **G**, unengorged and engorged female *Rhipicephalus* ticks (reprinted from Lewis T: Ticks and associated diseases. *Pet Focus* 1:21-23, 1989, with permission); **H**, *Pelodera* larva evident on skin scraping; **I**, cutaneous dirofilariasis—microscopic section from a dog with dirofilariasis. Note microfilaria in capillary (*arrow*).

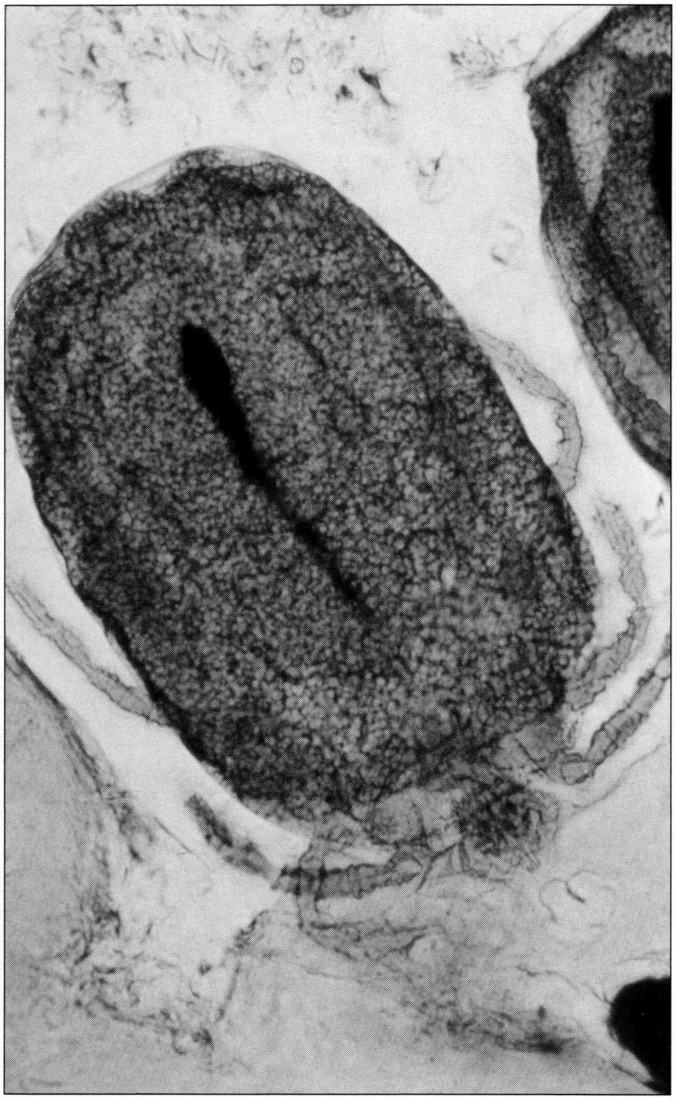

F

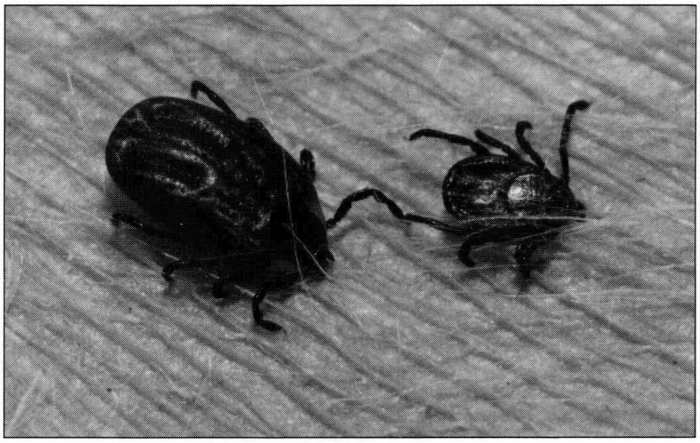

G

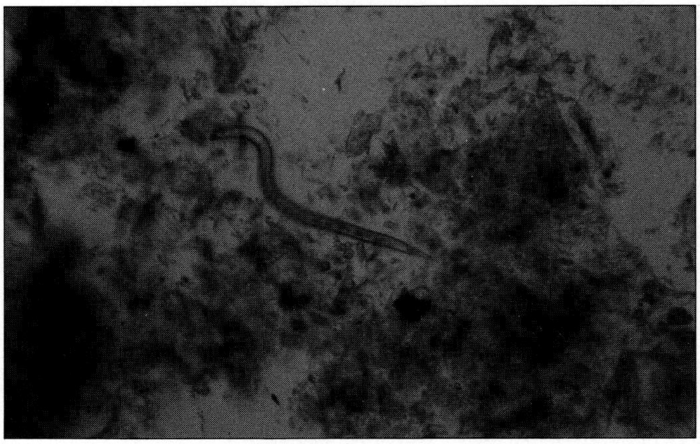

H

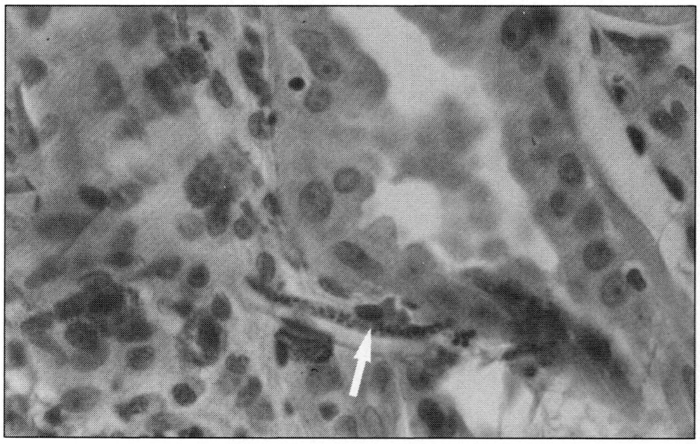

I

Fecal material is also suggestive. Multiple negative scrapings, however, do not rule out sarcoptic mange.

Two other methods described for identifying mites are the plastic box method and the centrifuge flotation method. The plastic box method involves placing a crust in a plastic box or petri dish and allowing it to set at room temperature for 12 hours. Close examination using a 4× magnifying glass may reveal mites on the floor of the dish. In the centrifuge flotation method, a large amount of material from scrapings is placed in a small tube or beaker. Then, 10% potassium hydroxide (KOH) is added, and the mixture is stirred and heated gently. This mixture is then added to a saturated sugar solution and centrifuged. A drop of the surface solution is examined for mites and eggs. The plastic box and the centrifuge flotation methods should be reserved for those cases in which skin scrapings are negative. Occasionally, cross-sections of mites will be observed in cutaneous biopsies.

Treatment

The environment should be thoroughly cleaned. The infested animal(s) should be isolated. Before specific treatment is started, long-haired dogs should be clipped. After the eyes are protected with a bland ophthalmic ointment, the dogs should be bathed with an antiseborrheic shampoo, such as tar and sulfur, to help remove the surface scale and crusts. While the dog is still wet, a miticidal dip is applied, being careful to saturate all of the surface of the body, including the pinnae and face.

Amitraz (Mitaban® —Upjohn) used at 0.025% concentration every 2 weeks for three treatments is effective and safe, although treatment for sarcoptic mange is an extra-label use. Organophosphates have been routinely used on adult animals. Sulfurated lime is recommended for dogs less than 3 months old or for the debilitated dog (see Table 3-5). If there is poor response after three or four insecticide dips, a different one should be tried because resistance to insecticides can occur.

Ivermectin is very effective although it is not approved for use in dogs as a scabicide. Ivermectin is administered orally or subcutaneously at a rate of 0.2 to 0.4 mg/kg every 14 days for two treatments. Ivermectin should not be administered to collies or collie mix breeds. The dog must be heartworm-negative before treating for sarcoptic mange with ivermectin.

All asymptomatic dogs on the premises should be given one prophylactic dip with amitraz, two to three prophylactic dips with organophosphates, or one dose of ivermectin to prevent contagion. Corticosteroids (see Table 3-9) can be used concurrently with parasiticides to help alleviate pruritus and self-trauma. They should be discontinued as soon as possible because immunosuppression can delay clinical response. Tranquilizers can be used to help control pruritus because of their sedative effect, but they usually are much less effective. Secondary pyoderma should be treated concurrently with antibiotics (see Table 3-11).

Prognosis

The prognosis for sarcoptic mange is good. Occasionally a dog will not respond as expected; however, sarcoptic mange should be considered a curable disease with minimal permanent side effects. Reinfection can occur if there is reexposure to the mites.

NOTOEDRIC MANGE

Notoedric mange, or feline scabies, is an uncommon parasitic disease of cats caused by *Notedres cati*, a sarcoptiform mite. It can also affect rabbits, dogs, and humans.

History

Notoedric mange is characterized by intense pruritus about the head and neck. There is often a history of an epidemic amongst a litter of young kittens. Concurrent human contagion may be reported. There may be a poor response to low-dose corticosteroids.

Clinical Signs

Lesions often appear on the ear margins, and then spread to the rest of the ear, face, and neck (Plate III-4). The feet and perineum also may become involved. The lesions consist of crust, scales, erythema, excoriation, alopecia, and in chronic disease, lichenification. In kittens the abdomen may be more severely involved than the head.

Diagnosis

A history of intense pruritus of the head and neck is suggestive, as are crusts and excoriation on the ear margins, face, and neck.

Before treatment, numerous mites usually are observed on skin scraping. A good clinical response to a therapeutic trial with a parasiticide is also considered diagnostic.

Treatment

Infested animals should be isolated and the contaminated environment thoroughly cleaned. The cats should be clipped and crusts and debris removed by gentle washing. A weekly sulfurated lime solution (2 to 3%) should be applied as a total body dip (see Table 3-5). This should be continued until 2 weeks beyond clinical remission, usually 6 to 8 weeks. Concurrent corticosteroids and antibiotics may be indicated to prevent self-trauma and secondary infection. Ivermectin at a dose of 0.3 to 0.4 mg/kg is reported to be safe and effective although it is not approved for use in cats in the United States. All other animals in the environment should be dipped at least twice at weekly intervals.

CHEYLETIELLOSIS

Cheyletiella-induced mange, or cheyletiellosis, is caused by *Cheyletiella yasguri* in dogs and by *C. blakei* in cats.

Pathogenesis

Cheyletiella mites are transmitted by direct contact. Young puppies and kittens, 2 to 8 weeks old, usually have the largest number of mites. Adult dogs and cats normally have a small number of mites even if there is direct contact with more heavily infested young animals, suggesting that an immune mechanism may be involved. The mites do not burrow into the skin, but live in the keratin layer of epidermis and are not associated with hair follicles. The mites move rapidly in pseudotunnels in epidermal debris. They periodically attach firmly to the epidermis, pierce the skin, and become engorged with a clear colorless fluid.

Life Cycle

The entire life cycle of the mite is spent on the host. Ova are laid and stick to the hair or surface debris. The incubation period is approximately 4 days, and the larval stage is approximately 7 days, after which there are two nymphal stages each lasting 4 to 5 days. The adult (Fig. 6-4B) has a short life of approximately 14 days. The larvae, nymphs, and adult males die within 48 hours after leaving the host. It has been reported that the adult females can live up to 10 days separated from the host if refrigerated; therefore, the infestation may exist longer in cooler climates than in warmer ones.

History

Mild to marked dandruff on the dorsum of a puppy or kitten with no irritation and variable pruritus is often reported. Occasionally, there will be a report of family members developing a pruritic rash shortly after obtaining the dog or cat. Asymptomatic carrier animals may be associated with human contagion. A drug history of clinical response to flea powders, shampoos, sprays, or dips is often elicited.

Clinical Signs

Puppies usually have a moderate to marked dandruff that starts over the caudal back and then progresses anteriorly; however, dandruff may only be observed about the dorsal neck area. There is a notable absence of any primary morphologic lesions. Scales are often the only secondary lesions observed. Close examination may reveal "walking dandruff," especially if the hair is clipped. Some dogs are asymptomatic. Cats may have dandruff similar to that seen in puppies (Plate III-5), a miliary dermatitic eruption of crusts and papules, or they may be asymptomatic carriers.

Diagnosis

Several techniques are used to identify *Cheyletiella* mites. The use of a strip of clear acetate tape pressed onto the hair in multiple sites picking up scale and hair is often rewarding. The tape is placed on a microscope slide and examined. Collecting debris with a flea comb and placing in mineral oil before microscopic examination is also recommended.

A positive skin scraping of any stage of the mite life cycle is diagnostic (Fig. 6-4B). In long-haired animals, it is helpful to clip the hair in the area to be scraped.

The adult *Cheyletiella* mite is identified by the hooks of the accessory mouthparts and a typical saddle-shaped body (Fig. 6-4B). *C. yasguri* is approximately twice the size of *Sarcoptes scabiei*. Occasionally, mites and/or eggs are found in fecal flotations.

Treatment

Most parasiticides are effective in controlling cheyletiellosis (see Table 3-5). Pyrethrins, carbamates, organophosphates (dog only), and sulfurated lime are routinely used in the form of dusts, sprays, or dips. Treatment must be continued for several weeks to eliminate the infection. Ivermectin at a dosage of 0.2 to 0.4 mg/kg repeated once in 2 weeks has been reported to be effective and safe. Ivermectin is not approved for this use in dogs or cats in the United States or Canada.

All animals on the premises must be treated, whether symptomatic or not. The premises should be kept clean and disinfected, especially the kennels or catteries. All new animals should be dusted, sprayed, or dipped before exposure to other animals.

Prognosis

The prognosis for cheyletiellosis is good; however, reinfestation can occur whenever there is direct contact with mites.

OTODECTIC MANGE

Otodectiasis, or otodectic mange, one of the most commonly encountered parasitic diseases of dogs and cats, is caused by *Otodectes cynotis*, a psoroptid ear mite.

Pathogenesis

Otodectes cynotis is transmitted by direct contact. Pruritus associated with the infestation may be caused by a combination of factors, including mechanical irritation by the mite, toxic materials produced by the mite, and the secretion of allergenic substances to which the host becomes sensitized. The mites live on the surface of the skin and feed on epidermal debris. There is evidence that Type 1 and Type 3 hypersensitivity reactions may play a role in the pathogenesis of ear mite infestations.

Acute ear mite infestations are associated with hyperplasia of the ceruminous glands and a mild mononuclear cell infiltrate in the external auditory canal. In chronic otodectic otitis, the gross canal change is a crusted layer formed from dried sebum, ceruminous secretions, and exfoliated epithelium. Microscopic findings include parakeratotic and hyperplastic epithelium, squamous metaplasia of duct epithelium, hair follicle atrophy, and increased inflammatory infiltrate. Dilated venules and edema of subcutaneous tissue also are common.

Life Cycle

The adult *O. cynotis* can live for 2 months, laying eggs on the ceruminous substrate of the ear canal or skin. Larvae are hatched after 4 days of incubation. The larvae feed for 3 to 10 days, rest 1 day, and then hatch to protonymphs. After feeding for 3 to 10 days and resting for another day, the protonymph molts to a deutonymph. After another feeding and resting cycle, a male attaches to the deutonymph. If a female adult is hatched, copulation takes place immediately. The entire life cycle takes about 3 weeks.

History

Pruritus and head shaking are the most common clinical signs noted by the owner, or the primary complaint may be self-trauma about the head and neck. A dark waxy discharge is often observed at the external orifice of the ear canal. Dogs frequently are more sensitive to ear mite infestations than are cats. The infestation may be associated with generalized multifocal dermatitis.

Clinical Signs

Otoscopic examination of the external ear canal reveals varying amounts of dark wax, usually with small white ear mites on the surface of the debris. The medial aspects of the pinnae may be normal, erythematous, or excoriated. Excoriation posterior to the base of the ear is common. The infestation and secondary trauma may be unilateral or bilateral. There is commonly a secondary bacterial or yeast infection, especially in dogs. Exudation is variable. Focal alopecic, erythemic, and excoriated lesions may be observed on the head, neck, and lower back. Some dogs and many cats may be asymptomatic carriers of ear mites.

Diagnosis

The most common way to diagnose otodectic mange is by visualizing the mites on otoscopic examination. Ear swabs and direct microscopic examination of the ear debris is sometimes necessary. Occasionally, it is necessary to flush the ears and collect and examine the debris. Scrapings of the lesions on the head, neck, or trunk may reveal *O. cynotis* mites or eggs (Fig. 6-4C). A therapeutic trial with otic miticides and flea parasiticides (see Table 3-5) resulting in 100% clinical response is suggestive of primary otodectic mange.

Treatment

The ear canals should be flushed and all wax and debris removed. An acaricidal preparation should be used either daily or every other day for a minimum of 2 weeks. Effective miticides include pyrethrins, rotenone, thiabendazole, and carbaryl. Ivermectin at a single dose of 0.2 to 0.4 mg/kg has been safe and effective although ivermectin is not approved for this usage in dogs and cats in the United States and Canada. Most acaricidal otic preparations incorporate antibiotics, antifungals, corticosteroids, and/or ceruminolytic agents to relieve acute inflammation and infection. Concurrent whole body treatment with a parasiticide must be done weekly. All animals in the environment must be treated, both locally (in the ears) and the whole body.

CANINE DEMODECTIC MANGE

Canine demodectic mange (demodicosis, red mange, follicular mange) is caused by the follicular mite, *Demodex canis*.

Pathogenesis

The pathogenesis of demodicosis is still not completely understood. *D. canis* is a normal inhabitant of the skin. A large percentage (estimates vary from 30 to 80%) of the normal canine population are asymptomatic carriers of the mites; there is an apparent genetic predisposition in dogs. Puppies acquire the infection during the first 72 hours of life while nursing the dam. If the puppies are delivered by cesarean section and not allowed to nurse, they will be free of demodectic mites.

Immunologic factors play a role in demodicosis. A serum factor is present that causes a suppression of T lymphocytes as measured by in vitro blastogenesis. There is some question as to whether this factor originates from the demodectic mites or concurrent bacterial infection. Antilymphocyte serum can precipitate the onset of demodicosis as can chronic corticosteroid administration. A skin graft of the infected skin adjacent to normal skin on a puppy can produce localized disease. A generalized form is not observed. A spontaneous clinical remission often is observed in animals less than 1 year of age.

The mites apparently feed on the sebum in the hair follicles. Clinical disease is observed when the demodectic mites reproduce in sufficient numbers to cause alopecia. A mild microscopic follicular and perifollicular inflammatory response may be observed in the unruptured hair follicle. The specific factors causing this reaction have not been identified. If the hair follicle ruptures, there is a more severe intrafollicular and perifollicular inflammatory response most likely caused by the mites or their metabolic products.

Life Cycle

The life cycle of *D. canis* is not completely understood. The mite spends the entire life cycle on the host. They are ingested during the neonatal period (within 72 hours of birth) and migrate from the stomach to the regional lymph nodes, probably by way of the lymphatics. In 2 to 3 months the mites reach the hair follicles. The mites live in the hair follicles and are occasionally found in sebaceous glands and apocrine sweat glands.

The stages of mites observed in the hair follicles include fusiform eggs, six-legged larvae, eight-legged protonymphs and deutonymphs, and eight-legged adults.

History

There appears to be an age predilection between 3 and 12 months for dogs; however, the mature dog (1 to 15 years) can be clinically infected, often in association with chronic pyoderma. A breed predilection also exists in short-haired breeds, including the dachshund, Doberman pinscher, beagle, Boston terrier, dalmatian, Great Dane, English bulldog, Chihuahua, boxer, Chinese shar pei, pug, and pointer. Other breeds at risk include the Old English sheepdog, collie, Afghan hound, German shepherd, and cocker spaniel. Demodicosis can be observed in any breed.

The distribution of lesions in the young animal is often localized to the head and feet. The owner usually observes focal, nonpruritic alopecic areas which may regress spontaneously without treatment. At times there is a history of focal lesions that progress to a more generalized distribution. There may be pruritus associated with superficial or deep pyoderma. The older dog is often examined for chronic interdigital pyoderma, which may be responsive to antibiotics and recurrent, or only partially responsive to antibiotics. Many of the generalized alopecic dogs with no secondary pyoderma have a drug history of poor response to hormonal therapy, such as L-thyroxine. It is common to see an exacerbation of clinical signs after corticosteroid therapy. A higher incidence of relapse of clinical signs is associated with estrus. Demodicosis is not a contagious disease among healthy puppies.

Clinical Signs

Two clinical forms of demodicosis are recognized. The localized or squamous form is characterized by a few (one to six) small, circumscribed erythematous or hyperpigmented, scaly, nonpruritic, alopecic macules or patches, usually located periorbitally, facially, or on the forelegs. Inflammation varies from none to moderate, and there may be an occasional papule or pustule. Alopecia varies from partial to complete.

The generalized form is characterized by large, multifocal areas of alopecia, erythema, hyperpigmentation, edema, and scaling (Plates III-6 and III-7). At times there is only alopecia and scaling without signs of acute inflammation. Superficial or deep secondary pyoderma is common. The ventral chin, face, and feet are the usual sites for the pyoderma. Peripheral lymphadenomegaly is common. Occasionally a young dog is examined for signs of septicemia, including fever and shock. Demodectic mites also have been found in the ear canals of dogs with otitis externa.

Diagnosis

Demodectic mange is often suspected on the basis of a history of focal, nonpruritic, alopecic areas on the face and forelimbs. Chronic pyoderma of the feet or ventral chin, which is recurrent or only partially responsive to antibiotics, also is suggestive. Skin scraping is the screening and definitive diagnostic test. The area to be scraped should first be squeezed to force the mites out of the hair follicles. The scraping should be done on a small focal area and should be deep enough to draw a small amount of blood. Any or all stages of the demodectic mites may be observed (Figs. 6-4D, 6-4E). If several lesions are present on physical examination, positive scrapings from multiple sites are diagnostic. If only one or two mites are found in scrapings from multiple areas, a diagnosis of active demodicosis must be questioned and scrapings should be repeated in 1 to 2 weeks.

The results of clinical laboratory testing, including complete blood counts and biochemical testing, usually are normal. If severe active pyoderma is present, there may be mild leukocytosis, elevated total protein, and elevated globulins. Some workers report a high degree of correlation between demodicosis and hypothyroidism based on baseline triiodothyronine (T_3) and thyroxine (T_4) serum levels or thyroid-stimulating hormone (TSH) stimulation tests. A direct cause-and-effect relationship has not been verified. These values usually return to normal after resolution of the demodicosis.

Demodicosis also can be diagnosed by means of a routine cutaneous biopsy. If demodectic mites have not been found on scrapings and are reported in biopsies, scrapings should be repeated. The pathologic findings include dilated hair follicles filled with keratin and mites. The degree of inflammation associated with dilated hair follicles varies from none to rupture of the follicle and total destruction of the individual pilosebaceous unit.

Treatment

Many young animals with either localized or generalized demodicosis have a spontaneous remission at maturity. Therefore, some consideration must be given to supportive treatment only until the animal is approximately 1 year old. Local application of benzoyl peroxide or rotenone may have some beneficial effect. If pyoderma is present, antibiotics should be used. Antiseborrheic shampoos to remove the scale are indicated (see Table 3-6). None of the aforementioned supportive therapy will prevent the localized type from progressing to generalized demodectic mange.

Amitraz (Mitaban® —Upjohn) at a 0.025% dilution is the treatment of choice for generalized demodicosis (see Table 3-2). The time required to see a good response to amitraz varies from 6 weeks to 6 months. A small percentage of animals with generalized demodicosis will never have a clinical cure. The manufacturer's recommended frequency of treatment is once every 2 weeks; however, in the healthy animal without an active pyoderma, the drug has been used safely at weekly intervals with a faster clinical response. If there is a poor response to the initial weekly or biweekly protocol, the concentration of amitraz has been doubled with better response observed.

It is recommended to clip the entire haircoat before the first dipping. All amitraz dips should be preceded with a benzoyl peroxide or tar and sulfur bath. The diluted amitraz must be used immediately because it is very unstable and deteriorates rapidly by oxidation and exposure to ultraviolet light.

The most common side effect of amitraz treatment is a transient sedation lasting up to 72 hours. A small number of dogs will have transient pruritus. Other reported side effects include hypothermia, elevated blood glucose, seizures, and acute death. Dry skin and flaking are minor problems which can be controlled with the addition of 1 or 2 capfuls of a bath oil rinse to the amitraz solution. Amitraz in mineral oil or propylene glycol, in a 1:15 to 1:60 dilution, has been used on localized areas, either on dogs with a few residual lesions after the series of general dips or on dogs with large lesions associated with the localized form of demodicosis. The solution is used daily or on alternate days.

All concurrent problems must be treated. An active pyoderma should be treated aggressively with bactericidal antibiotics (see Table 3-11) and topical antibacterial shampoos, such as benzoyl peroxide or tar and sulfur (see Table 3-6). If there are large areas of damaged skin as a result of pyoderma or self-trauma, it may be indicated to treat the concurrent problems initially, allowing the lesions to dry before starting the amitraz dips to avoid excessive absorption and toxicity. Tranquilizers and/or antihistamines, such as hydroxyzine HCl (see Table 3-15), can be used to minimize pruritus associated with the pyoderma. Corticosteroids should not be used.

Ovariohysterectomy is recommended for two reasons. First, there is a potential for a higher incidence of relapse of clinical signs associated with estrus. Second, there is a hereditary predisposition associated with demodicosis.

The course of the disease should be monitored by scraping the dog every 2 to 4 weeks and recording the ratio of the mature to the immature mites. If the disease is responding to treatment, there will be a gradual increase in the ratio of mature to immature and dead to live mites. Treatment should be continued until there are multiple negative scrapings 2 to 3 weeks apart. Vitamin E has been recommended as adjuvant therapy at doses from 100 IU to 400 IU at least four times daily but reported effectiveness has been variable.

Prognosis

It is estimated that 60 to 65% of the dogs treated with amitraz will have a clinical cure for at least one year. Many of the dogs that still have scrapings positive for mites will look nearly normal or have either partial or near total regrowth of hair in problem areas or they may be asymptomatic. Dogs that have scrapes that are chronically positive for mites but are showing minimal clinical signs are often maintained with amitraz dips every 3 to 4 weeks.

FELINE DEMODECTIC MANGE

Feline demodectic mange (demodicosis) is a rare disease caused in most cases by *Demodex cati*; another species, as yet unnamed, also has been reported. The pathogenesis and life cycle of *D. cati* are assumed to be similar to that of *D. canis*, with the entire life cycle spent on the host. Immunosuppression has been suspected but there is no experimental evidence to support this theory. Generalized demodicosis has been associated with diabetes mellitus, respiratory infection, feline immunodeficiency virus infection, and feline leukemia virus infection.

History

There is no sex predilection. Siamese and Burmese cats may have a higher incidence than other breeds. Young cats are more commonly affected. The initial complaint is usually of focal alopecia with variable pruritus; concurrent systemic disease also may be present.

Clinical Signs

Clinical signs associated with *D. cati* may be localized or generalized. The localized form is characterized by single or multiple areas of alopecia and erythema. Scaling, crusting, papules, and secondary pyoderma are variable. The localized form usually affects the head, ears, and neck. The generalized form is characterized by similar lesions that are not localized to the head and neck. Ceruminous otitis also may be present.

The clinical signs of the new species of *Demodex* are reported to be relatively mild, with pruritus, erythema, broken hairs, and alopecia with a predilection for the hindlimbs, flank, and ventral abdomen.

Diagnosis

Skin scraping is the definitive diagnostic test. The area to be scraped should first be squeezed, and multiple scrapes should be done. *D. cati* is found in the follicles while the new species has been recovered from the stratum corneum. *D. cati* is morphologically similar to *D. canis*. The new species of *Demodex* in cats is similar to *D. criceti* of hamsters, with a broad, blunted abdomen. In cases of ceruminous otitis, the contents of the ear canal should be removed with an ear swab and examined microscopically for mites (see Figs. 6-4D, 6-4E). Demodectic mites may be seen in histopathologic specimens with folliculitis, perifolliculitis, and superficial perivascular dermatitis observed. A workup to rule out systemic diseases should be done.

Treatment

As in dogs, many young cats with the localized form have spontaneous remission. Rotenone ointment (Goodwinol® —Goodwinol Products) can be used daily on localized lesions. Other successful treatments include 2.0% lime sulfur dips and carbaryl shampoos. Amitraz (250 ppm) has been used in cats with good response, although it is not approved for use in cats in the United States. In young kittens, amitraz may be associated with anorexia, depression, and diarrhea.

TROMBICULIASIS

Canine and feline trombiculiasis is caused by the third-stage larvae of the North American chigger, *Eutrombicula alfreddugesi*.

Pathogenesis

Lesions follow attachment of the parasitic larvae to the skin. The mite injects saliva containing proteolytic enzymes, which hydrolyze the stratum corneum and allow the tissue fluids to be sucked up by the mite. The larvae stay attached for several hours and then drop off. Pruritus occurs within a few hours of the bite and may persist for several days. A hypersensitivity reaction to the components of the mite saliva is suspected.

Life Cycle

Adult chiggers are free-living or prey on other arthropods. The eggs are laid in the moist ground. The six-legged orange larvae hatch and usually parasitize such hosts as snakes, lizards, wild rodents, or birds, but can parasitize dogs, cats, or humans when there is direct contact with larvae-infected foliage in fields or forests. The larvae drop to the ground and develop into nymphs. The free-living adults live on decaying vegetable material. The life cycle is completed in 50 to 70 days; however, adult females can survive more than 1 year.

History and Clinical Signs

Pruritus is the most common signs. Pinhead-sized, orange-red mites may be observed tightly adhered to the skin. Local irritation is characterized by erythematous papules, scaling, and alopecia. The most common distribution is on the head, neck, axillary regions, and feet; however, lesions of trombiculiasis can be generalized.

Diagnosis

A history of a dog or cat having been exposed to an endemic chigger area lends support to the diagnosis. The definitive diagnostic test is identification of the six-legged larvae on skin scrapings (Fig. 6-4F). A good response to a therapeutic trial with a parasiticidal shampoo or dip (see Table 3-5) is highly suggestive if the history and clinical signs are consistent with trombiculiasis.

Treatment

If there is much scaling or crusting, a bath with an antiseborrheic shampoo should be given followed by a parasiticidal dip (see Table 3-5). In endemic areas, dips should be repeated every 10 to 14 days.

TICK INFESTATIONS

Based on taxonomic classifications, ticks are generally divided into two classes: hard and soft ticks.

HARD TICKS (IXODID)

The majority of ticks that cause clinical dermatologic problems in dogs are ixodid or hard ticks. Ixodid tick infestations are seldom reported in cats. Several species are capable of infesting dogs and cats, including *Rhipicephalus sanguineus* (brown dog tick), *Dermacentor andersoni* (Rocky Mountain wood tick), *D. variabilis* (American dog tick), *Amblyomma maculatum* (Gulf Coast tick), and *A. americanum* (Lone Star tick).

Incidence

The incidence of tick infestations is dependent on many factors, including environmental temperature, moisture, and availability of the hosts.

Pathogenesis

The tick attaches itself to the host, buries its mouthparts deeply into the tissues of the host to feed, and remains attached until it is engorged with blood. An inflammatory reaction occurs at the site of penetration. Crusting at the penetration site often follows removal of the tick. A tick bite hypersensitivity is occasionally reported (see Chapter 4).

Life Cycle and Diseases Transmitted

Rhipicephalus sanguineus is a three-host tick but can complete its life cycle on one animal as a host. After engorgement, the tick drops off the host and molts on the ground. Because of its low moisture requirement, it often is found in kennels and houses.

The stages of the life cycle of ticks are listed in Table 6-1. Eggs are laid in sheltered spots, such as under stones and in crevices of walls. The newly hatched larvae or seed ticks climb onto grass and shrubs and then attach to a host. *R. sanguineus* can transmit several viral, rickettsial, protozoan, and bacterial diseases (Table 6-2), and may cause tick paralysis.

TABLE 6-1

Life Cycles of Ticks

Tick	*Stage*	*Activity*	*Duration*
Rhipicephalus sanguineus	Adult female	Engorge: lays 2000–3000 eggs	6–21 days
	Adult male	Engorge	6 days to months
	Adults	Nonengorge	Survive up to 19 months
	Eggs	Hatch	17–30 days or longer
	Larvae	Engorge	2–6 days
		Molt	5–23 days
		Nonengorge	Survive up to 6 months
	Nymphs	Engorge	4–9 days
		Molt	11–73 days
		Nonengorge	Survive up to 6 months
Dermacentor spp.	Adult female	Engorge: lays 4000–6000 eggs	8–14 days
	Eggs	Hatch	15–57 days
	Larvae	Engorge	3–14 days
		Molt	6–87 days
	Nymphs	Engorge	3–9 days
		Molt	21 days
Ixodes dammini/I. pacificus	Adult female	Engorge: lays thousands of eggs	Approximately 30 days
	Eggs	Hatch	2–36 weeks
	Larvae	Engorge	2–6 days
		Molt	4–51 weeks
	Nymphs	Engorge	3–7 days
		Molt	8–28 weeks
Otobius megnini	Adult female	Lays 500–600 eggs	
	Adult	Nonparasitic (do not feed)	
	Eggs	Hatch	
	Larvae	Engorge	10 days to 8 weeks 5–10 days after attaching to external ear canal
		Nonengorge	Survive for 2–4 months
	Nymphs	Engorge	1–7 months in ear
		Molt	Few days after dropping off host

Dermacentor andersoni and *D. variabilis* are three-host ticks. The stages and duration of the life cycle are listed in Table 6-1. The larvae and nymphs can attach to most small mammals, especially rodents. The unfed adults can live for 3 years, but engorged adults only live for a few weeks. *D. variabilis* is more sensitive to dryness but is resistant to cold. Diseases transmitted by *Dermacentor* spp. are listed in Table 6-1. They also can cause tick paralysis.

Amblyomma spp. have similar life cycles to those of the other ixodid ticks (Table 6-1). Diseases transmitted by these ticks are listed in Table 6-2.

History

No age, breed, or sex predilection is found for ixodid tick infestation. The animal's exposure to tick-infested vegetation or to rodents acting as hosts of tick larvae or nymphs are the major factors promoting infestation. During routine grooming or examination, ticks usually are observed on the dorsum, especially about the ears, head and neck, or in the feet; however, they can be found on any part of the body. Pruritus usually is minimal and localized to the site of the tick attachment.

Clinical Signs

Ticks in various stages of the life cycle can be observed attached to the skin (Plate III-8). Focal erythema of the skin adjacent to the attached tick is commonly seen. After the tick is removed, crusting and the development of a firm cutaneous nodule usually is observed. If pruritus has been present, mild excoriation and alopecia may be seen. The local lesions tend to persist for several days to

TABLE 6-2

Diseases and Organisms Transmitted by Ixodid Ticks

Disease or Organism	*Rhipicephalus sanguineus*	*Dermacentor andersoni*	*Dermacentor variabilis*	*Amblyomma americanum*	*Amblyomma maculatum*	*Ixodes dammini*
Babesia gibsoni	X					
Babesia canis		X				
Hepatozoon canis	X					
Coxiella burnetii	X	X				
Ehrlichia canis	X					
Pasteurella tularensis	X		X			
Rocky Mountain spotted fever		X	X	X		
Western equine encephalitis		X				
St. Louis equine encephalitis			X			
Leptospira pomona					X	
Borrelia burgdorferi				X		X

weeks, depending on the degree of local irritation present.

Diagnosis

The observation of ticks is diagnostic (Fig. 6-4G). A history of tick infestation, focal crusty lesions, or cutaneous nodules is suggestive.

Management

The two objectives in the control of tick infestations are (1) breaking the tick life cycle in the environment and (2) minimizing infestation of all animals. Eliminating ticks from the indoor or kennel environment requires repeated spraying of the premises, including all cracks and crevices, with parasiticides (see Table 3-5). Infested animals should be isolated in areas that can be disinfected easily. In many endemic areas, repeated treatment at 2-week intervals is necessary. Eliminating ticks from the outdoor environment is difficult. An attempt should be made to eliminate or decrease the number of rodent hosts and to destroy or spray tick-infested vegetation. Avoidance of known infested vegetation is also helpful.

The control of ticks on animals is easier to accomplish than the environmental control. After soaking the tick with alcohol or ether, the tick should be mechanically removed with forceps by grasping it near the head. The dog or cat should then be dipped in an approved parasiticide to remove any ticks missed on physical examination. Tick control on all animals should be maintained by using powders, sprays, dips, or insecticide collars (see Table 3-5).

SOFT TICKS (ARGASID)

The only soft tick of clinical importance is the spinose ear tick, *Otobius megnini*, which is found only in warm, moist climates.

Pathogenesis

The larval and nymphal stages can be found in the ears of most mammals. The larvae feed on lymph while nymphs suck blood. Severe irritation and inflammation of the external ear canal occurs because of mechanical attachment and piercing of the mucosa.

Life Cycle

Otobius megnini is a one-host tick. Only the larvae and nymphal stages are parasitic (Table 6-1).

History and Clinical Signs

The dog or cat may be examined for a history of head shaking, pain about the ears, and localized pruritus of the ear region. On physical examination, a waxy or oily exudate, together with larval and nymphal ticks, usually is found in the external ear canal. After removing the wax, acute otitis externa is observed. Excoriations often are found at the base of the ears as a result of the pruritus.

Diagnosis

The observation of ticks during an otic examination confirms the diagnosis. A history of severe head shaking and pruritus around the ears is suggestive, especially if the animal lives in an endemic area.

Management

Ticks are mechanically removed with forceps, and tick powders or sprays are used on external surfaces (see Table 3-5). The otitis externa is treated locally with antibiotics and corticosteroids. Spraying the premises helps to control reinfestation.

PELODERA DERMATITIS

Pelodera, or rhabditic dermatitis, is an uncommon disease of dogs caused by the larvae of the free-living nematode, *Pelodera strongyloides*. Parthenogenetic adult females also may be found in the hair follicles.

Pathogenesis

Pelodera dermatitis is associated with unsanitary conditions and damp bedding. Most lesions are secondary to pruritus. The larvae penetrate the skin causing microscopic subcutaneous inflammation. Previously injured skin may be predisposed to infection.

Life Cycle

The life cycle of *P. strongyloides* is direct. Adults live in damp soil or in decaying organic matter. Female adults are parthenogenetic or oviparous.

History and Clinical Signs

Dogs with pelodera dermatitis usually are intensely pruritic. There is often a history of exposure to damp bedding, such as straw. Lesions usually are confined to the ventral contact areas of the body. The primary lesions are papules and pustules, which usually progress to secondary crusts and scales. Erythema may be intense. Alopecia is more variable depending on severity and duration of the pruritus.

Diagnosis

A history of intensely pruritic ventral dermatitis in a dog that sleeps on damp bedding is suggestive of pelodera dermatitis. A definitive diagnosis can be made by observing nematode larvae with a rhabditiform esophagus on scraping (Fig. 6-4H). Sections of larvae or adult females may be seen in cutaneous biopsy. Bedding also may be infested with larvae or adults.

Treatment

Complete removal and destruction of infested bedding is imperative. The premises should be washed and then disinfected with organophosphates or chlordane. The infested dog should be bathed with an antiseborrheic and antibacterial shampoo to remove crusts and surface infection and then dipped weekly for 3 weeks with a parasiticide (see Table 3-5).

HOOKWORM DERMATITIS

Hookworm dermatitis, or ancylostomiasis, in dogs is caused by the larvae of *Ancylostoma caninum* or *Uncinaria stenocephala*.

Pathogenesis

The third-stage larvae enter the skin of the distal extremities. Local tissue inflammation occurs which results in intense pruritus. Clinical signs appear within 16 hours of the hookworm larvae penetration and may persist for 1 month. Microscopic examination of the resulting lesion suggests an immune-mediated reaction.

History

Intense pruritus and inflammation of all feet is observed. A history of exposure to a hookworm endemic environment generally is reported. The fecal examination often is positive for hookworm ova.

Clinical Signs

There is moderate to severe erythema. The feet are edematous, painful, and warm to touch. The pads are soft and spongy in the acute stage. If the dermatitis is chronic, the footpads become hyperkeratotic, dry, and cracked. Paronychia also is reported.

Diagnosis

A presumptive diagnosis of hookworm dermatitis is based on history of exposure, concurrent intestinal hookworm parasitism based upon fecal examination, and pedal dermatitis. A therapeutic trial with a hookworm anthelmintic resulting in clinical improvement of the pedal dermatitis is further support for the diagnosis.

Treatment

Specific treatment involves appropriate anthelmintic therapy, such as pyrantel pamoate or fenbendazole. The environment must be cleaned and the premises kept dry to minimize hookworm infestation in the soil. Borax should be applied to dirt or gravel runs.

CUTANEOUS DIROFILARIASIS

Cutaneous dirofilariasis in dogs is caused by the microfilariae of *Dirofilaria immitis*, the heartworm larvae.

Pathogenesis

The pathogenesis of lesions associated with microfilarial infection caused by *D. immitis* is not known; however, a hypersensitivity reaction is suspected.

History and Clinical Signs

Skin lesions are nonspecific. The clinical signs associated with cutaneous dirofilariasis include erythematous and alopecic eruptions, or multiple ulcerating nodules on the head, neck, trunk, and proximal limbs. Pruritus is often associated with the lesions.

Diagnosis

A positive test for circulating microfilariae and a cutaneous biopsy of a lesion that reveals microfilariae within vessels surrounded by a pyogranulomatous infiltrate (Fig. 6-4I) are diagnostic. A response to heartworm therapy supports the diagnosis of cutaneous dirofilariasis.

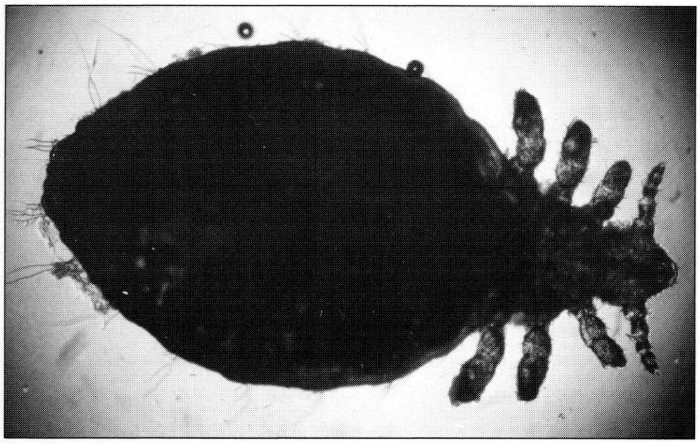

Figure 6-5. *Linognathus setosus* (sucking louse) of dogs.

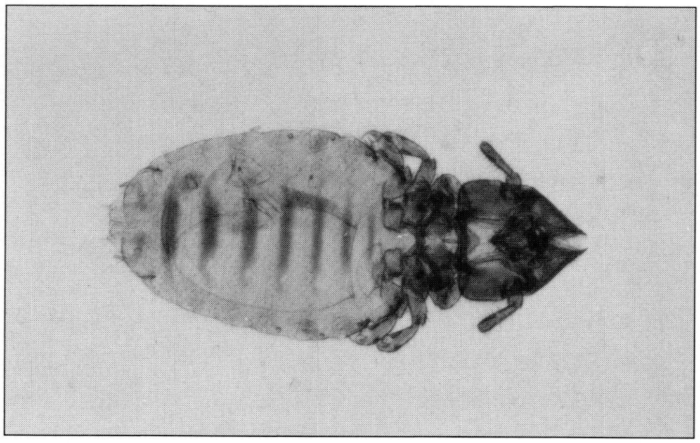

Figure 6-6. *Felicola subrostratus* (biting louse) of cats.

Treatment

The standard protocol for heartworm treatment with thiacetarsamide and dithiazanine is recommended.

LICE INFESTATION (PEDICULOSIS)

Lice are wingless, dorsoventrally flattened insects that are host-specific and spend their entire life cycle on the host. The incidence of pediculosis in the United States is low, and is more commonly associated with cool climates.

The two types of lice that affect dogs are the biting and sucking types. The most common biting louse is *Trichodectes canis*. *Heterodoxus spiniger* occasionally is found in warm climates. The common sucking louse is *Linognathus setosus* (Fig. 6-5). Cats are only affected by biting lice, most commonly *Felicola subrostratus* (Fig. 6-6). *Trichodectes canis* rarely affects kittens.

Pathogenesis

Lice can be transmitted directly by mechanical means (for example, grooming tools). Biting lice cause an irritation at the attachment site. Sucking lice extract blood and thus potentially can cause anemia. Pruritus is caused by the release of proteolytic enzymes in the oral secretions of lice or after mechanical trauma associated with penetration of the tissue.

Life Cycle

Operculate eggs or nits are deposited and cemented to the hair. The eggs hatch into nymphs which molt three times before becoming adults. The entire life cycle lasts 2 to 3 weeks.

History and Clinical Signs

Owners may report observing lice. Often there is a complaint of mild pruritus. The most common clinical finding is white, glistening nits attached to the hair. Lice may be found accidentally after clipping in the absence of a history of infestation or pruritus. Mild to moderate inflammation may be accompanied by scales, papules, or small crusts.

Treatment

Lice are susceptible to most parasiticides (see Table 3-5). It is necessary to treat all animals on the premises. All new dogs and cats should be dusted, sprayed, or dipped before exposure to other animals.

MYIASIS

Myiasis is caused by two families of flies: the calliphorids, or blowflies, and the sarcophagids, or flesh flies.

Pathogenesis

Flies are attracted to moist, traumatized areas. Fly larvae cause marked destruction of the skin by secreting proteolytic enzymes. Secondary fly larvae infections can occur, causing more severe lesions. Deep tunnels can form in the subcutaneous tissue. Toxemia may be seen in dogs and cats with neglected myiasis, which is likely caused by metabolic breakdown products of the necrotic tissue.

Life Cycle

Calliphorid eggs are laid in clusters on moist skin lesions. The larvae hatch in 8 hours to 3 days. Within the next 2 to 19 days, two ecdyses follow. The larvae drop off the host and become pupae. The pupae persist for a minimum of 3 to 7 days before becoming adults which live for 1 month or longer.

The sarcophagids are larviparous, thus they deposit larvae rather than eggs on the skin. The rest of the life cycle is similar to that of the calliphorid flies.

History

Myiasis usually occurs in a chronically neglected wound or on skin that is persistently moist and covered by soiled hair, such as is associated with a debilitated animal. There may be a history of previous trauma or injury. There is often a complaint of a foul odor from a large open wound.

Clinical Signs

Myiasis is characterized by the presence of a large number of fly larvae in solitary or multiple ulcerated lesions, which are often associated with marked tissue necrosis (Plate III-9). In the acute phase of myiasis the larvae may be found in fistulous tracts as well as in the body orifices, including the vagina and anus. There is often a large area of acutely erythematous moist skin in the infected area.

Diagnosis

The definitive diagnosis is based on finding larvae in a wound.

Treatment

The wounds and surrounding area must be cleaned by clipping and scrubbing and removing all larvae. It is best to use an iodine solution and hydrogen peroxide to clean the wound. Insecticide sprays may be absorbed too rapidly through the traumatized tissue, resulting in toxicity as well as potential local irritation. Insecticide sprays or powders should be used on the rest of the body for continuous fly control. Most animals with myiasis require local wound treatment as well as general supportive care. The debilitated animal must be kept in a fly-free environment.

SELECTED READINGS

Ackerman L: Demodicosis in cats. *Mod Vet Pract* 65:751–753, 1984.

Dryden MW, Long GR, Gaarar SM: Effects of ultrasonic flea collars on *Ctenocephalides felis* on cats. *JAVMA* 195:1717–1718, 1989.

Folz SD: Canine scabies (*Sarcoptes scabiei* infestation). *Compend Contin Educ Pract Vet* 6:176–180, 1984.

Hoskins JD, Cupp EW: Ticks of veterinary importance. Part I. The Ixodidae family: Identification, behavior and associated diseases. *Compend Contin Educ Pract Vet* 10:564–580, 1988.

Hoskins JD, Cupp EW: Ticks of veterinary importance. Part II. The Argasidae family: Identification, behavior and associated diseases. *Compend Contin Educ Pract Vet* 10:699–708, 1988.

Kwochka KW: Mites and related diseases. *Vet Clin North Am [Small Anim Pract]* 17(6):1263–1281, 1987.

Kwochka KW, Bevier DE: Flea dermatitis. In: Nesbitt GH (ed): *Dermatology. Contemporary Issues in Small Animal Practice*, vol 8. New York, Churchill Livingstone, 1987, pp 21–51.

Kwochka KW, Kunkle GA, Foil CO: The efficacy of amitraz for generalized demodicosis in dogs: A study of two concentrations and frequencies of application. *Compend Contin Educ Pract Vet* 7:8–17, 1985.

Melman SA, Hutton P: Flea control on dogs and cats indoors and in the environment. *Compend Contin Educ Pract Vet* 7:869–887, 1987.

Moriello KA: Common ectoparasites of the dog. Part 1: Fleas and ticks. *Canine Pract* 14:6–18, 1987.

Moriello KA: Common ectoparasites of the dog. Part 2: *Sarcoptes scabiei* var *canis* and *Demodex canis*. *Canine Pract* 14:25–41, 1987.

Moriello KA: Dermatologic manifestations of internal and external parasitism. *Compan Anim Pract* 2:12–17, 1988.

Moriello KA: Oh, no! Not fleas again! *Vet Focus* 1:19–28, 1989.

Paradis M, Villeneuve A: Efficacy of ivermectin against *Cheyletiella yasguri* infestation in dogs. *Can Vet J* 29:633–635, 1988.

Paradis M, Scott D, Villeneuve A: Efficacy of ivermectin against *Cheyletiella blakei* infestation in cats. *JAAHA* 26:125–128, 1990.

Chapter 7

BACTERIAL DISEASES

Gene H. Nesbitt, DVM, MS
Lowell Ackerman, DVM

Bacterial diseases (pyoderma) represent one of the most common dermatologic problems encountered in dogs, but are much less common in cats. Diagnostic Keys 5 and 6 (see end of Chapter 2) list the most pertinent historical and clinical findings and definitive diagnostic tests necessary to differentiate the common bacterial diseases in dogs and cats.

CLASSIFICATION

Pyoderma is the term commonly used to denote bacterial infection of the skin. Such infection may be either primary or secondary. In dogs, infection is more commonly secondary to another dermatologic problem, such as pruritus, abnormal keratinization, or parasitic infestation. Other than abscesses resulting from bite wounds or scratches, bacterial disease is uncommon in cats.

Bacterial disease is subdivided into three types based on the depth of involvement of the skin: surface, superficial, and deep. Surface pyoderma is characterized by superficial overcolonization of the skin in an area where inflammation is the inciting cause. The infection is only as deep as the inflammation. Pyotraumatic dermatitis (acute moist dermatitis, "hot spots") and intertrigo (skin fold pyoderma) are classified as surface pyodermas.

Superficial pyoderma is localized to the epidermis and manifests as subcorneal pustules or as a microabscess within the epithelium and lumen of an intact hair follicle. Impetigo, superficial folliculitis, and dermatophilosis are included in the superficial pyoderma classification.

Deep pyoderma is characterized by bacterial involvement of the dermis and subcutis, and includes the clinical entities of furunculosis, cellulitis, hidradenitis suppurativa, cat-bite abscesses, mycobacterial infections, and actinomycotic mycetoma (nocardiosis and actinomycosis).

ETIOLOGIC FACTORS

The normal bacterial flora of canine and feline skin include nonpathogenic coagulase-negative *Micrococcus* spp., alpha-hemolytic streptococci, *Corynebacterium* spp., and *Staphylococcus epidermidis*. *Clostridium* spp. are frequently isolated anaerobically from canine skin. Transient cutaneous bacteria of dogs and cats include *Proteus* spp., *Pseudomonas* spp., *Corynebacterium* spp., and coagulase-positive *Staphylococcus* spp.

Staphylococcus intermedius is the most commonly isolated pathogen in dogs; *S. aureus* is isolated in a small number of dogs. *Streptococcus* spp. may be isolated concurrently with *S. intermedius*. It may be an opportunist in some animals and may not contribute to the disease process. *Pseudomonas* spp. and *Proteus* spp. are most commonly isolated from surface lesions and from acute and chronic otitic ear canals. *Pasteurella multocida* is the most common isolate from cat-bite abscesses. *Nocardia* and *Dermatophilus* have been isolated from both dogs and cats. Mycobacteria are uncommon in both species. Cutaneous tuberculosis usually is caused by *Mycobacterium bovis*, but infections with the human tubercular agent, *M. tuberculosis*, have been reported. Feline leprosy (atypical mycobacterial granuloma) is probably caused by *M. lepraemurium*, the cause of murine leprosy. Another group of mycobacteria (Group IV, fast growers) that does not cause either tuberculosis or leprosy has been reported to cause a disease in dogs and cats termed *cutaneous atypical mycobacteriosis*.

PATHOGENESIS

Three major factors are involved in the pathogenesis of pyoderma: the pathogenic properties of the organism, the portal of entry, and the host response to microbial invasion. The important pathogenic properties of staphylococci include the antiphagocytic properties of the capsule and protein; the presence of a protease, leukocidin, which acts on the cytoplasmic membrane of neutrophils and macrophages to cause cell lysis; an alpha hemolysin (necrotizing toxin), which is highly toxic to macrophages and epithelial cells; and lipase and esterase, which permit the bacteria to survive the antibacterial action of lipids on the skin. Beta-lactamases destroy the beta-lactam ring of penicillin and related drugs.

Bacteria can gain entrance into the skin by several routes: through the hair follicles, through the epidermal barrier near the surface of the skin, by focal penetration directly into the deeper layers of skin, or systemically by way of the blood or lymph vessels. Hyperkeratosis and follicular plugging, which are commonly observed in many chronic skin conditions, predispose to the entrance and colonization of bacteria in the follicles. The increased epidermal cell turnover time associated with abnormal keratinization, as seen in seborrheic syndromes and endocrine disease, increases the permeability of the epidermal barrier. The physical irritation of external parasites and the secretions of parasites and bacteria also alter the epidermal barrier. Direct penetration through the epidermis into the dermis and subcutis by way of bite wounds, trauma, or penetrating foreign bodies can cause tissue damage resulting in a more favorable environment for colonization of the bacteria in the deeper tissues. A systemic origin of bacterial skin infections, such as cutaneous feline tuberculosis, is rare.

Host response to the invasion of bacteria varies among dogs and cats. Both cellular and humoral factors are probably involved. It is generally accepted that alterations in the cell-mediated (Type IV) hypersensitivity reactions play a role in the development of generalized pyoderma.

Both resident and transient bacteria can act as pathogens. Primary bacterial pathogens initiate disease in normal skin. Secondary pathogens ordinarily do not initiate the disease, but do contribute to the disease process. Many bacteria will colonize on the skin but do not contribute to the disease process or elicit a host response. The differentiation of the latter two is often difficult.

Many concurrent factors can influence the predisposition to bacterial infection, including external parasites, especially fleas and demodectic mites; allergic dermatitis; hypothyroidism; chronic internal parasitism; systemic diseases; and corticosteroid therapy.

CANINE BACTERIAL DISEASES

General History

The history is variable and depends on primary and secondary etiologic factors, duration and distribution of lesions, and previous therapy. Historical data commonly include (1) no systemic involvement (excluding peripheral lymphadenopathy); (2) mild to marked pruritus; (3) partial to good response to antibacterial therapy, often with an exacerbation of signs following withdrawal; (4) concurrent external parasites or allergic dermatitis; and (5) offensive odor.

If the bacterial dermatitis is primary, pruritus usually will follow the onset of clinical signs. If the infection is secondary to parasites or allergic disease, pruritus will be observed before or concurrently with the signs of pyoderma. Deep pyoderma usually is persistent or recurrent. Many superficial pyodermas recur rapidly, most commonly because of inadequate treatment time.

General Clinical Signs

The lesions associated with primary and secondary bacterial infection are variable. Primary morphologic lesions commonly observed with staphylococcal infections are papules, pustules, and macules. Secondary lesions include scale, crust, excoriation, and hyperpigmentation. Erythema and alopecia are variable.

History and Clinical Signs by Depth of Lesion

Surface Pyodermas

Pyotraumatic Dermatitis. Pyotraumatic dermatitis (acute moist dermatitis, "hot spots") is characterized by an acute onset of a pruritic, focal or multifocal eroded area with an erythematous, moist surface (Plate IV-1). In most cases the role of bacteria in pyotraumatic dermatitis is that of a secondary pathogen. A deep furunculosis has been observed in a high percentage of golden retrievers and St. Bernards with pyotraumatic lesions.

The primary causes usually are parasitic (fleas) or allergic, such as atopy. Otitis externa and matted hair can predispose to the pyotraumatic lesions. A seasonal occurrence coinciding with flea infestations and seasonal atopy are common.

The distribution of pyotraumatic dermatitic lesions is variable; they are most commonly found on the flanks, dorsal caudal back, lateral thighs, neck, and face.

Skin Fold Pyoderma. Skin fold pyoderma (intertrigo) is a lifelong problem of breeds anatomically predisposed. Spaniels and setters have a higher incidence of lip fold pyoderma (Plate IV-2). Facial fold pyodermas are seen most commonly in brachycephalic breeds and shar peis. Bull dogs and Boston terriers have tail fold pyodermas. Vulvar fold pyodermas are seen in obese spayed females of any breed.

The deep skin folds lead to increased moisture, bacterial growth, and odor. Erythema and erosions are variable. Excoriation, hyperkeratosis, and hyperpigmentation are commonly observed around the involved skin folds as a result of pruritus.

Superficial Pyoderma

Impetigo. Impetigo (puppy pyoderma) is a disease of young puppies 2 to 16 weeks old. It is associated with crowding and unsanitary conditions. There is seldom any pruritus or discomfort observed.

Impetigo is characterized by small superficial pustules that are not associated with hair follicles. The distribution usually is inguinal and axillary. The pustules are easily ruptured, leaving a characteristic yellow crust.

Superficial Folliculitis. Superficial folliculitis (recurrent pyoderma) is the most common form of pyoderma affecting dogs. The lesions can be primary or secondary (see Tables 2-3 and 2-4). Breeds predisposed to primary superficial folliculitis include the Doberman pinscher, dalmation, boxer, English bulldog, dachshund, Great Dane, weimaraner, Shetland sheepdog, collie, Irish setter, Labrador retriever, Chesapeake Bay retriever, and golden retriever.

Superficial folliculitis lesions are characterized by pustules and papules. The following sequence of clinical signs is characteristic of superficial folliculitis (Plate IV-3): (1) an erythematous papule with minimal peripheral erythema; (2) a pustule; (3) a flattened crust, 5 to 10 mm in diameter—if the crust is removed, a moist erythematous lesion remains; (4) the crust loosens, the center falls off, and a thin layer of epidermal scale remains on the periphery of the lesion with an alopecic dry center (epidermal collarette); and (5) a hyperpigmented macule. Papules and pustules frequently are observed on the abdomen or other sparsely haired areas of the body, while the lesions that characterize the more mature stages, such as crusts and hyperpigmented macules, are found on the dorsal and lateral trunk as well as ventrally.

Dermatophilosis. Dermatophilosis (cutaneous streptothricosis) is associated with animals that are exposed to large amounts of moisture so the hair and skin stay damp. Other predisposing factors usually are present, such as fleas, chronic folliculitis, or seborrheic dermatitis.

Dermatophilosis lesions are most commonly seen on the hairy or glabrous skin of the dorsum and thigh. The lesions are characterized by exudate beneath crusts in haired areas. They may start as papules and pustules and subsequently develop into larger crusts. Dry crusts, scaling, hyperpigmentation, and alopecia are seen in the later stages of dermatophilosis.

Deep Pyoderma

Primary deep pyoderma usually is seen in middle-aged to older dogs. In deep pyoderma lesions, the bacterial infection has spread to the perifollicular tissue after rupture of the hair follicle. Furunculosis, a pyogranulomatous dermal reaction, characterizes deep pyoderma. The lesions may be focal, multiple, or generalized (Plate IV-4). Cellulitis is characterized by diffuse soft-tissue swelling following rupture of the hair follicle and subsequent infection in the dermis. There may be heat, pain, and erythema, and the animal's hair may epilate easily. Fever and peripheral lymphadenomegaly may be observed. In the acute stages, the surface usually is moist with crusts, alopecia, and erythema. Exudate usually can be expressed from dermal tracts. Chronic deep pyodermic lesions are characterized by thickened skin, hyperpigmentation, hyperkeratosis, and frequent scarring. Pyothorax, osteomyelitis, septic arthritis, and septicemia can be sequelae. Leukocytosis and neutrophilia also are common findings.

Deep pyoderma occurs secondary to demodectic mange, immunodeficiency problems, immunosuppression, foreign bodies, and severe pruritic conditions. Regardless of the underlying cause of deep pyoderma, the clinical findings are similar.

Deep pyodermas are commonly classified by distribution patterns, including muzzle and chin, nasal, interdigital, pressure points, and generalized.

Muzzle and Chin Folliculitis and Furunculosis (Acne). Uncomplicated acne is common in young dogs; it usually is asymptomatic and often spontaneously resolves as the dog reaches maturity. Follicular plugs or comedones characterize acne. If the hair follicles become infected, papules and pustules are observed. In a small number of dogs, the hair follicles rupture, resulting in deeper lesions characterized by hemorrhagic bullae, furuncles, and draining tracts. These are observed most commonly in the mature English bulldog, boxer, Great Dane, and Doberman pinscher. The lesions often are a lifelong problem.

Nasal Pyoderma. Nasal pyoderma is characterized by painful erosions, ulceration, and crusting on the dorsum of the nose. Erythema and alopecia are variable. In the chronic stages, scarring is common. The majority of nasal pyoderma lesions are secondary to other diseases, including demodicosis, pemphigus foliaceus, pemphigus erythematosus, and lupus erythematosus. These diseases should be ruled out before a diagnosis of primary nasal pyoderma is made.

Interdigital Pyoderma. Interdigital pyoderma is characterized in the active stages by deep draining tracts or large, deep pustules between the interdigital spaces of one or more feet. Often there are pustules between the pads. The feet are usually moist and erythematous secondary to foot licking. In the chronic stages, pyogranulomas are observed as are pain and lameness.

Interdigital pyoderma often is chronic and recurrent. Many concurrent or predisposing factors must be ruled out, including demodicosis, dermatophytosis, hypothyroidism, allergic dermatitis, sterile pyogranulomas, and foreign bodies.

Pressure Point Pyoderma. Pressure point pyoderma usually is associated with ulceration and draining tracts on the elbows, lateral stifles, hocks, and digits. Persistent matting of hair, erosions, and crusting result from constant irritation and friction. Large-breed dogs are most commonly affected.

Generalized Deep Pyoderma. Generalized deep pyoderma is a chronic disease characterized by multifocal distribution. Lesions vary from erythematous, moist, alopecic, erosive areas to deep furunculosis and cellulitis (Plate IV-5) with multiple draining tracts (Plate IV-4). In the acute stages, the hair often is matted such that the lesions are not recognized until the hair is clipped. Deep generalized pyoderma can occur in any breed; however, it is observed most frequently in German shepherds, Irish setters, and Doberman pinschers. Perianal pyoderma is common in German shepherds (Plate IV-6). Initially, cases of hidradenitis suppurativa as reported in collies and Shetland sheepdogs may have been cases of bullous pemphigoid.

Acute exacerbation of deep pyoderma may be associated with a history of anorexia and lethargy. Pain and lameness are common in dogs with cellulitis of the extremities.

Mycobacterial Infections (Mycobacterial Granulomas). Mycobacterial infections are uncommon. They are characterized by cutaneous nodules and draining tracts and a poor response to antibiotic therapy. Mycobacterial infections in dogs are divided into two categories: cutaneous tuberculosis and atypical mycobacteriosis.

Cutaneous tuberculosis lesions can be solitary or multiple nodules, ulcers, or abscesses. Weight loss, anorexia, fever, and lymphadenopathy often accompany the cutaneous lesions. Because of the public health aspects of tuberculosis, care should be exercised in the handling of suspect animals and laboratory specimens.

A dog or cat with pulmonary infection and subcutaneous draining nodules is a prime suspect for nocardiosis or the systemic mycoses.

Cutaneous atypical mycobacteriosis is characterized by draining tracts and subcutaneous nodules. Plaques and ulcerations also may be seen. The head, extremities, and ventral trunk are sites that are predisposed. Discomfort is minimal and there are no systemic signs. Many mycobacteria have been implicated, including *M. fortuitum, M. chelonei, M. phlei, M. balnei,* and *M. smegmatis.*

A successful diagnosis may prove challenging. Cultures are helpful in fast-growing mycobacteria, but are more difficult in slow-growing and tubercular mycobacteria, and are not possible for feline leprosy. Special media, such as Lowenstein-Jensen and blood agar, must be used to recover most mycobacteria. Skin biopsies or cytology specimens can be processed with acid-fast or Ziehl-Neelsen stains.

Caution is always warranted when treating mycobacteriosis. Treatment should involve surgical excision if the lesion is localized. Recurrence and dehiscence is common. Medical therapy should be based on culture and sensitivity data if available, although this does not ensure success. Aminoglycosides, dapsone, and doxycycline have all been reported to be effective in selected cases. Treatment for tuberculosis is not recommended because of the serious public health risk, and in these cases, public health officials should be notified.

Miscellaneous Pyodermas

Botryomycosis (Bacterial Pseudomycetoma, Cutaneous Bacterial Granuloma). Botryomycosis is a granulomatous dermatitis caused by several species of bacteria, with coagulase-positive staphylococci being the most frequently reported. The bacteria usually are inoculated by bite wounds or other trauma, and the ensuing granuloma is believed to result from immunologic incompetence on the part of the host. Lesions are firm nodules that can drain to the skin surface and exude tissue "grains" (Plate IV-7).

Culture and sensitivity of the exudate or tissue grains is diagnostic. Differentiation from mycobacteria and fungal infections can be made with histopathology and special stains. Complete surgical excision is the treatment of choice, although antibiotic therapies (for example, rifampin, cephalosporins, trimethoprim sulfas) may be effective.

Actinomycotic Mycetoma. Actinomycotic mycetoma is a granulomatous process resulting from infection (usually caused by trauma) with species of *Nocardia*, *Actinomyces*, and occasionally *Streptomyces*. The lesions associated with nocardiosis include cellulitis, ulcerated dermal nodules, and fistulous tracts with a brownish red exudate. Sulfur granules are not observed. The extremities are most often affected. Systemic signs associated with *Nocardia* pulmonary infection may be seen.

FELINE BACTERIAL DISEASES

History and Clinical Findings

Surface and Superficial Pyoderma

Surface pyoderma, associated with "mouthing" by the queen, has been observed in young kittens. Lesions are characterized by alopecia, papules, and crusts on the dorsal neck, occasionally progressing caudally on the trunk. Systemic signs are unusual.

There is no breed, sex, or age predilection for feline folliculitis, which is commonly observed on the chin and associated with feline acne (see Plate VII-9). The clinical signs vary depending on the depth of skin involvement. Alopecia, erosions, ulcers, crusts, and occasionally fistulous tracts and cellulitis have been reported. Pain and pruritus are variable. Peripheral lymphadenomegaly may be observed in cats with deep folliculitis.

Subcutaneous Abscesses

Most bacterial infections are associated with a history of cat scratches or bites that result in abscesses or cellulitis. The highest incidence occurs in intact males, with no breed or age predilection. Lesions are most commonly seen on the extremities, face, dorsal tail, and back. The history is variable. Acute pain, fever, anorexia, and lameness may be noted. In some cats, focal or diffuse soft-tissue swelling or a ruptured abscess is the first sign observed by the pet owner.

Physical examination may reveal varying degrees of focal erythema and swelling, and evidence of a puncture or bite wound may be observed. If an abscess has not ruptured, a thick white to reddish-brown odoriferous exudate is seen on aspiration or drainage.

Cellulitis

Cellulitis is characterized by diffuse soft-tissue swelling, which usually occurs on one limb. There may be heat, pain, and erythema, and the animal's hair may epilate easily. Fever and peripheral lymphadenomegaly may be observed. Pyothorax, osteomyelitis, septic arthritis, and septicemia may be sequelae to cat-bite abscesses and cellulitis. Leukocytosis and neutrophilia also are common findings.

Miscellaneous Pyodermas

Actinomycotic Mycetoma. Feline actinomycotic mycetoma is most often caused by *Nocardia* organisms that enter via penetrating wounds. Thoracic infection is more common than cutaneous manifestions but dermatologic eruptions usually present as indurated to papulonodular lesions, often with draining tracts (Plate IV-8). The hallmark of mycetoma is granuloma formation, fistulation, and the presence of "grains."

Feline Cutaneous Tuberculosis. Feline cutaneous tuberculosis is a disease of young adult cats (average age 2 years) living in geographic areas of the world in which tuberculosis is endemic in cattle. Even though *Mycobacterium bovis* is the most common cause, *M. tuberculosis* can be contracted from infected humans. Feline tuberculosis is frequently asymptomatic without signs or outward evidence of disease. Cutaneous lesions are characterized by single or multiple ulcers, abscesses, plaques, and nodules. Thick, yellow to green exudate usually can be discharged from the lesions. Lesions are most commonly distributed on the head, neck, and extremities. Regional lymphadenopathy and pyrexia also may be present.

Feline Leprosy (Atypical Mycobacterial Granuloma). Feline leprosy is a disease with no age, breed, or sex predilection. The probable cause is *M. lepraemurium*; feline infection is most likely contracted from the bite of an infected rat. Solitary and occasionally multiple subcutaneous nodules or abscesses with or without draining tracts are the lesions most commonly seen (Plate IV-9). If the nodule is at the dermoepidermal junction, ulceration is observed. The head, neck, and limbs are most frequently involved.

DEFINITIVE DIAGNOSTIC TESTS

Bacterial Culture and Sensitivity Testing

Bacterial culture is the diagnostic test of choice for most chronic bacterial diseases. The isolation of pathogenic bacteria from a lesion does not differentiate between primary and secondary pyoderma. Cultures are not routinely recommended for mild or first-occurrence surface or superficial pyodermas; however, they are indicated for all dogs and cats with chronic or frequently recurring superficial pyodermas or deep pyodermas, and for animals with a history of poor or partial response to antibiotics.

The sampling techniques for bacterial cultures are described in Chapter 2. The techniques for bacterial culture and in vitro antibiotic sensitivity testing also are described in Table 2-8. Bacterial cultures are seldom indicated for surface pyodermas.

Valid results may be obtained when the animal is still undergoing treatment if there is bacterial resistance to the antibiotic being used. If there is partial antibiotic inhibition of the bacterial growth in vivo, however, in vitro growth on the medium may be completely suppressed. Therefore, if possible, it is recommended to withhold all antibiotics for 2 to 4 days before culturing.

All bacteria that grow on the culture medium should be identified because it is common to have both pathogenic and nonpathogenic bacteria in a mixed culture. Gram-negative bacteria (*Pseudomonas* or *Proteus*) should be suspected to be primary opportunistic surface bacteria when isolated from superficial pyodermal lesions. If *Escherichia coli* is isolated from any cutaneous lesion, it should be considered a contaminant.

In vitro antibiotic sensitivity testing is routinely performed on all bacterial isolates. Tests should be run on individual isolates, inasmuch as testing performed on a mixed culture is not valid because of overgrowth of one of the bacteria. The antibiotic disks should include both bacteriostatic and bactericidal antibiotics. As with many diagnostic tests, results of in vitro antibiotic sensitivity testing must be considered in concert with the other historical, physical, and laboratory findings. Several factors may influence the in vivo antibiotic response. Animals with secondary bacterial infections may not respond well to antibiotics based on sensitivity testing because of another primary problem. Antibacterial disks and zones of inhibition have been standardized based on blood levels of antibacterials in people, exerting an effect on a standard number of bacteria. The antibacterial drug must reach the site of bacterial infection, contact a standardized number of bacteria, and be fully potent when it does contact the bacteria. Abscesses and granulomas tend to "wall off" infectious agents, making them less accessible to antimicrobials. Some drugs are inactivated by contact with blood, pus, or damaged tissue and thus may have less antibacterial effect.

Cutaneous Biopsy

Cutaneous biopsies are sometimes definitive and often supportive of a diagnosis of bacterial dermatitis. They are necessary to determine the depth and extent of dermal and adnexal involvement, data that are useful for establishing treatment protocols and prognosis. The techniques for cutaneous biopsy are described in Table 2-9.

The microscopic findings of a surface bacterial lesion mainly involve the upper epidermis. Erosion of the stratum corneum is observed in pyotraumatic dermatitis and many skin fold pyodermas. In superficial pyoderma the surface is often intact. Epidermal changes include hyperkeratosis, variable acanthosis, spongiosis, and microabscesses with neutrophils traversing the stratum spinosum (diapedesis). The dermal changes are limited to the adnexa and upper dermis (dermoepidermal junction). Mild hyperkeratosis and edema of the follicular epithelium often are seen. Perifollicular or periglandular involvement can include a mixed inflammatory cell infiltrate and edema. The upper dermal infiltrate that consists of a variable number of mixed inflammatory cells is most often focal or perivascular, but it may be diffuse.

Chronic superficial pyoderma is characterized by hyperkeratosis, variable hypergranulosis, acanthosis, and a mild to moderate mononuclear cell infiltrate at the dermoepidermal junction. The perifollicular and periadnexal changes include a minimal to moderate number of mononuclear leukocytes and variable fibrosis. There may be proliferation of upper dermal blood vessels.

The epidermal changes in a deep pyoderma are similar to those of severe superficial pyoderma. Usually moderate to severe crusting is observed. The dermal changes may involve all of the dermis, and sometimes extend into the panniculus. Frequently there is a focal to diffuse mixed inflammatory infiltrate. As the lesion becomes chronic, fibroplasia increases. In many microscopic sections, multifocal pyogranulomatous lesions are observed in the dermis, characterized by a central core of mixed inflammatory infiltrate surrounded by histiocytes and an occasional multinucleated giant cell. Follicular and perifollicular involvement varies (Fig. 7-1). Often there is partial to total destruction of the follicle and replacement with fibrous tissue. The adnexal glands usually are

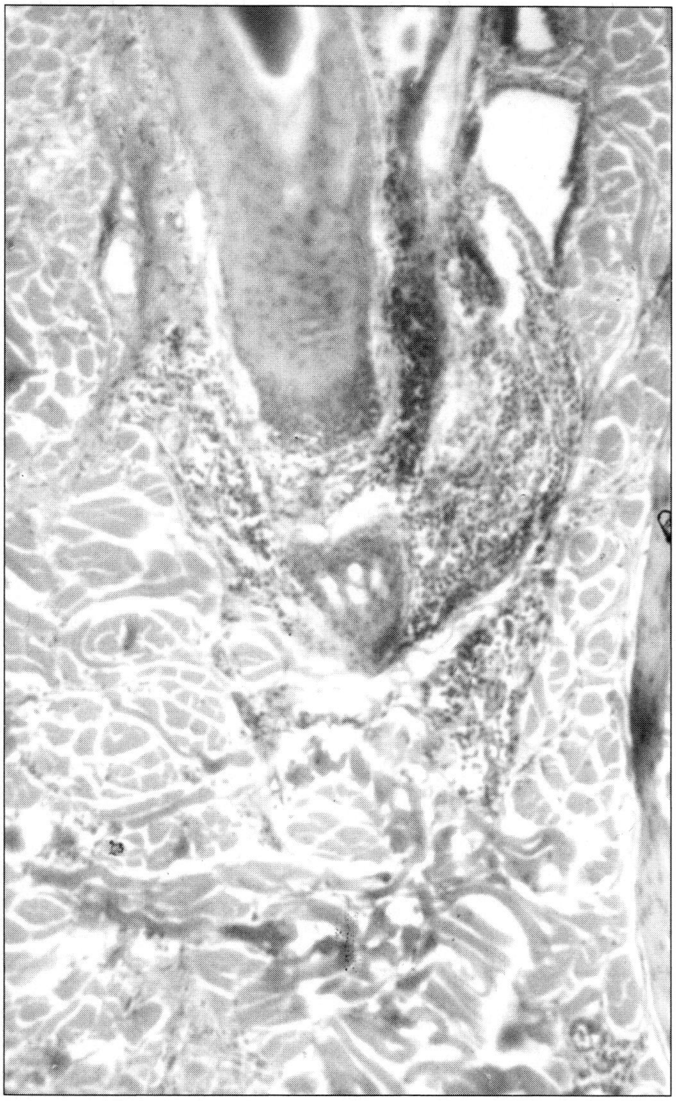

Figure 7-1. Deep pyoderma. Microscopic section with edema and dense perifolliculitis.

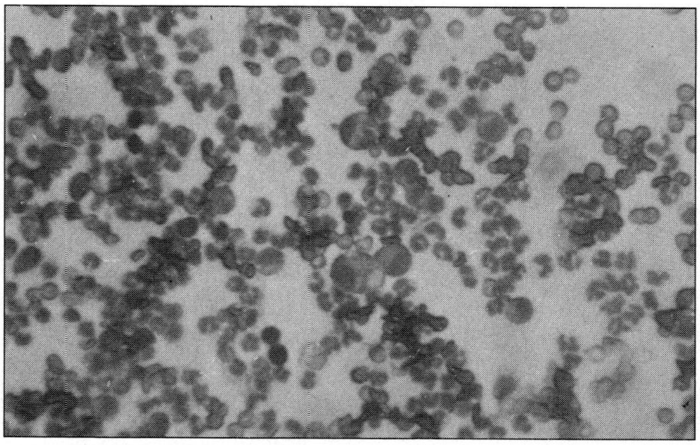

Figure 7-2. Direct smear of exudate with pyogranulomatous infiltration of neutrophils, histiocytes, and fibrin.

few in number and apocrine gland ducts may be dilated.

Microscopic lesions of feline tuberculosis and feline leprosy are granulomas with acid-fast organisms sometimes identified by using special stains.

Direct Smears

Direct smears are helpful in differentiating superficial bacterial disease from nonbacterial bullous disease. A direct smear (see Table 2-9) of the contents of a pustule stained with Wright's or Giemsa stain will reveal a predominance of neutrophils (Fig. 7-2). The number of free or phagocytized bacteria observed varies from none to many. Almost all bacteria seen will be cocci because *Pseudomonas* and *Proteus* spp. seldom manifest as isolated pustules.

Dermatophilosis is easily diagnosed with the direct smear. Several parallel rows of gram-positive cocci will be observed when stained with Wright's or Giemsa's stain.

Diagnostic Interpretation

The subjective or definitive confirmation of bacterial dermatitis is based on several factors, including history (response to antibiotics), clinical signs (pustules), and diagnostic tests (direct smears, cultures, biopsy). The major challenge is to interpret the diagnostic findings in order to formulate therapeutic protocols and to improve the prognostic acumen. Interpretation should include determination of primary versus secondary bacterial disease, depth of infection (surface, superficial, or deep), and chronicity.

TREATMENT

Several guidelines should be kept in mind when selecting the treatment protocol to be used. First, the proper antibiotic should be selected (see Table 3-11). In general, bacteriostatic antibiotics, such as erythromycin and lincomycin, are effective in treating most mild superficial pyodermas. In treating first-occurrence superficial pyoderma, most antibiotics are effective, including lincomycin, erythromycin, and chloramphenicol. For deep or chronic pyoderma and frequently recurring superficial pyoderma, bactericidal antibiotics should be used initially.

The second general guideline should be the use of therapeutic dosages of the drug(s) for a minimum of 7 to 10 days after there is a complete clinical response. This often results in a treatment time of 4 to 6 weeks. If there is minimal response to a specific antibiotic after 5 to 7 days of therapy, a different antibiotic should be tried and/or the initial diagnosis should be questioned. If long-term administration of antibiotics is required, it may be advantageous to use more than one antibiotic during the course of the treatment.

Third, topical therapy using antibacterial and antiseborrheic shampoo (see Table 3-6) or water soaks is indicated for most pyodermas. Removing crusts, debris, and excess sebum from the skin surface reduces the surface bacterial population, helps prevent follicular plugging, and helps restore normal keratinization. Clipping the hair and local cleansing, soaking, or washing with an antibacterial solution is helpful when there are lesions of deep pyoderma. Astringents (see Table 3-2) are indicated for use in areas that remain persistently moist, such as skin folds and between digits.

Fourth, concurrent problems, such as primary allergic or parasitic diseases (see Diagnostic Keys 2 and 4 at end of Chapter 2), must be treated symptomatically or specifically at the same time as the pyoderma. If there is marked pruritus causing exacerbation of clinical signs, an antihistamine (see Table 3-15), such as hydroxyzine (for example, Atarax® —Pfizer), may be effective.

Biological management is indicated in chronic or recurrent pyoderma and in deep pyoderma in dogs. The products currently available are nonspecific immune stimulators (see Table 3-16). Clinical response is variable. These drugs should be considered as adjunct therapy to be used concurrently with antibiotics initially, and then continued as prophylactic therapy.

Feline bacterial infections often respond to penicillin, amoxicillin, ampicillin, and hetacillin. All abscesses must be drained. Flushing with hydrogen peroxide and antibacterial agents also is recommended. Castration of intact male cats is an effective preventive measure.

SELECTED READINGS

Ackerman L: Cutaneous bacterial granuloma (botryomycosis) in five dogs. *Mod Vet Pract* 68:404–409, 1987.

Berg JN, Wendell DE, Bogelweid C, et al: Identification of the major coagulase-positive *Staphylococcus* sp. of dogs as *Staphylococcus intermedius*. *Am J Vet Res* 45:1307, 1984.

DeBoer DJ, Moriello KA, Thomas CB, Schultz KT: Evaluation of a commercial staphylococcal bacterin for management of idiopathic recurrent superficial pyoderma in dogs. *Am J Vet Res* 51:636–639, 1990.

Ihrke PJ: Therapeutic strategies involving antimicrobial treatment of the skin in small animals. *JAVMA* 185:1165, 1984.

Kunkle GA, Gulbas NK, Fadok V, et al: Rapidly growing mycobacteria as a cause of cutaneous granulomas-report of 5 cases. *JAAHA* 9:513, 1983.

White SD, Ihrke PJ: Pyoderma, in Nesbitt GH (ed): *Dermatology. Contemporary Issues in Small Animal Practice*, vol 8. New York, Churchill Livingstone, 1987, pp 95–119.

White SD, Ihrke PJ, Stannard AA, et al: Cutaneous atypical mycobacteriosis in cats. *JAVMA* 182:1218, 1983.

Chapter 8

FUNGAL SKIN DISEASES

Lowell Ackerman, DVM
Gene H. Nesbitt, DVM, MS

Fungal diseases can be divided into three major groups: superficial, intermediate, and systemic. Diagnostic Key 7 (see end of Chapter 2) lists the most pertinent historical and clinical findings and diagnostic tests necessary to differentiate the common etiologic factors of canine and feline fungal disease.

SUPERFICIAL MYCOSES

Dermatophytosis (Dermatomycosis, Ringworm)

Dermatophytosis describes the superficial fungal infections that remain limited to the cornified (keratinized) parts of the skin and claws.

Etiologic Factors

Three species of fungi (*Microsporum canis, M. gypseum, Trichophyton mentagrophytes*) are responsible for over 95% of all ringworm cases in pets.

Microsporum canis is the most common cause of ringworm in pets, and cats are the natural reservoir. Cats can be carriers of infection without manifesting the disease themselves and therefore can transmit it to other unsuspecting animals and humans. The fungus can also be contracted from spores in the environment or on contaminated objects (for example, brushes, combs, toys, furniture).

Microsporum gypseum normally is a soil inhabitant and can be found transiently on the hair and skin of outdoor animals. Infection usually is acquired from direct contact with contaminated soil, and once infected, an animal can transmit the fungus to other animals and humans.

Rodents are the natural reservoir for the fungus *Trichophyton mentagrophytes*. Infections thus can occur from contact with infected rodents or exposure to contaminated areas.

Less common causes of dermatophytosis in dogs and cats include *Microsporum persicolor, M. nanum, M. vanbreuseghemii, Trichophyton verrucosum, T. terrestre, T. rubrum, T. equinum, T. schoenleinii*, and *Epidermophyton floccosum*.

The relative incidence of each fungus varies in different geographic areas. Warm, moist climates are more favorable for a high incidence of dermatophytosis.

Classification

The individual type of fungus is classified according to its preferred habitat: zoophilic fungi have animals as their natural host; anthropophilic fungi (for example, athlete's foot fungus) are normally adapted to people; and geophilic fungi have the soil as their natural habitat.

Pathogenesis

Dermatophytes normally do not invade, nor can they survive in living tissue. They only parasitize keratinized structures, which include the horny layer (stratum corneum) of the epidermis, the hair, and the claws. Dermatophytes invade hair only in the anagen or growing stage.

When a dermatophyte contacts the skin of an animal, one of several alternatives will ensue. The fungus may be removed mechanically by cleaning or brushing and pose no real concern; it may persist on the skin but be prevented from invading the skin because of host resistance; it may invade the skin, but not produce disease; or it may invade the skin and produce disease. In addition, the fungus must grow downward at a rate greater than the normal desquamation of the epidermis or the organism will be shed.

Dermatophytes can cause cutaneous manifestations in a number of ways:

(1) Dermatophytes can invade the hair shaft and weaken it, making the hair susceptible to breakage.

(2) Metabolic products are produced by fungi. When these soluble, irritant toxins or allergens reach the dermal blood vessels, they cause an inflammatory response which is detrimental to further fungal growth.

(3) An irritant reaction to the metabolic products can occur, resulting in an irritant contact dermatitis manifested by erythema and scaling.

(4) An allergic reaction can occur, with associated edema, suppuration, and necrosis.

(5) The inflammatory reaction to the fungal growth causes hypertrophy of the corneal layer of the hair follicle and epidermal surface (hyperkeratosis), resulting in increased scale formation and plugging of the hair follicle. If bacteria are trapped in the follicle, bacterial folliculitis can develop.

(6) Finally, in some cases, a hypersensitivity reaction known as an "id" reaction, or autosensitization, may be associated with dermatophytosis.

Young, debilitated, or immunocompromised animals appear to be more likely to develop fungal infections. Some circumstantial evidence in cats indicates that certain breeds (especially the Persian) also might be predisposed to fungal infection. Poor nutritional status and contaminated environmental conditions also can be associated with an increased incidence of dermatophytosis.

History

Young dogs and cats often are seen with a history of a slowly progressive focal or multifocal alopecic, proliferative skin disease. Pruritus is variable. Older animals may have chronic dermatoses with variable degrees of alopecia, inflammation, and pruritus. Frequently these cases are characterized by a poor response to antibiotics and corticosteroids. Some animals may have a drug history of long-term immunosuppressive therapy with corticosteroids or chemotherapeutic agents prior to the onset of the fungal disease.

A history of contagion between animals or between animals and humans may be reported and this obviously is important information. A history of human dermatophyte infection while all animals in the same household are asymptomatic also may be revealed. It is important not to jump to the conclusion that any fungal infection must have been contracted from animals. People can contract anthropophilic and geophilic fungi on their own, and can even transmit these infections to animals.

Clinical Signs

Clinical presentation may vary from being asymptomatic, to patchy hair loss (Plates V-1 and V-2), to a papulocrustous eruption, to an exfoliative dermatosis (Plate V-3), to erythematous plaques, and to a suppurative nodular disorder (kerion reaction). The degree of scaling, crusting, and pruritus is extremely variable. In general, *T.*

mentagrophytes causes the most severe inflammatory response on both dogs and cats. *M. gypseum* infection usually is characterized by proliferative hyperkeratotic lesions, mainly about the face and feet. Lesions caused by *M. canis* infection in dogs and cats vary from a mild, alopecic, slightly focal lesion to marked generalized scaling or severe crusting. Onychomycosis is manifested by distorted claws that break easily and grow improperly. The nail bed often is inflamed and painful when palpated.

Dermatophytosis can mimic many other diseases, such as parasitism, bacterial infections, allergies, immunologic diseases, nutritionally related dermatoses, hormonal disorders, some skin cancers, and disorders of keratinization (seborrhea).

Figure 8-1. Distorted hair shaft on direct microscopic examination. Numerous fungal spores and hyphal structures are evident on higher magnification.

Diagnosis

Dermatophytosis can be diagnosed by Wood's lamp evaluation, microscopic examination of hairs, fungal culture, or skin biopsy but cannot be confirmed by visual examination alone.

Wood's Lamp Evaluation. A Wood's lamp uses ultraviolet light filtered through nickel oxide to cause some fungi to glow green in a darkened room. A tryptophan metabolite is the fluorescing material. Only *M. canis* fluoresces (also *M. distortum* and *M. adouinii* in humans), and then only about 50% of the time.

Direct Microscopic Evaluation. The microscopic examination of hairs to identify characteristic spores and hyphae (Fig. 8-1) is a relatively specialized test in animals and is not commonly performed in general veterinary practices. Specimens can be sent to a laboratory and when viewed by an experienced technician, a diagnosis may be rendered about 60 to 70% of the time. The inexperienced may find it difficult to distinguish spores from pigment and hyphae from keratin. In animals, direct microscopic examination can be made with mineral oil alone, potassium hydroxide (KOH), KOH-dimethyl sulfoxide (DMSO), or a solution of KOH, DMSO, and chlorazol fungal stain. This last stain is often helpful in practice because hyphae stain green against a gray background and thus are clearly visible.

Fungal Culture. Fungal cultures on dermatophyte test medium (DTM) are relatively easy to use but the fungi occasionally take up to 2 weeks to grow (although most commence growth in 3 to 7 days). Dermatophytes produce alkaline metabolites which react with the phenol red in the medium to change the color of the medium from yellow to red with the growth of ringworm fungi (Plate V-4). Most contaminants do not grow as fluffy white colonies (Plate V-5) and usually only change the medium from yellow to red after 14 or more days (unless the medium has become heavily contaminated). It is important that hairs be chosen carefully, correctly applied to the medium, and the cap not tightened because dermatophytes are aerobic and need a supply of oxygen. Broken or "sick"-looking hairs are the best choice and are frequently found around the periphery of lesions. One must not put too much material on the medium or contaminants are likely to grow; the material should not be embedded in the medium but gently placed on the surface. Whatever grows and regardless of whether the medium has changed color, any fungal growth should be examined microscopically and identified (Fig. 8-2). This is easily done by taking some transparent tape and touching it to some of the growth and then applying the tape to a clean microscope slide to which has been added either a drop of water or lactophenol cotton blue (Fig. 8-2A–I). Most fungal culture kits provide a guide to the microscopic identification of fungi.

Biopsy. Cutaneous biopsy is sometimes used to diagnose dermatophytosis. Biopsy is indicated if a fungal infection is suspected but no pathogenic growth is obtained on fungal culture, or if a skin condition is not suspected of being fungal and is being biopsied for further diagnostic clues. Although the fungi are often evident on hematoxylin and eosin (H&E) sections, visualization of organisms is facilitated with either periodic acid–Schiff (PAS) or acid Orcein Giemsa (AOG) staining.

Management

Four therapeutic principles must be considered when treating dermatophytosis, including disinfecting the environment, preventing recontamination of the environment, and using topical and systemic fungicides (see Tables 3-2 and 3-12). The aggressiveness of treatment varies with the particular clinical evaluation of each individual animal. Some infections are mild and self-limiting

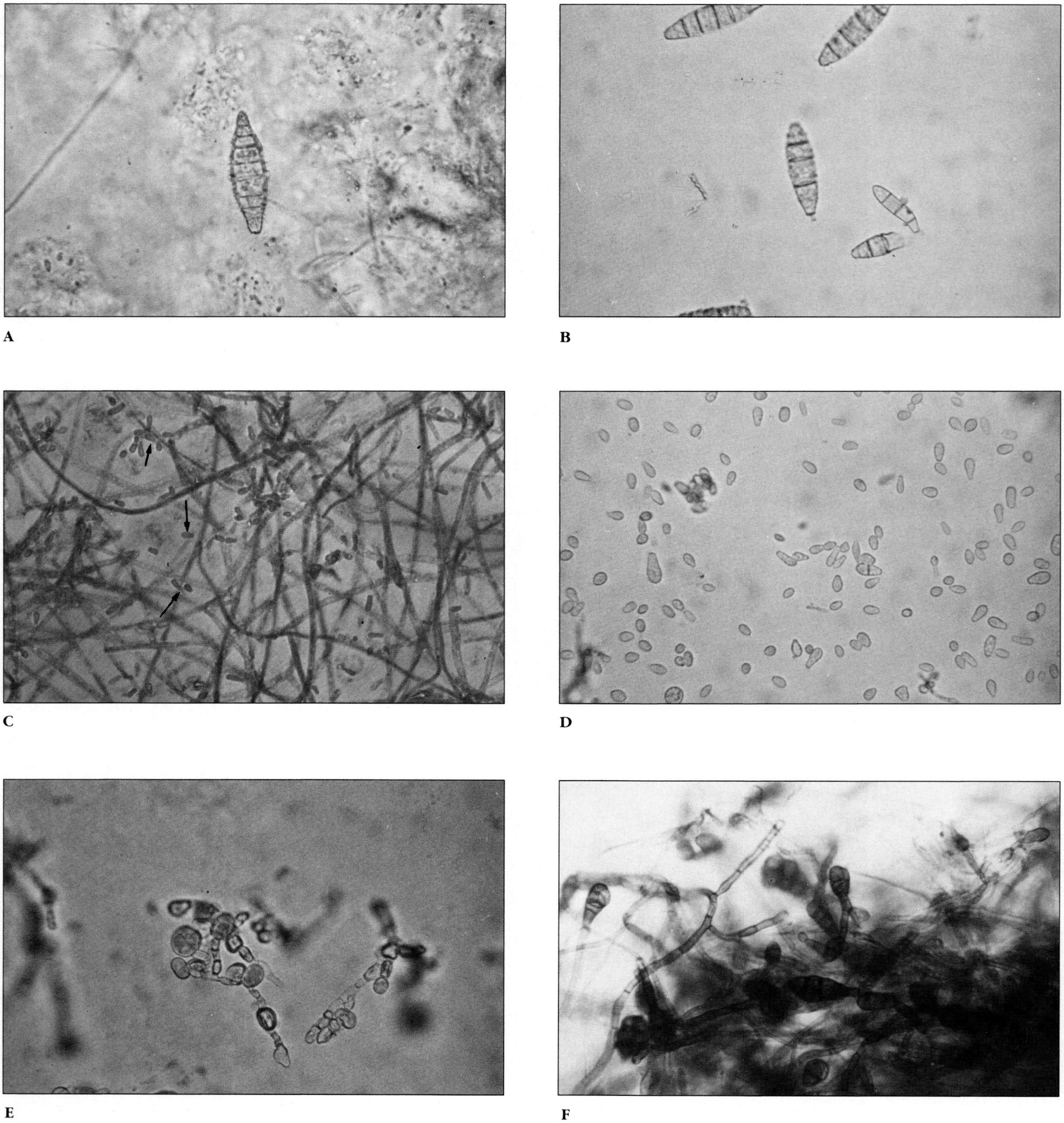

Figure 8-2. Fungal organisms that may be recovered on dermatophyte test medium (DTM). **A**, *Microsporum canis*: macroconidia with a thick wall and more than six cells; **B**, *Microsporum gypseum*: macroconidia with a thin wall and six or less cells; **C**, *Trichophyton mentagrophytes*: tear drop–shaped microconidia (*arrows*); **D**, *Trichophyton terrestre*; **E**, *Epidermophyton floccosum*; **F**, *Alternaria*; **G**, *Aspergillus*; **H**, *Cladosporium*; **I**, *Trichothecium*.

and may spontaneously regress, while others are chronic, debilitating, and respond poorly to therapy.

The environment can be disinfected by using tamed iodine or hypochlorite solutions on all washable surfaces. Furniture and carpets should be vacuumed well, washable bedding should be laundered, and thorough cleaning is recommended. Environmental decontamination is essential because such fungi as *M. canis* can per-

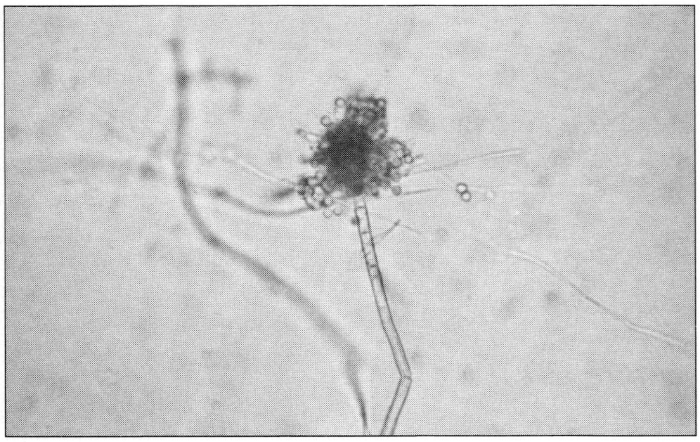

G

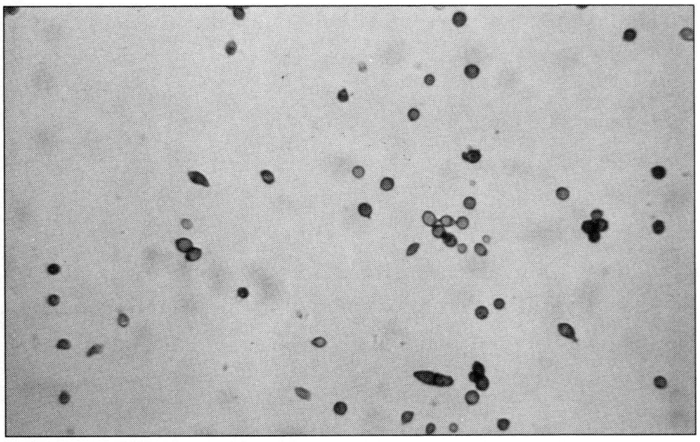

H

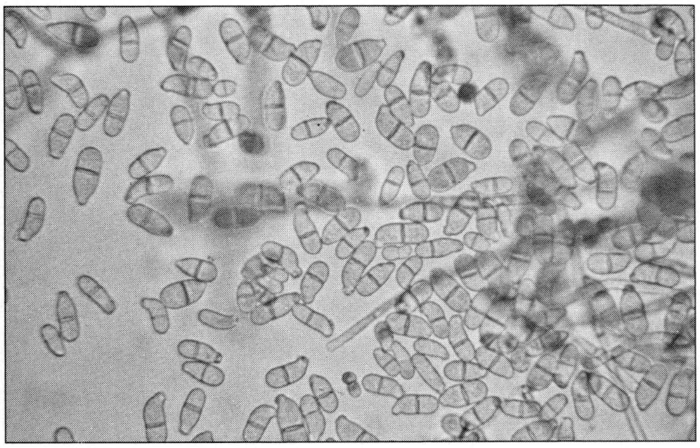

I

sist in the environment for over a year. A new compound, enilconazole (Clinafarm® —Janssen), has recently become available in Europe for environmental cleaning of dog kennels; cats appear to be more susceptible to toxicity with this compound than dogs.

Preventing recontamination of the environment can be partially achieved by frequent vacuuming and disinfecting the environment, by isolating the animals to an area with a washable surface, and by using topical fungicidal agents. Routinely clipping the hair from local lesions and totally clipping the body of dogs and longhaired cats with generalized lesions will help reduce contamination of the environment. Bathing weekly with a tamed iodine, lime sulfur, captan, or chlorhexidine solution is recommended to prevent reinfecting the dog or cat as well as recontaminating the environment. In Europe, enilconazole (Imaverol® —Janssen) can be used as a wash, in a dilution of 1:50 for dermatophyte infections in dogs, on four occasions at 3-day intervals; cats are prone to toxicity. Topical fungicidal agents, such as miconazole, clotrimazole, thiabendazole, cuprimyxin, and ketoconazole, are helpful for treating localized lesions (see Table 3-2).

Griseofulvin (Fulvicin-U/F® —Schering), a fungistatic drug, is the systemic treatment of choice for dermatophytosis (see Table 3-12). Better intestinal absorption of the drug is achieved with the addition of fat to the diet. Griseofulvin may be administered as a microsize form at dosages of 50 to 150 mg/kg daily. An ultramicrosize form of griseofulvin (Gris-PEG® —Dorsey) requires half the dosage and is absorbed without additional dietary fat supplementation. Griseofulvin usually is administered for a period of 6 weeks, but at least until 2 weeks beyond apparent clinical cure. The drug has an unpleasant taste and may cause vomiting in many animals. The product should never be given to pregnant animals because it has been proven to cause birth defects.

More potent antifungals, such as ketoconazole, may be helpful in unresponsive patients. Additional therapies that have not been thoroughly investigated include hyperthermia and immunotherapy.

INTERMEDIATE MYCOSES

Intermediate mycoses are caused by those fungal organisms found in the environment that are considered opportunistic rather than pathogenic and are usually traumatically introduced into the subcutaneous space, inhaled, or ingested. These conditions usually are named for their causative agent (for example sporotrichosis, aspergillosis), their clinical appearance (mycetoma), or their histopathologic presentation (phaeohyphomycosis).

Aspergillosis

Etiologic Factors

Aspergillosis is a rare cause of fungal infection in dogs and cats. Two species, *Aspergillus fumigatus* and *A. flavus*, are among the most common fungi found in the environment. Aspergillosis is frequently listed as a cause of hyalohyphomycosis because of its histopathologic presentation.

Pathogenesis

The respiratory tract is the most common site of infection by *Aspergillus* organisms; other areas of involvement include the eyes and gastrointestinal tract. Involvement of the skin is usually a manifestation of generalized aspergillosis. Aspergilli are considered to be opportunistic invaders, only colonizing traumatized skin or patients that have defective immune systems. Thus, cutaneous infections normally occur following immune suppression caused by disease, drugs, or other causes of debilitation. Such infections are the result of direct contact with the fungal spores. The specific mechanisms involved with the production of lesions vary and depend on predisposing factors, such as immune status, integrity of epidermal barriers, and concurrent disease.

History and Clinical Signs

Aspergillus spores are not uncommon causes of rhinitis and inhalant allergy. With more generalized infections, animals often are examined for a history of sneezing for several weeks, usually accompanied by a nasal discharge. Neurologic signs, weight loss, diarrhea, conjunctivitis, and blepharitis may be seen on physical examination. When *Aspergillus* organisms affect the skin or the mucous membranes of the nose they normally appear as nodules or ulcers and this usually represents a form of the disease in which internal spread may have already occurred.

Diagnosis

The finding of septate hyphae and characteristic conidiophores on examination of direct smears of lesions in KOH preparations supports the diagnosis, but because *Aspergillus* organisms are so common in the environment, a firm diagnosis of aspergillosis requires not only a positive fungal culture but supportive histopathology as well. Specimens for culture should be obtained as aseptically as possible and should normally be grown on Sabouraud's agar rather than dermatophyte test medium because aspergilli are sensitive to the cycloheximide found in DTM.

Ancillary diagnostic tests might include radiography of the skull (increased soft tissue density in affected areas) and serology.

Treatment

No satisfactory treatment exists for generalized cutaneous aspergillosis. Focal lesions can be surgically excised. The nasal form is treated with surgery and amphotericin B. Alternative therapy includes administration of potassium iodide, 5-fluorouracil, nystatin, and thiabendazole (see Table 3-12).

Eumycotic Mycetoma

Etiologic Factors

Eumycotic mycetomas are caused by several different fungi, such as *Curvularia geniculata, Petriellidium (Pseudoallescheria) boydii, Acremonium hyalinum, Madurella* spp., and others.

Pathogenesis

The normal habitat of the fungi is soil or plants. Penetration of the skin usually follows traumatic injury to the extremities. Once the fungi penetrate the subcutaneous tissue, they elicit an inflammatory reaction characterized by swelling, abscessation, fistulous tracts, and the presence of tissue "grains." The fungi can invade deeper into the periosteum.

History and Clinical Signs

The classic triad of clinical signs includes the formation of a nodule (tumefaction), with draining tracts, in which are found "grains" of fungal mycelia. The condition may resemble a chronic abscess that does not respond to antibiotic therapy. Lesions usually are found on the extremities, especially on the feet.

Diagnosis

Wet mounts of crushed granules examined in 10 to 20% KOH reveal hyphae and chlamydospores. The granules should be washed several times in sterile saline solution, crushed, and streaked onto Sabouraud's agar. A biopsy of the lesions may reveal a pyogranulomatous reaction with mycelial elements. The fungi are best demonstrated with PAS, methenamine silver, and Gridley's stains.

Treatment

Eumycotic mycetoma is best treated by radical surgical excision. If left untreated, the infection usually becomes deeper and may involve the muscle and bone.

Phaeohyphomycosis

Etiologic Factors

Phaeohyphomycosis is caused by several different fungi including *Dreschlera spicifera*, *Curvularia* spp., and *Phialophora verrucosa*, which normally invade the subcutaneous tissue without imparting much damage to the epidermis and dermis.

Pathogenesis

The agents responsible for causing phaeohyphomycosis are normal outdoor fungi that usually are traumatically introduced into the subcutaneous fat. The distinguishing feature of the organisms that cause phaeohyphomycosis is pigmentation of hyphae on H&E–stained sections.

History and Clinical Signs

Because phaeohyphomycosis normally results from traumatic inoculation, the condition often presents as a solitary lump that is painless to the touch and may exude pus.

Diagnosis

Diagnosis is accomplished by fungal culture and biopsy. Because these fungi are pigmented, they are easily visualized in routine histopathology sections stained with H&E, methenamine silver, PAS, or Gridley's stains. Fungal cultures on Sabouraud's agar provide identification of the causative organism.

Treatment

The only truly curative treatment is wide surgical excision. Most cases occur on the extremities and thus surgical options may be limited. Amphotericin B or ketoconazole are considered the drugs of choice, although successful treatment is unlikely (see Table 3-12).

Pythiosis (Oomycosis)

Etiologic Factors

Pythiosis results from infection with a member of the genus *Pythium* (formerly *Hyphomyces destruens*), itself a member of the Protista rather than a fungus. Many early cases initially diagnosed as phycomycosis were actually cases of pythiosis.

Pathogenesis

Pythium spp., of the class Oomycetes, live in warm, wet environments, which thereby limits their distribution preferentially to the southeastern United States. *Pythium* has aquatic motile zoospores which are the presumed infective stage. Pythiosis can cause cutaneous or gastrointestinal disease.

History and Clinical Signs

Animals with subcutaneous pythiosis normally present with a papulonodular dermatitis, induration, ulceration, and often draining fistulous tracts. The clinical presentation is essentially indistinguishable from zygomycosis.

Diagnosis

Diagnosis of pythiosis relies on histopathologic evaluation and culture on blood or Sabouraud's dextrose agar. Cultural identification normally requires an experienced mycologist because sporulation is not evident with standard cultural techniques and may be reported simply as a phycomycete. Histopathologic evaluation is most likely to render a diagnosis. Hyphae are not readily apparent with H&E preparations, are enhanced by Gomori's methenamine silver, and can often be confirmed by an indirect peroxidase technique.

Treatment

Wide surgical excision is the treatment of choice for pythiosis. Medical treatment with amphotericin B and ketoconazole (see Table 3-12) is rarely effective, a reflection of the fact that *Pythium* is a member of the kingdom Protista rather than a fungus. Another option being evaluated is immunotherapy with autogenous products.

Prognosis

The prognosis varies according to how amenable the lesion is to complete surgical removal. Generalized systemic spread has been reported.

Sporotrichosis

Sporotrichosis is caused by a dimorphic soil saprophyte, *Sporothrix schenckii*. The saprophytic form exists in nature and the parasitic form is an oval or elongated budding yeast in the tissues. Sporotrichosis has been reported as a zoonotic infection transmissible from cats to people, and must be treated as an important public health concern.

Pathogenesis

The fungus usually penetrates the skin after a traumatic injury that breaks the epidermal barrier; there also have been reports of infection caused by inhalation or ingestion of the fungus. The saprophytic form lives in the soil, on plants, in water, and on small insects, and is commonly found in warm, moist climates.

After entrance of the organism, tissue invasion occurs with penetration into the subcutis and often into the lymphatic vessels, with subsequent spread to the regional lymph nodes. Further spread may occur by way of the lymphatics from the regional lymph nodes to most organs of the body. The fungus elicits a chronic inflammatory response with shallow cutaneous ulcers, nodules, and granulomas.

Clinical Signs

Sporotrichosis is characterized by three distribution patterns: cutaneous, cutaneolymphatic, and disseminated. The skin lesions include firm, round, tender nodules and crusted ulcers in the subcutis associated with a traumatized site (Plate V-6). A thick, brownish-red exudate may be present. Often the nodules are found along the lymphatics. The regional lymph nodes may be swol-

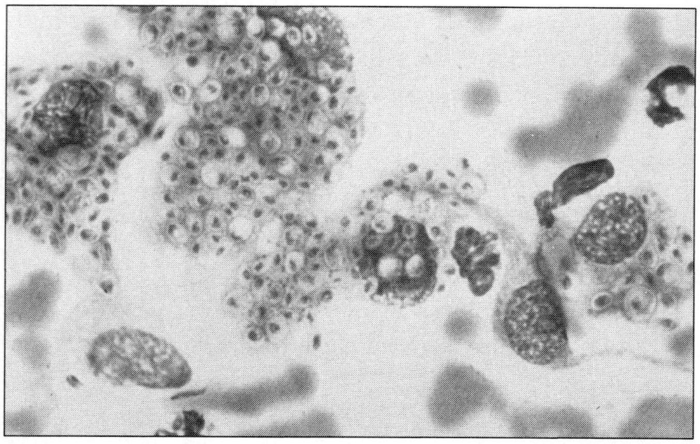

Figure 8-3. *Sporothrix schenckii*: Direct smear of exudate from sporotrichosis lesion with numerous phagocytized yeast bodies (high power). (Courtesy of Nita Gulbas, Phoenix, Arizona)

len and ulcerative. In both dogs and cats the disseminated form may be seen with involvement of many organs, especially the lungs and liver.

Diagnosis

Aspirates of unopened lesions should be used for fungal culture, plated on Sabouraud's agar at 30 °C (86 °F), and kept at 37 °C (98.6 °F), which maximizes the mold and yeast phases. The yeast phase may be observed in direct smears of exudate, impression smears of tissue, or in microscopic sections from biopsy specimens using special fungal stains (Fig. 8-3).

Treatment

The treatment of choice for sporotrichosis is either sodium iodide or ketoconazole (see Table 3-12). A new antifungal, itraconazole, may also have applications in the treatment of sporotrichosis. A good response from animals with the cutaneolymphatic form is expected within 30 days; however, to prevent relapse, therapy should be continued for an additional 3 to 4 weeks. When treating with sodium iodide one must always be alert to the possibility of iodine toxicity, which usually is manifested by a dry coat, discharge from the nose and mouth, vomiting, depression, and occasionally cardiac collapse. Potassium iodide can also be given orally as a form of therapy.

Prognosis

The ultimate prognosis varies with the form of sporotrichosis, with the disseminated form having the worst outcome, despite therapy. When treating cats, it is important to remember the public health implication of their disease.

Zygomycosis

Etiologic Factors

Zygomycosis and *phycomycosis* were terms once used synonymously but it is now appreciated that phycomycosis encompasses two quite different etiologies (zygomycosis and pythiosis), so both are discussed independently. Infection by zygomycetes can result from organisms belonging to the order Mucorales (*Mucor, Rhizopus, Absidia*) or Entomophthorales (*Conidiobolus, Basidiobolus*).

Pathogenesis

Organisms causing zygomycosis can enter the system either through injury to the skin or via the digestive tract. Depending on the route of infection animals may have cutaneous and/or gastrointestinal symptoms.

History and Clinical Signs

Animals with zygomycosis may have systemic signs of vomiting, diarrhea, and weight loss, or strictly cutaneous manifestations of ulcers, nodules, and draining tracts. A regional lymphadenomegaly frequently is present.

Diagnosis

The diagnosis is made by finding broad, nonseptate hyphae in tissues or in tissue samples. Absolute identification requires fungal culture.

Treatment

To date all forms of therapy for this condition have been disappointing, although amphotericin B would probably be considered the drug of choice.

SYSTEMIC MYCOSES

Systemic mycoses are characterized by primary pulmonary infection with subsequent dissemination to other organs. The pulmonary infection may be subclinical and resolve without clinical signs. Inhalation is the route by which most infections are acquired. Although systemic mycoses are not considered contagious between animals and humans, a zoonotic potential exists in that the infective form (spores) can occur in secretions (such as cutaneous discharges or sputum).

Blastomycosis

Etiologic Factors

Blastomycosis is caused by *Blastomyces dermatitidis*, a dimorphic fungus endemic to areas drained by rivers in the eastern United States and parts of southern Canada.

Pathogenesis

In nature, the fungus is in the mycelial or saprophytic phase, which requires high humidity. Pulmonary infection occurs after inhalation of spores, and dissemination to the skin, eyes, and bone can occur by way of the blood or lymphatic vessels. Many animals are exposed to *Blastomyces* organisms but it is presumed that altered immune function, especially cell-mediated, appears to predispose to dissemination of the disease.

History and Clinical Signs

It is assumed that most cases of blastomycosis are subclinical and resolve spontaneously. Animals with the disseminated form of blastomycosis are affected with a chronic debilitating disease beginning with respiratory signs that are frequently followed by eye, bone, and skin lesions. Young animals appear to be predisposed and the hunting breeds are overrepresented. Clinical signs include pyrexia, emaciation, lethargy, coughing, dyspnea, and anorexia. Lymphadenomegaly is common, and draining lesions associated with lymph nodes may be evident. Skin lesions seen most frequently include nodular disorders of the skin and subcutaneous tissues (Plate V-7), abscesses, ulcers, and draining tracts.

Diagnosis

History of concurrent respiratory, skin, and eye lesions in an endemic blastomycosis area is suggestive. Specific diagnostic tests include direct smears of lesions demonstrating the large, thick-walled budding yeasts (5 to 20 μm in diameter) with double-contoured walls (Fig. 8-4) and cutaneous biopsies showing a pyogranulomatous reaction associated with the budding yeasts.

A tentative diagnosis can be reached on the basis of clinical findings, radiography, high complement fixation titers, and a positive agar-gel immunodiffusion (AGID) test. With complement fixation tests, cross-reactions between histoplasmosis and blastomycosis do occur. Isolation of the fungus on culture is diagnostic but growth is slow and the material poses a public health concern.

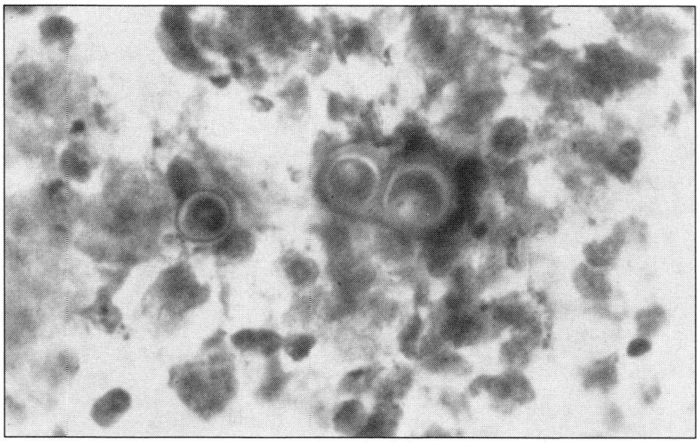

Figure 8-4. *Blastomyces dermatitidis*: Large thick-walled budding yeasts with double-contoured walls, seen on cytology. (Courtesy of Patrick McKeever, University of Minnesota, Minneapolis)

Treatment

Treatment is most often attempted with ketoconazole or amphotericin B (see Table 3-12).

Coccidioidomycosis

Etiologic Factors

Coccidioidomycosis (valley fever) is caused by the dimorphic fungus *Coccidioides immitis*, which is endemic to the arid Sonoran life zone of the southwestern United States and Mexico.

Pathogenesis

Coccidioides immitis exists in nature in the mycelial form. In tissue, it is a large, thick-walled spherule with endospores. The mycelial form grows in the soil during periods of rainfall. Infection then occurs by inhalation of spores associated with dust and other fomites, especially during dry periods of the year. Altered cellular immunity is believed to be a predisposing factor to dissemination of coccidioidomycosis.

History and Clinical Signs

The disease often remains localized to the respiratory system, and often resolves spontaneously. Only occasional generalization of the process is seen with dissemination to bones, eyes, and skin.

Coccidioidomycosis usually is seen in younger animals or those that are immunocompromised for one reason or another. Intermittent respiratory signs usually are observed before there is evidence of lesions. Episodes of coughing and intermittent pyrexia, anorexia, dyspnea, listlessness, weight loss, and lymphadenopathy with drainage of the lymph nodes often are reported. Lameness is common in the disseminated form.

Cutaneous lesions associated with coccidioidomycosis include ulcers, abscesses, nodules, and draining tracts. Abscesses and ulcers (Plate V-8) are most common in cats while granulomatous nodules are more common in dogs.

Diagnosis

A positive diagnosis of coccidioidomycosis can be made by cytology, biopsy, or fungal culture. Cytologic or histopathologic demonstration of thick-walled refractile spherules containing endospores are diagnostic (Fig. 8-5). Fungal cultures are time-consuming and create a potential public health hazard.

A presumptive diagnosis of coccidioidomycosis can be made with suggestive radiography, high complement fixation titers, or an AGID test in an animal with history of exposure to an endemic area. Early in the course of the disease, the AGID test usually is positive and the complement-fixation test is negative. With early active infection, both tests are positive. Later in the disease, the AGID test becomes negative while the complement-fixation test remains positive for many months.

Treatment

Coccidioidomycosis is best treated with ketoconazole, although intravenous amphotericin B is an alternative (see Table 3-12). Dosages are variable, with bone and brain lesions requiring higher doses and longer treatment.

Cryptococcosis

Etiologic Factors

Cryptococcosis is caused by a soil-borne fungus, *Cryptococcus neoformans*, which has a worldwide distribution. The fungus is associated with soil contaminated by excreta of bats, pigeons, and other birds.

Pathogenesis

The yeast form of *C. neoformans* is found in nature as well as in the tissue. It is 5 to 15 μm in diameter and surrounded by a polysaccharide capsule. Infection is attributed primarily to inhalation and in addition to respiratory symptoms, the fungi can spread to the skin, central nervous system, bone, and other areas. The means of dissemination is primarily by the blood and lymphatic vessels. Direct extension from the oropharynx has been suggested. Animals with an altered immune system may be predisposed to infection. Infection is seen more commonly in cats than in dogs.

History and Clinical Signs

The history often includes a chronic course of multiple facial lesions (nodules, ulcers, crusting) that are unresponsive to antibiotics and corticosteroids. The clinical signs are variable but skin lesions are normally found around the head or in the mouth or nose (Plate V-9). Central nervous system signs, such as incoordination or blindness, may be evident and herald a poorer prognosis.

Diagnosis

The diagnosis of cryptococcosis is confirmed by cytology, histopathology, and fungal culture. The large mucoid capsule of the cryptococcal organisms is often visible on impression smears (Fig. 8-6) and the addition of a few drops of diluted India ink to an air-dried slide facilitates visualization of the organisms. The organism remains unstained with India ink, and is silhouetted against a dark background. Fungal culture can also confirm a diagnosis but is slow and presents a potential public health concern. For suspected infection in cats, the cryptococcal antigen latex agglutination test is a very sensitive and specific diagnostic test for cryptococcosis.

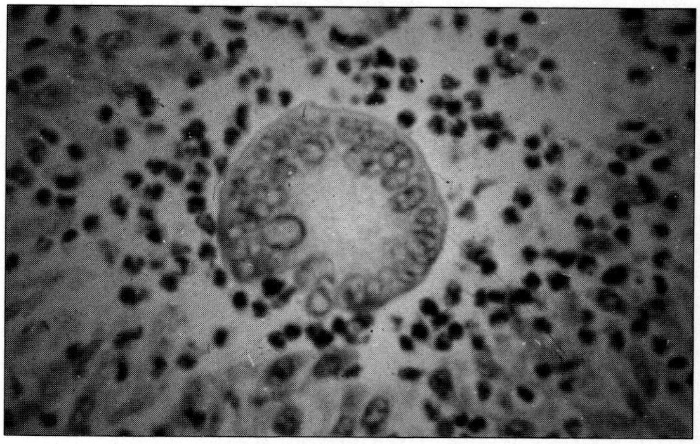

Figure 8-5. *Coccidioides immitis*: Spherules with endospores in an aspiration biopsy of a lymph node (high power). (Courtesy of Robert Wilkins, Cenvet Laboratories, New York, New York)

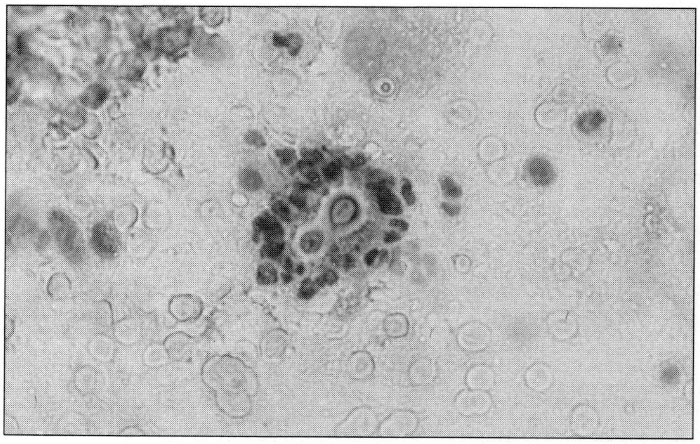

Figure 8-6. *Cryptococcus neoformans*: Budding yeast in a direct smear of exudate (high power). (Courtesy of Robert Wilkins, Cenvet Laboratories, New York, New York)

Treatment

Cryptococcosis is best treated with either ketoconazole or amphotericin B (see Table 3-12).

Histoplasmosis

Etiologic Factors

Histoplasmosis is caused by *Histoplasma capsulatum*, a dimorphic fungus most prevalent around the Great Lakes, Appalachian mountains, and the Mississippi, St. Lawrence, and Ohio river valleys. It has a worldwide distribution.

Pathogenesis

Histoplasma is found in nature in the mycelial or saprophytic form. It is often associated with soil contaminated by bird or bat feces. Infection occurs when small microaleuriospores are inhaled into the lungs, where they transform into tiny, intracellular oval bodies found within cells of the reticuloendothelial system. Dissemination from the lungs is uncommon, but when it does oc-

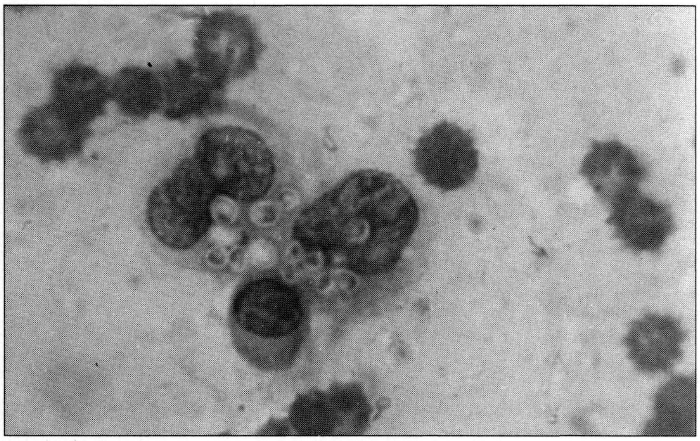

Figure 8-7. *Histoplasma capsulatum*: Yeast phase phagocytized by macrophages in aspiration biopsy of a lymph node (high power). (Courtesy of Robert Wilkins, Cenvet Laboratories, New York, New York)

cur the intestinal tract usually is involved. Dissemination to the skin occurs occasionally by way of the lymphatic or blood vessels.

History and Clinical Signs

Most animals with histoplasmosis have a history of chronic respiratory disease or chronic large bowel diarrhea. The clinical signs include chronic cough, gradual weight loss, persistent or intermittent diarrhea, lethargy, and anorexia. The skin lesions, which are uncommon, include cutaneous nodules, ulcers, abscesses, and fistulous tracts.

Diagnosis

The diagnosis of histoplasmosis is based on identifying the yeast within reticuloendothelial cells from lymph nodes or transtracheal aspirates or biopsies from gut, lung, or skin (Fig. 8-7). Organisms occasionally are found in peripheral blood cells. Fungal culture is also diagnostic but is a slow process and presents potential public health concerns. Serologic tests are supportive. Chronic pulmonary histoplasmosis is clinically and radiographically indistinguishable from blastomycosis.

Treatment

Histoplasmosis is best treated with ketoconazole or intravenous amphotericin B (see Table 3-12).

SELECTED READINGS

Ackerman LJ: Cutaneous coccidioidomycosis. *Proceedings of the Arizona Veterinary Specialists Seminar*, May 10-11, 1989, pp 12–13.

Ackerman LJ: Feline cryptococcosis. *Compend Contin Educ Pract Vet* 10:1049–1055, 1988.

Ackerman LJ: *Practical Canine Dermatology*. Goleta, CA, American Veterinary Publications, 1989, 369 pp.

Ackerman LJ: *Practical Feline Dermatology*. Goleta, CA, American Veterinary Publications, 1989, 264 pp.

Angarano DW, Scott DW: Use of ketoconazole in treatment of dermatophytosis in a dog. *JAVMA* 190:1433–1434, 1987.

Armstrong PJ, DiBartola SP: Canine coccidioidomycosis: A literature review and report of eight cases. *JAAHA* 19(6):937–946, 1983.

Beale KM, Pinson D: Phaeohyphomycosis caused by two different species of *Curvularia* in two animals from the same household. *JAAHA* 26(1):67–70, 1990.

Carakostas MC, Miller RI, Gossett KA: Clinical laboratory evaluation of deep mycotic diseases in dogs. *J Small Anim Pract* 25:687–693, 1984.

Clinkenbeard KD, Wolf AM, Cowell RL, Tyler RD: Feline disseminated histoplasmosis. *Compend Contin Educ Pract Vet* 11:1223–1233, 1989.

Chester DK: Superficial fungal infection of the skin. *Compend Contin Educ Pract Vet* 1(12):910–916, 1979.

Coyle V, Isaacs JP, O'Boyle DA: Canine mycetoma: A case report and review of the literature. *J Small Anim Pract* 25:261–268, 1984.

Ford RB: Canine histoplasmosis. *Compend Contin Educ Pract Vet* 2(8):637–642, 1980.

Jackson JA: Immunodiagnosis of systemic mycoses in animals: A review. *JAVMA* 188(7):702–705, 1986.

Kwochka KW, Calderwood Mays MB, Ajello L, Padhye AA: Canine phaeohyphomycosis caused by *Dreschlera spicifera*: A case report and literature review. *JAAHA* 20(4):625–633, 1984.

Legendre AM, Walker M, Buyukmihci N, Stevens R: Canine blastomycosis: A review of 47 clinical cases. *JAVMA* 178(11):1163–1168, 1981.

Medleau L, Greene CE, Rakich PM: Evaluation of ketoconazole and itraconazole for treatment of disseminated crptococcosis in cats. *Am J Vet Res* 151(9):1454–1458, 1990.

Miller PE, Miller LM, Schoster JV: Feline blastomycosis: A report of three cases and literature review (1961 to 1988). *JAAHA* 26:417–424, 1990.

Noxon JO, Monroe WE, Chinn DR: Ketoconazole therapy in canine and feline cryptococcosis. *JAAHA* 22(2):179–183, 1986.

O'Neill Foil CS, Short BG, Fadok VA, Kunkle GA: A report of subcutaneous pythiosis in five dogs and a review of the etiologic agent *Pythium* spp. *JAAHA* 20(11):959–966, 1984.

Pyle RL, Dunbar M, Nelson PD, et al: Canine blastomycosis. *Compend Contin Educ Pract Vet* 3(11):963–974, 1981.

Rachofsky MA, Chester DK, Conroy JD, Read WK: Sulfone-responsive subcorneal vesiculopustular dermatitis with characteristics of an id reaction in a dog. *JAAHA* 25(4):405–408, 1989.

Sharp N, Burrell MH, Sullivan M, Cervantes-Olivares RA: Canine nasal aspergillosis: Serology and treatment with ketoconazole. *J Small Anim Pract* 25:149–158, 1984.

Stampley AR, Barsanti JA: Disseminated cryptococcosis in a dog. *JAAHA* 24:17–21, 1988.

Troy GC: Canine phycomycosis: A review of twenty-four cases. *Calif Vet* 39(2):8–11, 1985.

COLOR PLATES

PLATE I

I-1. Acute atopic dermatitis: Alopecia, diffuse erythema, and excoriation of axillae and ventral thorax.

I-2. Periorbital distribution of hair loss, erythema, and scaling in a dog with inhalant allergies.

I-3. Lichenification and hyperpigmentation associated with chronic allergic disease.

I-4. Reactions seen 15 to 30 minutes after intradermal allergy testing in an allergic dog. (Reprinted from Ackerman LJ: Inhalant allergies. *Pet Focus* 1:4–9, 1989, with permission)

I-5. Feline allergic dermatitis associated with airborne allergens: Facial alopecia and excoriations.

I-6. Acute allergic contact dermatitis: Diffuse erythema of the ventral abdomen.

I-7. Facial swelling and erythema associated with an adverse food reaction in a Chinese shar pei.

I-8. Erosions, ulcerations, and excoriations associated with beef hypersensitivity in a cat. (Reprinted from Ackerman LJ: Food hypersensitivity: A rare, but manageable disorder. *Vet Med* 83:1142–1148, 1988, with permission)

I-9. Hair loss, erythema, and excoriations associated with fleabite hypersensitivity in a dog.

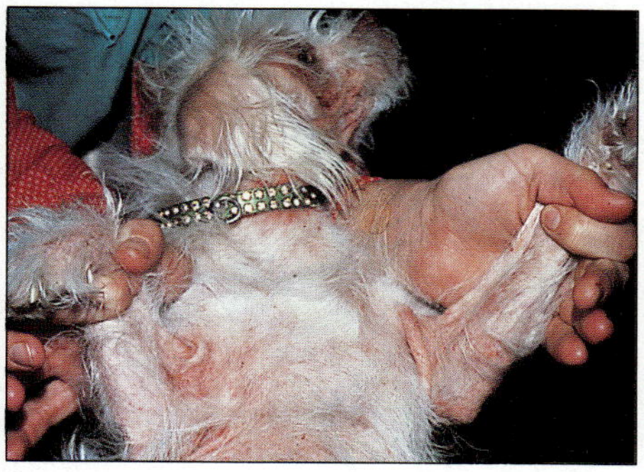
I-1

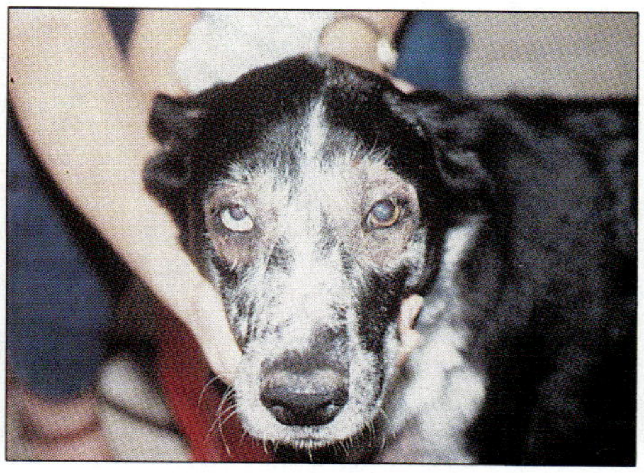
I-2

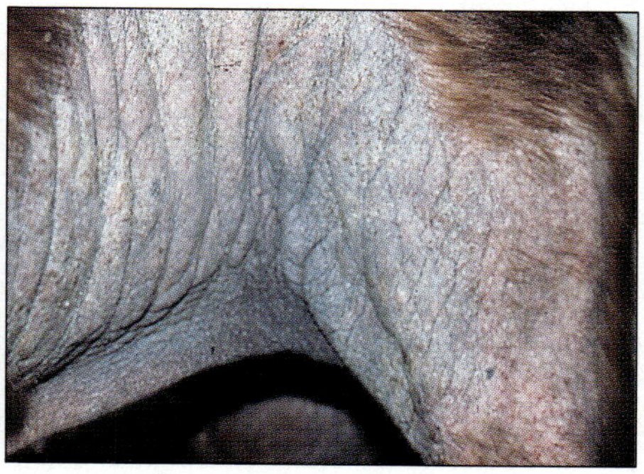
I-3

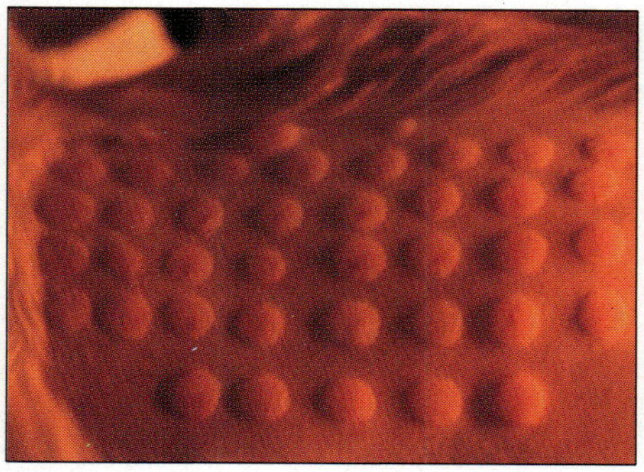
I-4

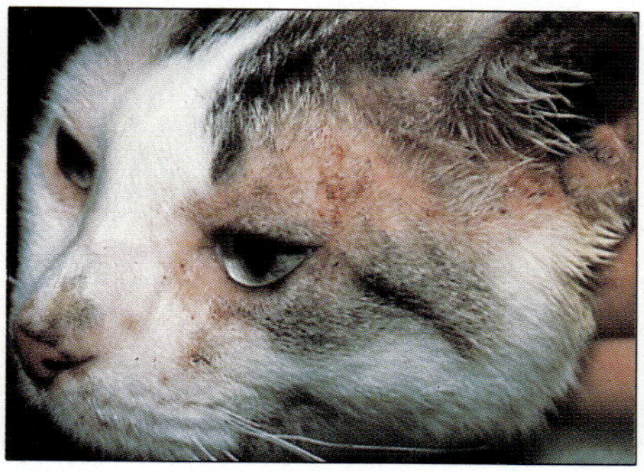
I-5

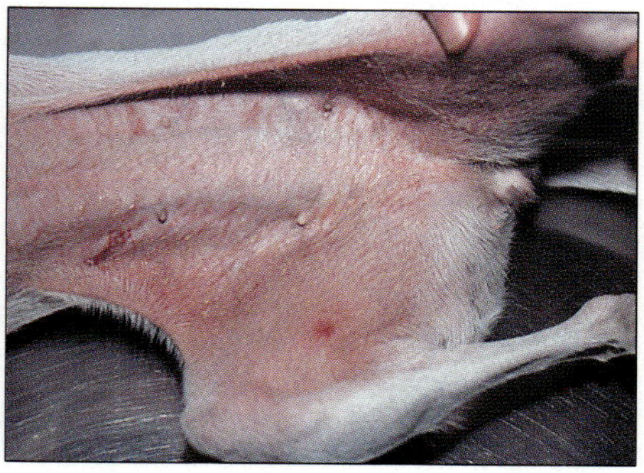
I-6

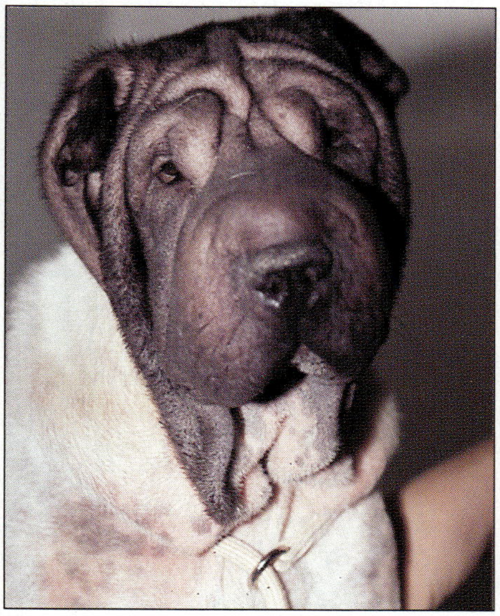
I-7

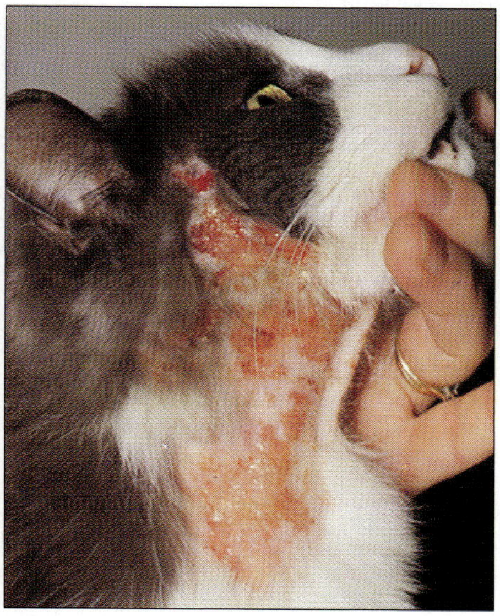
I-8

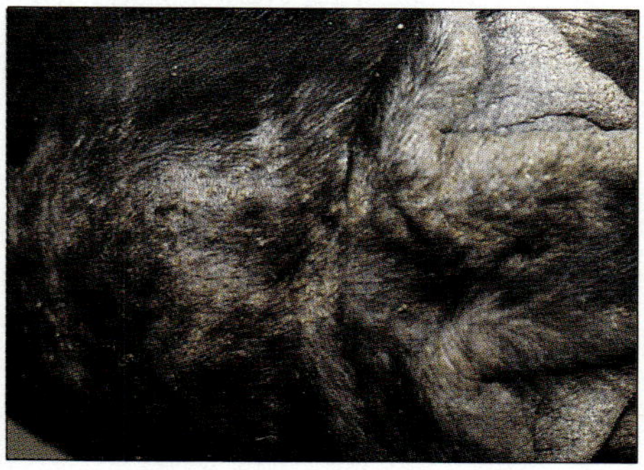
I-9

PLATE II

II-1. Systemic lupus erythematosus: Pronounced facial ulceration.

II-2. Cutaneous (discoid) lupus erythematosus: Hypopigmentation and ulceration of the planum nasale and anterior muzzle of a dog.

II-3. Pemphigus vulgaris: Crusting at the mucocutaneous junction.

II-4. Pemphigus foliaceus: Diffuse alopecia, excoriation, and crusting of the dorsal muzzle, anterior face, and medial pinnae of a dog.

II-5. Bullous pemphigoid: Ulceration on the ventrum of a dog.

II-6. Drug eruption: Adverse reaction to tetracycline resulting in ulceration of the footpad.

II-7. Toxic epidermal necrolysis: Dorsal crusting associated with total epidermal necrosis in a linear pattern.

II-8. Juvenile cellulitis: Erythema, induration, and erosions in a young dog.

II-9. Sterile pyogranuloma: Interdigital dermatitis of an immune-mediated nature.

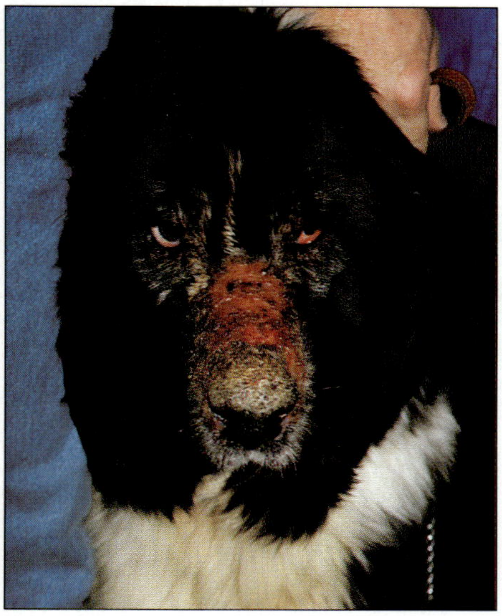

II-1

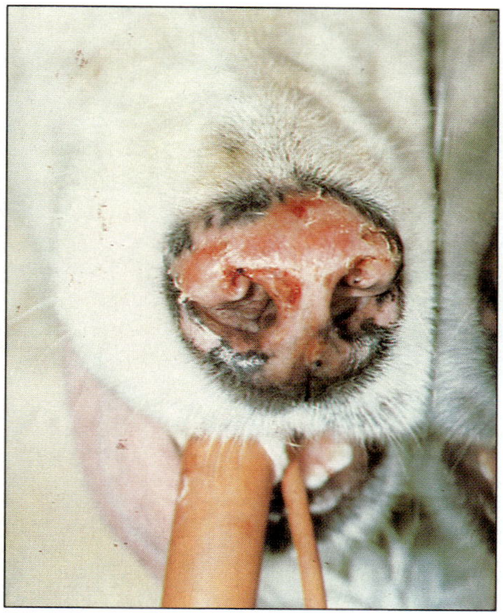

II-2

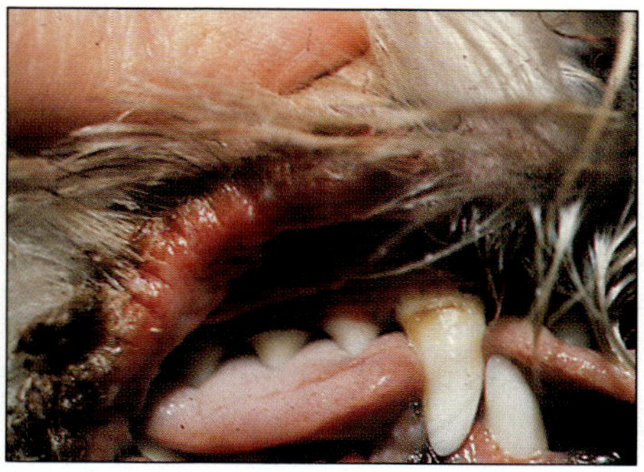

II-3

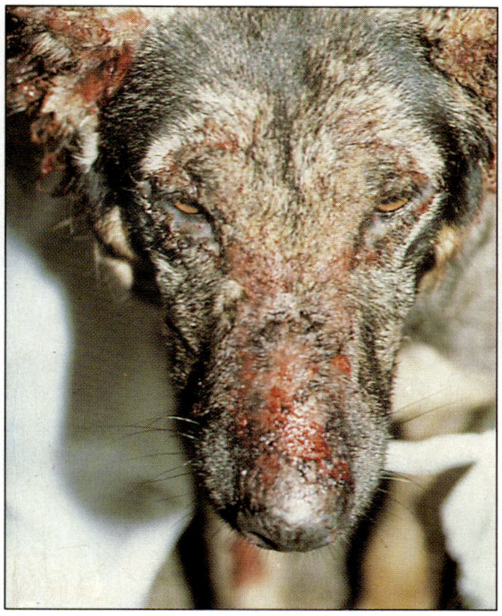

II-4

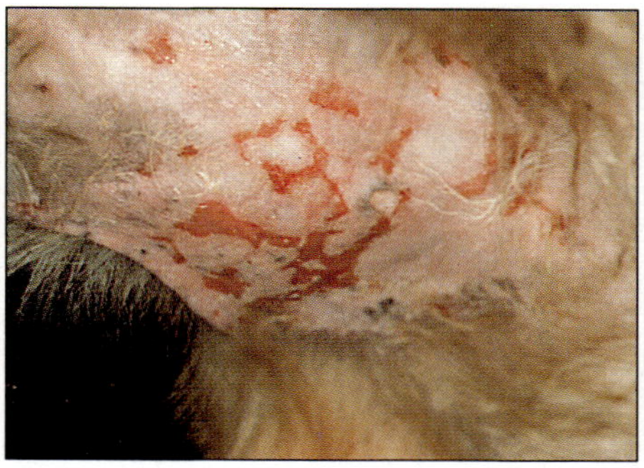

II-5

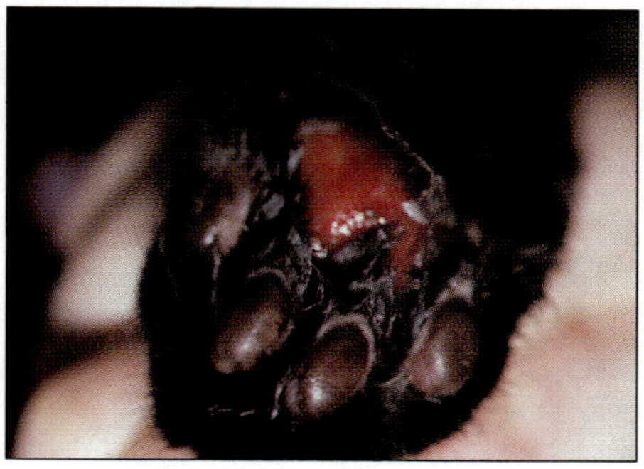

II-6

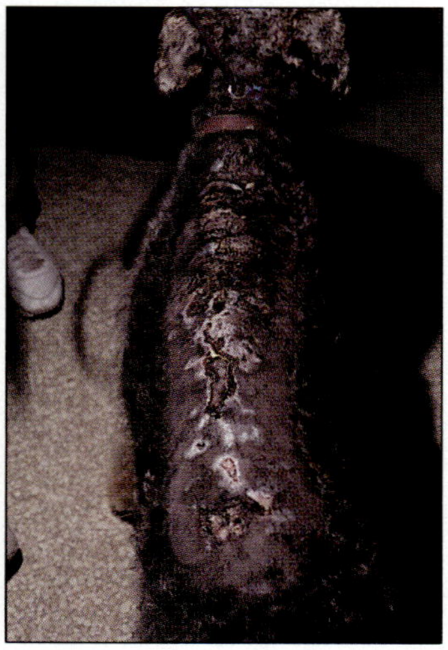

II-7

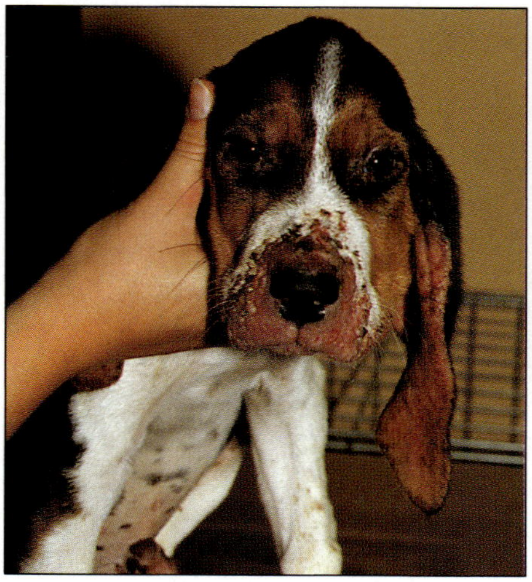

II-8

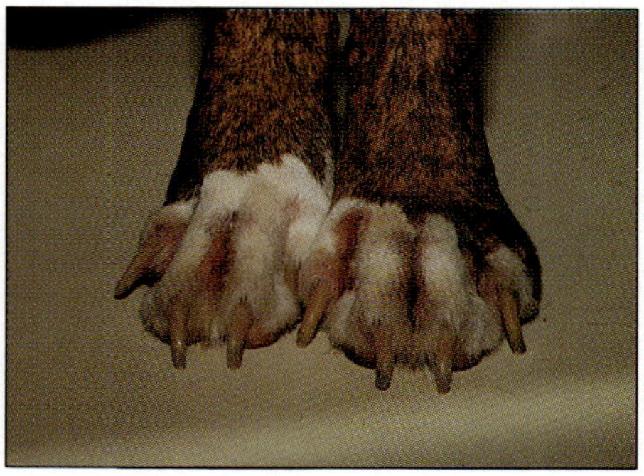

II-9

PLATE III

III-1. Flea dermatitis: Adult flea on an alopecic patch of dorsal caudal back.

III-2. Flea dermatitis: Multifocal, erythematous papules on the ventral abdomen.

III-3. Sarcoptic mange: Severe diffuse crusting of the face of a 3-month-old dog.

III-4. Notoedric mange: Diffuse alopecia with scales and crusts on the head and dorsal neck of a cat. (Courtesy of Tom Willemse, State University of Utrecht, Utrecht, The Netherlands)

III-5. Cheyletiellosis: Mild dandruff on the dorsum of a cat.

III-6. Generalized demodicosis: Patchy alopecia, hyperpigmentation, and focal excoriation with crusts on the face and neck of a 4-year-old dog.

III-7. Generalized demodicosis: Diffuse alopecia and erythema of the foot of a 6-month-old dog.

III-8. Adult *Rhipicephalus* ticks feeding in the ear of a dog. (Reprinted from Lewis T: Ticks and associated diseases. *Pet Focus* 1:21–23, 1989, with permission)

III-9. Myiasis: Multifocal ulcers after the removal of larvae from the lesions on the dorsal caudal back of a dog.

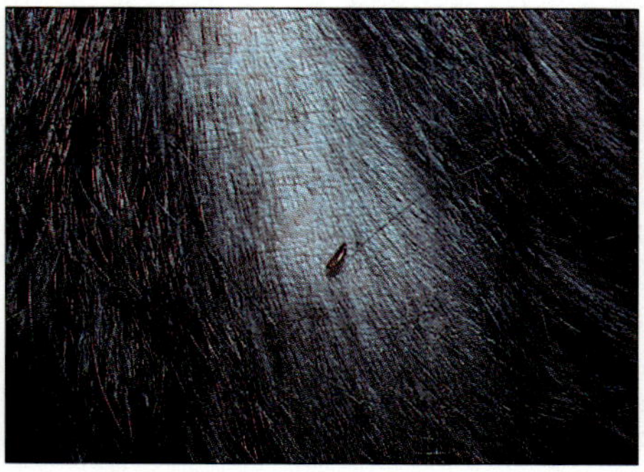
III-1

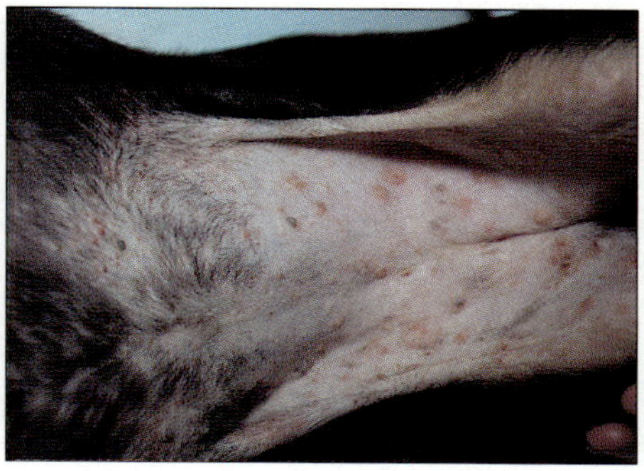
III-2

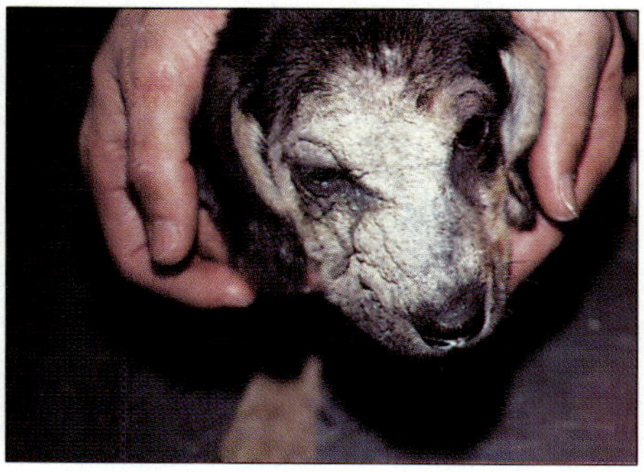
III-3

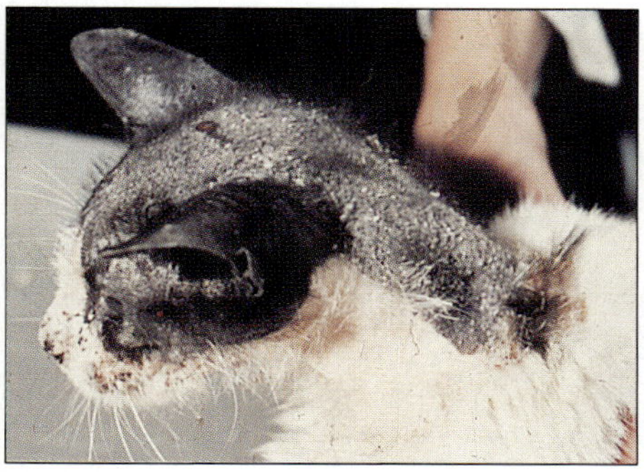
III-4

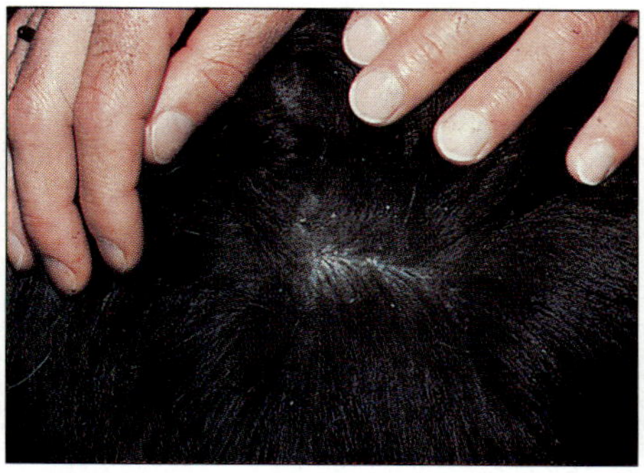
III-5

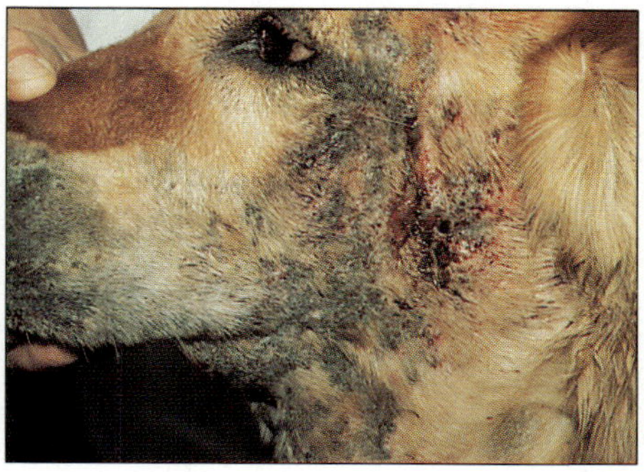
III-6

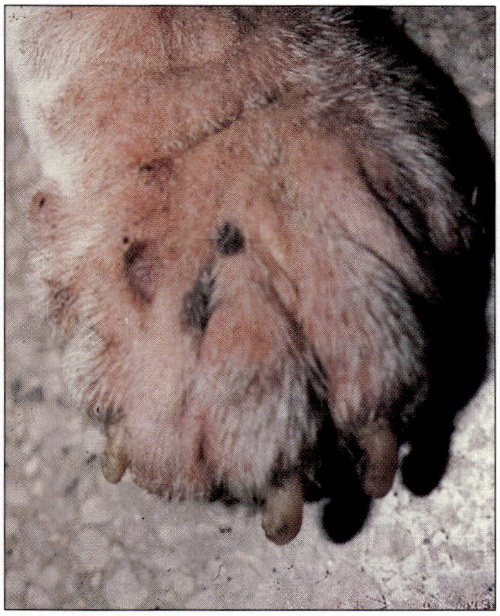
III-7

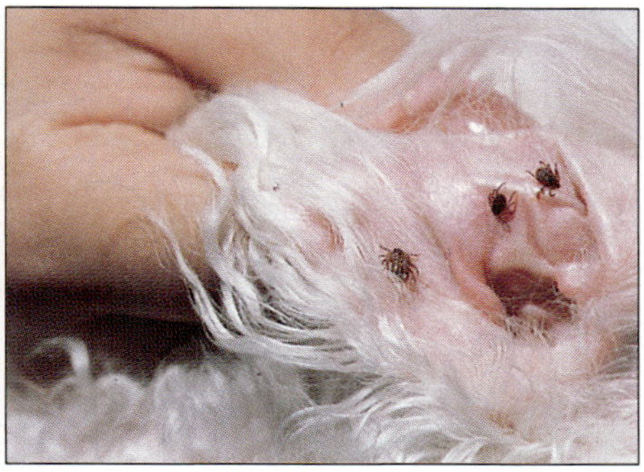
III-8

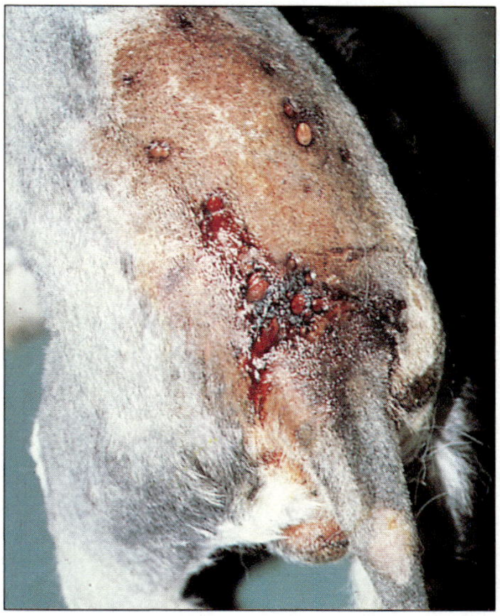
III-9

PLATE IV

IV-1. Pyotraumatic dermatitis: Erosion, erythema, and hair loss.

IV-2. Lip fold pyoderma: Focal erythema and erosion on the lower lip.

IV-3. Superficial folliculitis: Erythematous papules and pustules on the ventrum of a dog.

IV-4. Deep pyoderma: Generalized multifocal ulceration on the trunk associated with furunculosis.

IV-5. Cellulitis: Ulceration and swelling associated with a deep infection.

IV-6. Perianal pyoderma: Multiple fistulous tracts dorsolateral to the anus.

IV-7. Bacterial granuloma: Chronic nodular dermatitis associated with impaired resistance to staphylococcal infection.

IV-8. Actinomycotic mycetoma: Chronic induration, ulceration, and fistulation resulting from nocardiosis in a cat.

IV-9. Atypical mycobacteriosis: Nodular facial dermatitis in a cat.

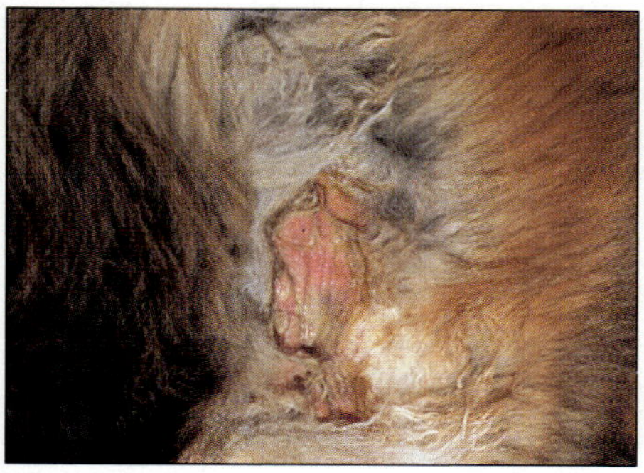
IV-1

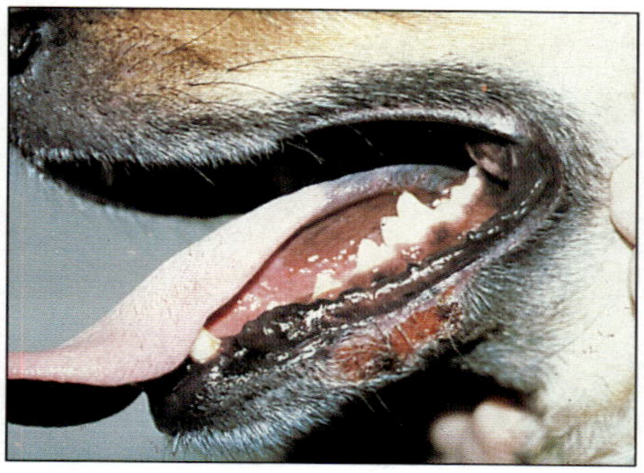
IV-2

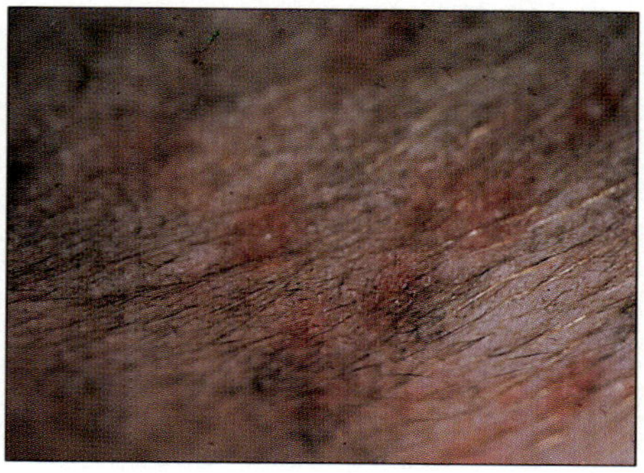
IV-3

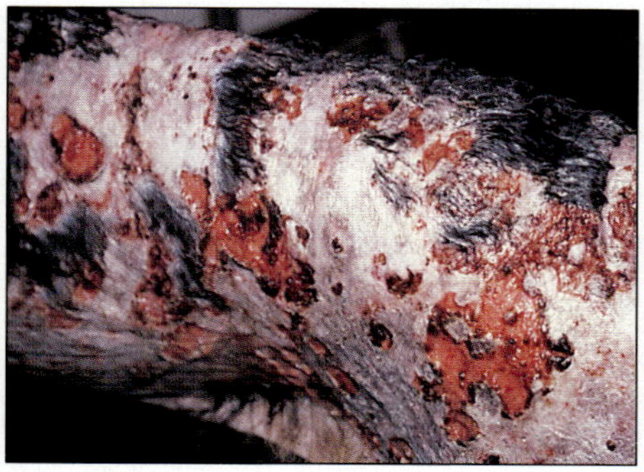
IV-4

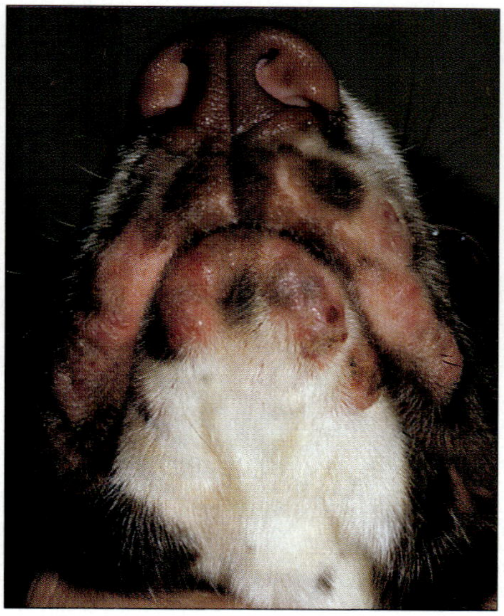
IV-5

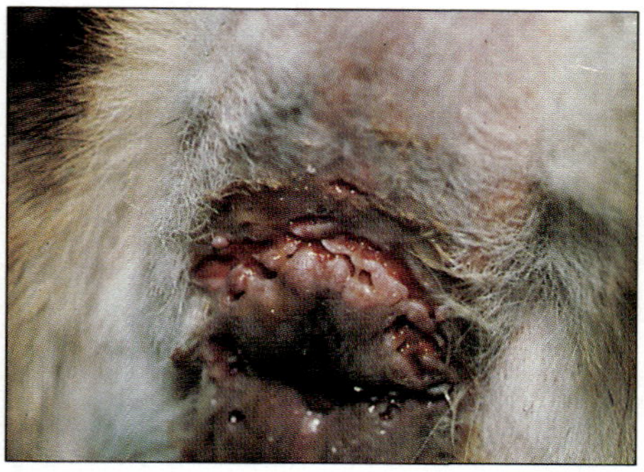
IV-6

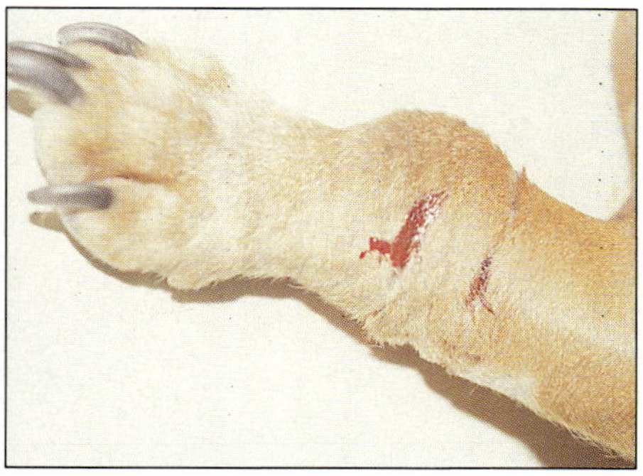
IV-7

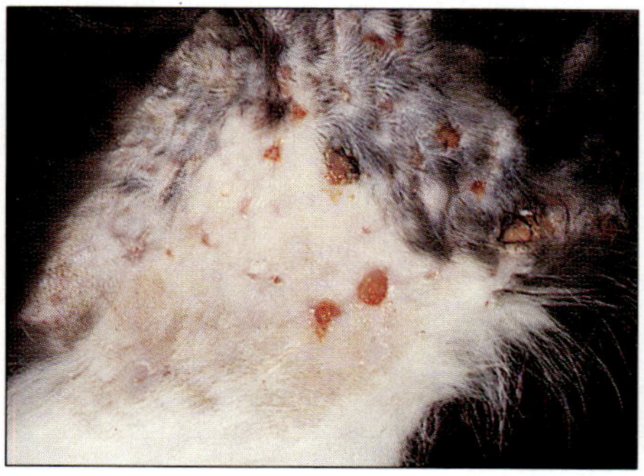
IV-8

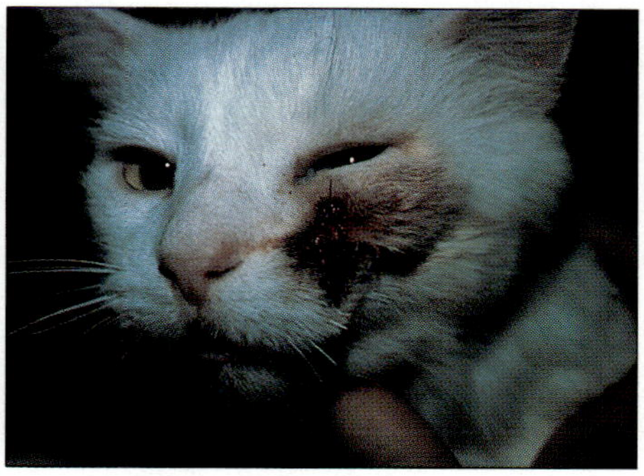
IV-9

PLATE V

V-1. Dermatophytosis: *Microsporum gypseum* infection with alopecia and mild erythema of the dorsal head, neck and shoulders of an adult dog.

V-2. Dermatophytosis: *Microsporum canis* infection causing hair loss and scaling on the dorsum of the head of a kitten.

V-3. Dermatophytosis: Scaling and hair loss as the only clinical signs in a cat.

V-4. Positive culture of a dermatophyte showing a white fluffy colony that turns the dermatophyte test medium red.

V-5. Contaminant growth on dermatophyte test medium in which the medium is red but the colony is not fluffy and white.

V-6. Sporotrichosis: Multiple subcutaneous ulcerated nodules and crusting on the distal extremities of a cat. (Courtesy of Nita Gulbas, Phoenix, Arizona)

V-7. Blastomycosis: Granulomatous nodule on the lateral surface of the foot of a dog. (Courtesy of Al Legendre, University of Tennessee, Knoxville)

V-8. Coccidioidomycosis: Ulceration and fistulation on the head of a cat.

V-9. Cryptococcosis: Multiple ulcerated granulomatous nodules on the face of a cat. (Courtesy of Nita Gulbas, Phoenix, Arizona)

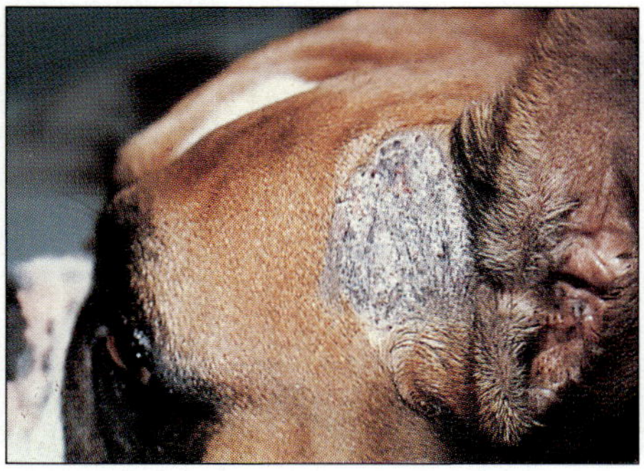

V-1

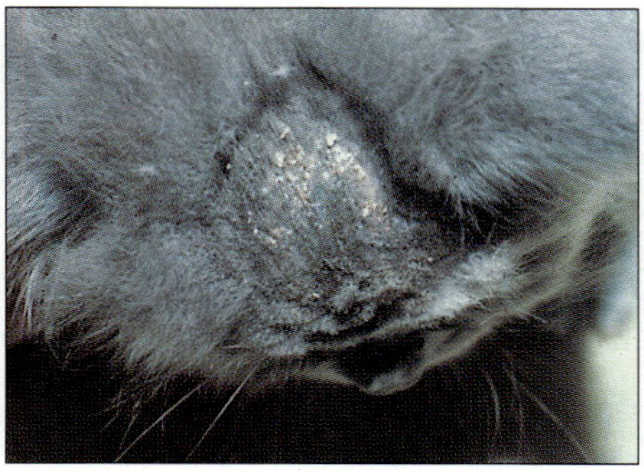

V-2

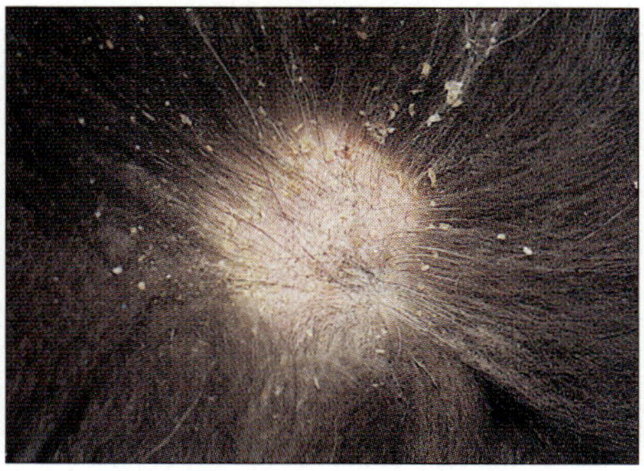

V-3

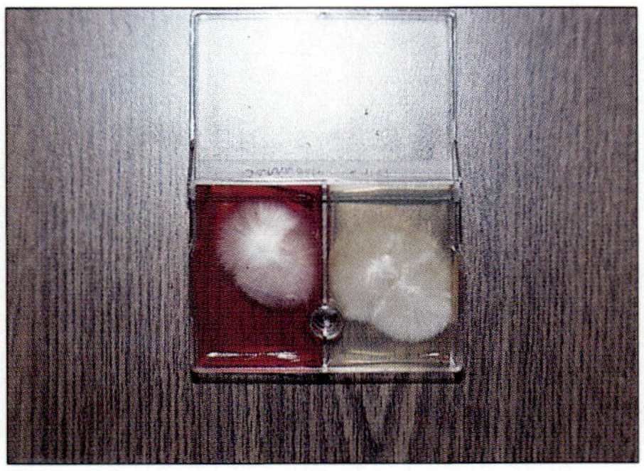

V-4

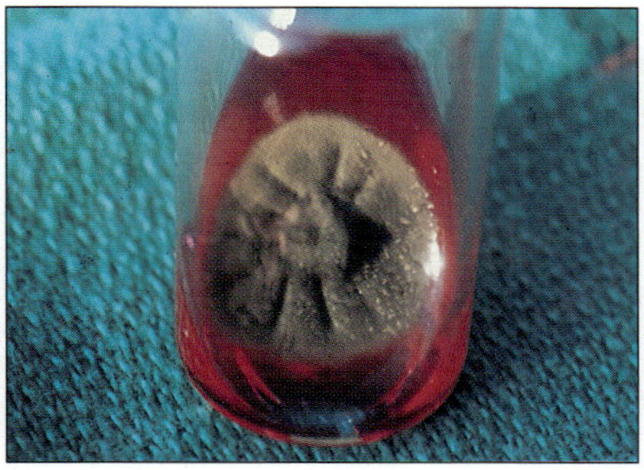

V-5

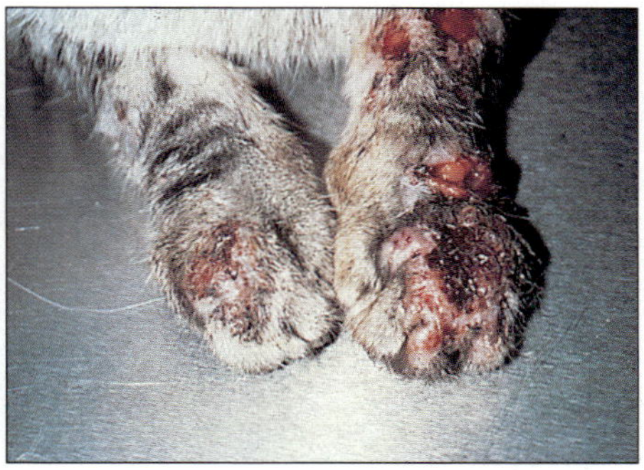

V-6

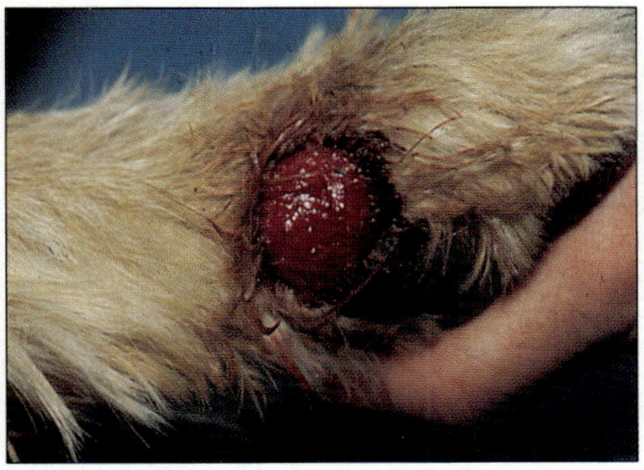

V-7

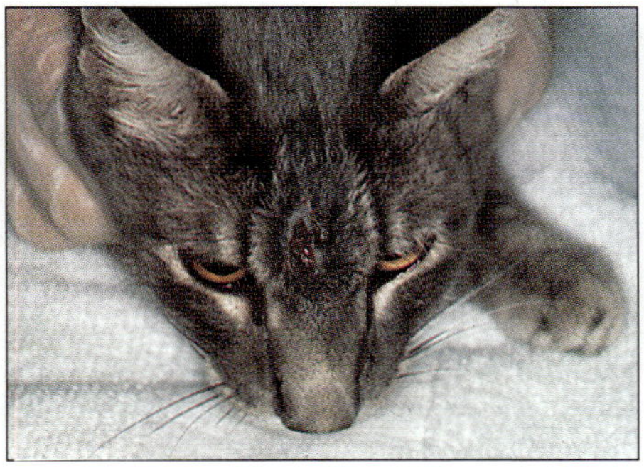

V-8

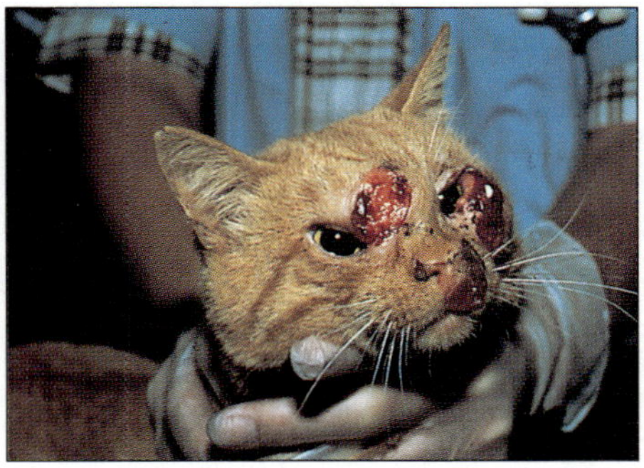

V-9

PLATE VI

VI-1. Hypothyroidism: Multifocal patches of hair loss and folliculitis.

VI-2. Hypothyroidism: Diffuse alopecia of perineum and posterior thighs of a dog.

VI-3. Hyperadrenocorticism: Total truncal alopecia and hyperpigmentation.

VI-4. Hyperadrenocorticism: Calcinosis cutis presenting as erythematous plaques in a dog.

VI-5. Pituitary dwarfism: 4-year-old German shepherd cross that had a progressive thinning of the haircoat and lethargy.

VI-6. Growth hormone-responsive dermatosis: Bilaterally symmetrical hair loss and intense hyperpigmentation.

VI-7. Hyperestrogenism: Partial alopecia and moderate hyperpigmentation of the perineum and posterior thigh of an intact female dog.

VI-8. Hypoestrogenism: Diffuse alopecia of ventrum and abnormally soft, smooth skin of a spayed Weimaraner.

VI-9. Male feminizing syndrome: Bilaterally symmetrical alopecia, hyperpigmentation, and pendulous prepuce in a dog with a testicular Sertoli cell tumor.

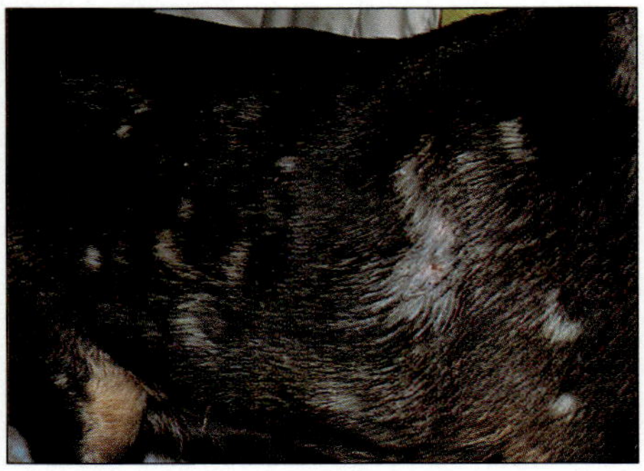
VI-1

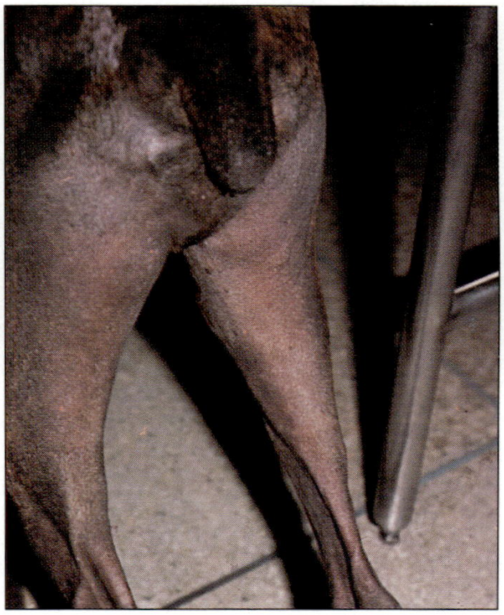
VI-2

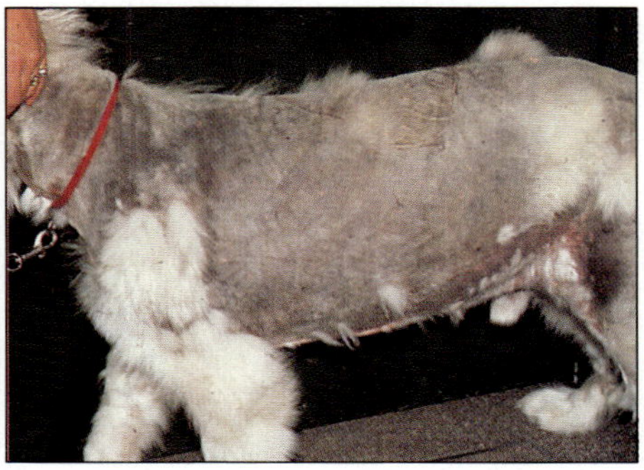
VI-3

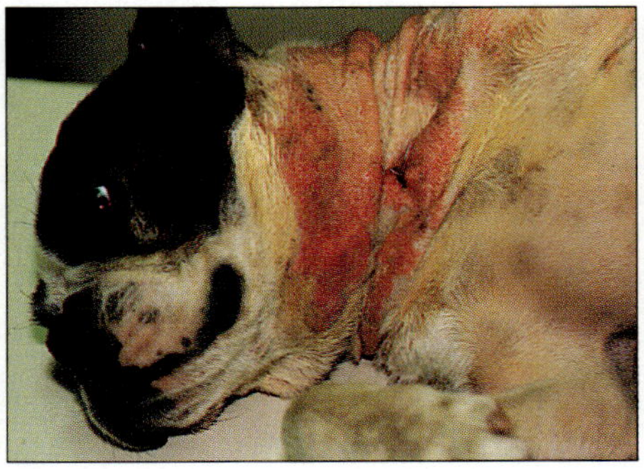
VI-4

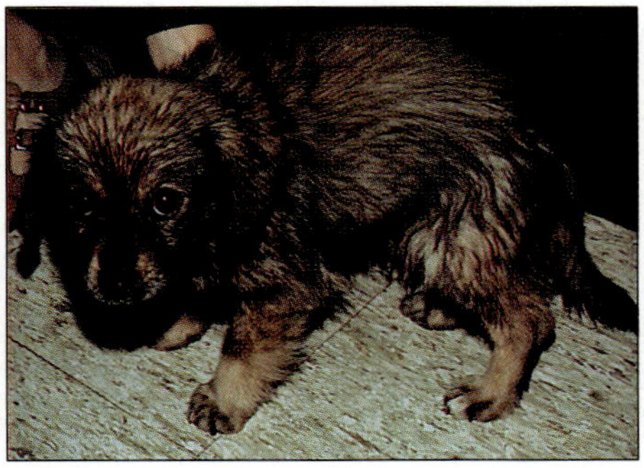
VI-5

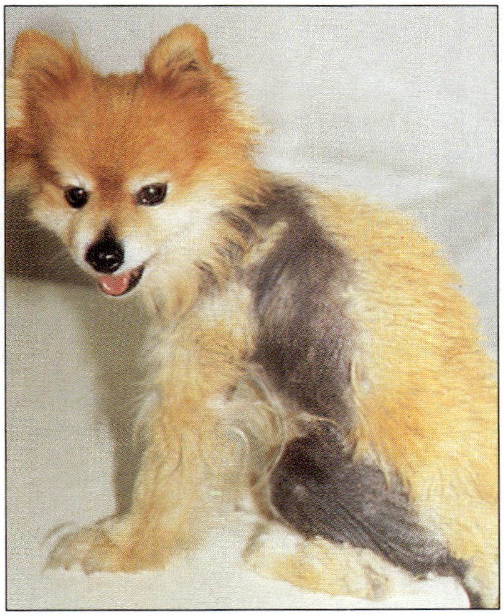
VI-6

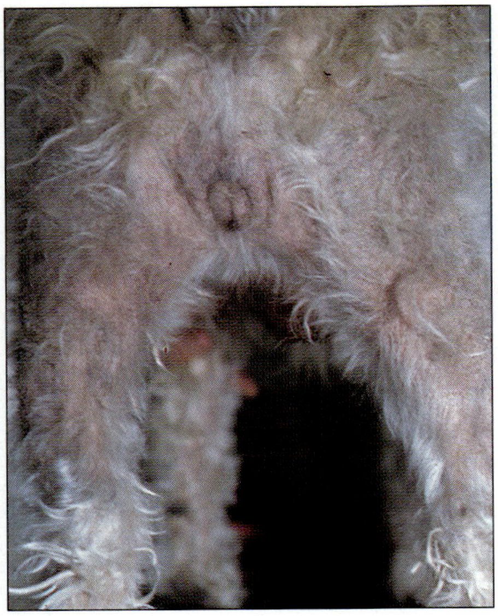
VI-7

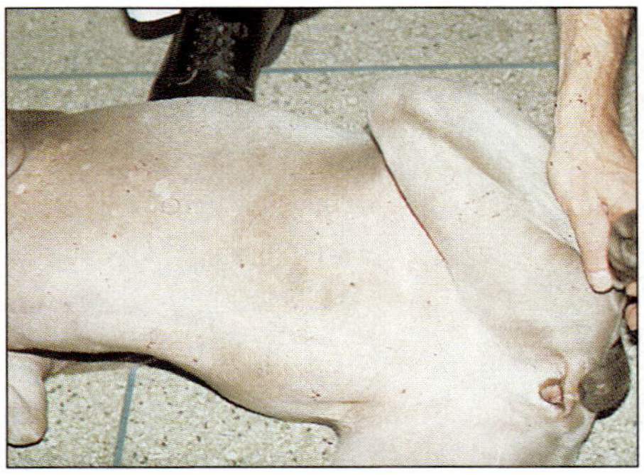
VI-8

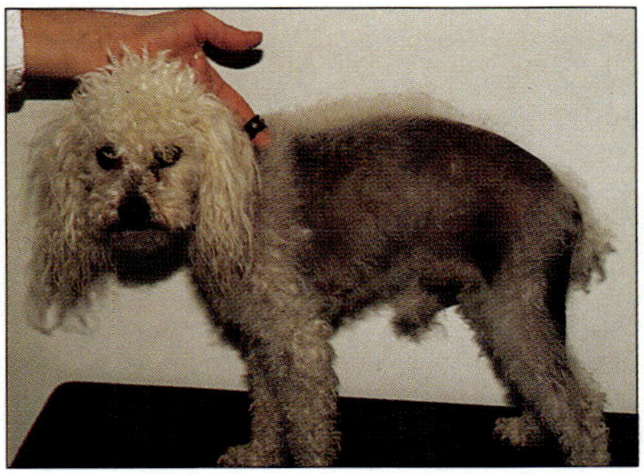
VI-9

PLATE VII

VII-1. Epidermal dysplasia: Extensive hair loss, exfoliation, and erythema in a young dog.

VII-2. Ichthyosis: Marked exfoliative dermatitis in a young dog with suspected ichthyosis. (Reprinted from Ackerman LJ: A new approach to dermatologic diagnosis in the dog. *Vet Focus* 1:6–11, 1989, with permission)

VII-3. Zinc-responsive dermatosis: Footpad hyperkeratosis and erythema.

VII-4. Periappendageal dermatitis: Marked erythroderma and hair loss.

VII-5. Footpad hyperkeratosis. Increased thickness of stratum corneum of the footpads.

VII-6. Psoriasiform-lichenoid dermatitis: Papulonodular dermatitis with plaques in a springer spaniel. (Reprinted from Ackerman LJ: A new approach to dermatologic diagnosis in the dog. *Vet Focus* 1:6–11, 1989, with permission)

VII-7. Follicular dysplasia: Hair loss on the head and ears of a young Doberman pinscher.

VII-8. Canine acne: Alopecia and comedones on the ventral chin accompanied by focal erythematous ulceration and furunculosis.

VII-9. Feline acne: Comedone formation on the anterior ventral chin. Note crust secondary to trauma at the posterior aspect of the lesion.

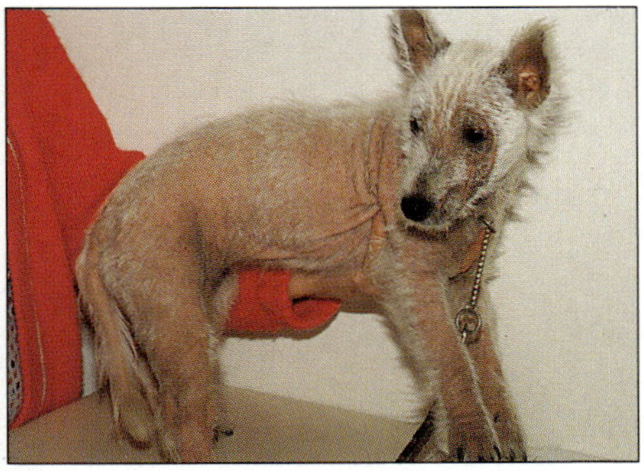
VII-1

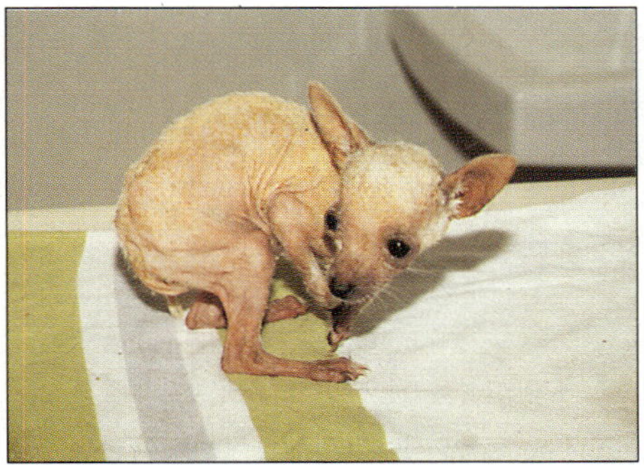
VII-2

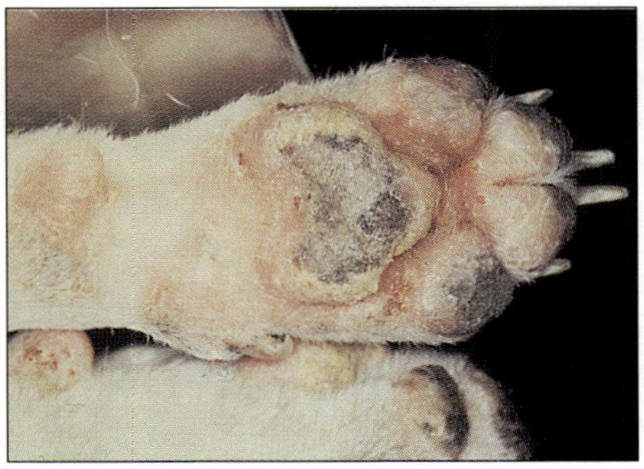
VII-3

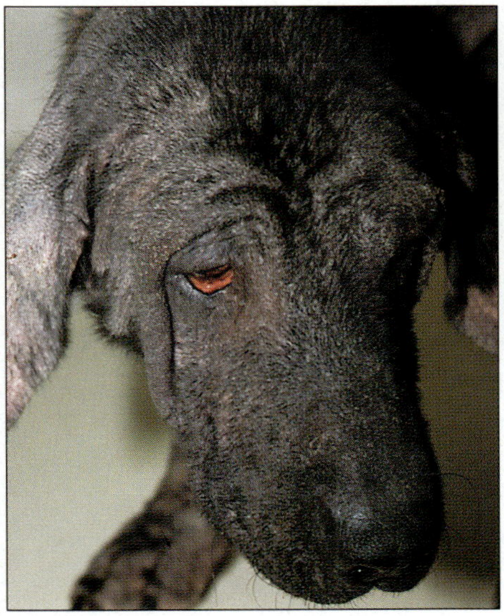
VII-4

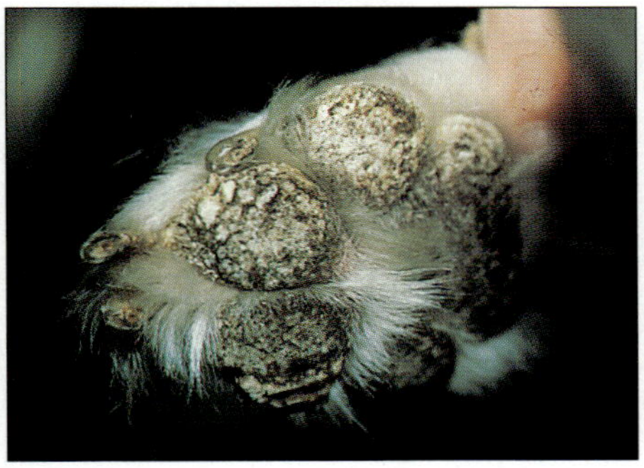
VII-5

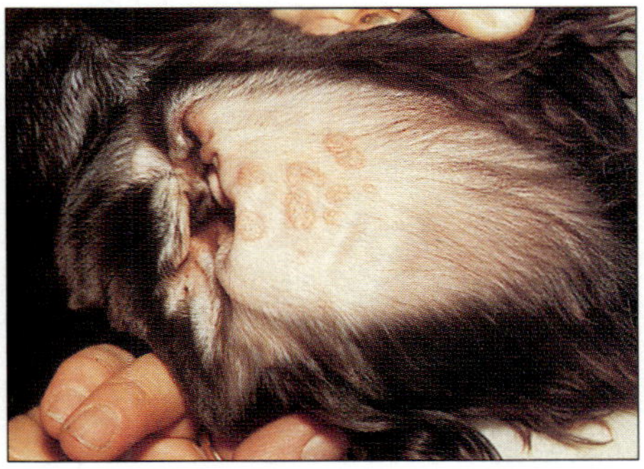
VII-6

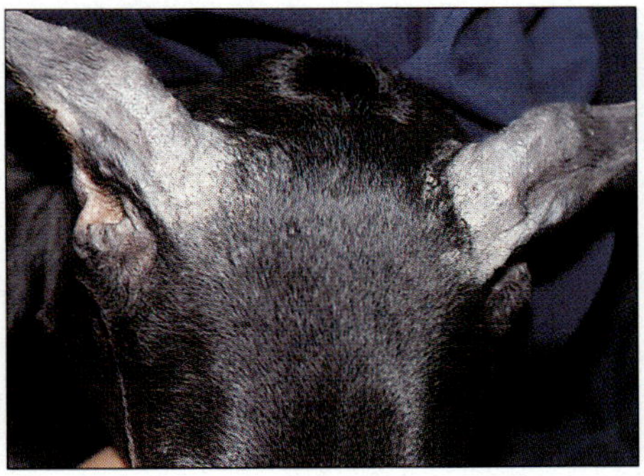
VII-7

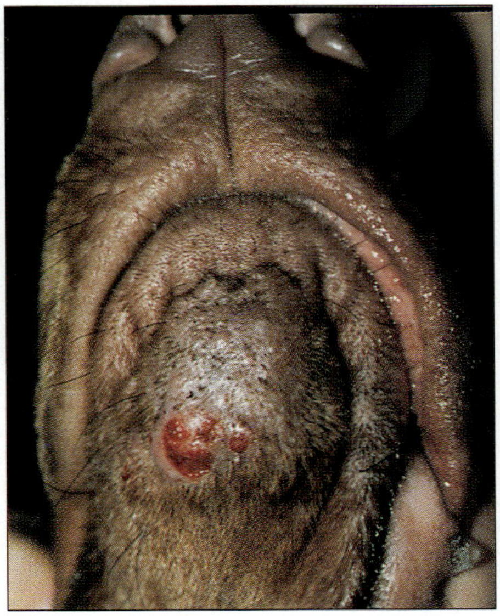
VII-8

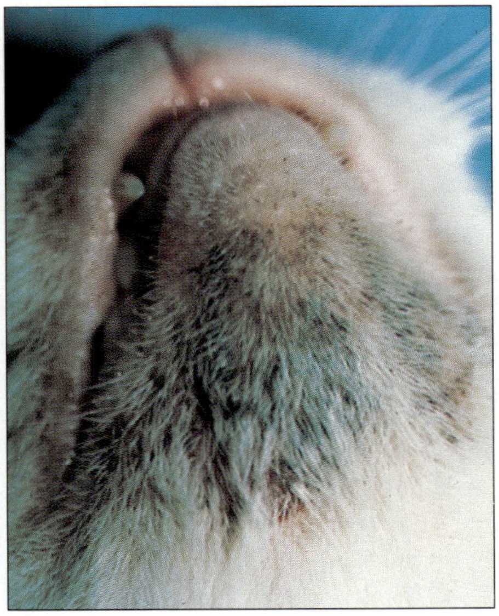
VII-9

PLATE VIII

VIII-1. Basal cell tumor: Solitary, circumscribed tumor with a smooth, glistening surface on the leg of a dog.

VIII-2. Sebaceous gland hyperplasia: Discrete lobulated tumor approximately 5 mm in diameter.

VIII-3. Squamous cell carcinoma: Erosion and crusting of the lower eyelid and face of a cat.

VIII-4. Fibrosarcoma: Large circumscribed mass with invasion into surrounding tissue on the dorsum of an aged cat. (Courtesy of Richard Bradley, Manassas, Virginia)

VIII-5. Cutaneous hemangiopericytoma on the rear limb of a dog.

VIII-6. Canine cutaneous histiocytoma: Small, circumscribed, smooth dermal tumor with mildly erythemic surface.

VIII-7. Canine lymphosarcoma: A dog with multiple, discrete dermal nodules over the trunk and extremities.

VIII-8. Canine mast cell tumor: Solitary circumscribed tumor with a smooth surface on the stifle.

VIII-9. Feline mast cell tumor: Rapidly growing, ulcerated tumor on the face.

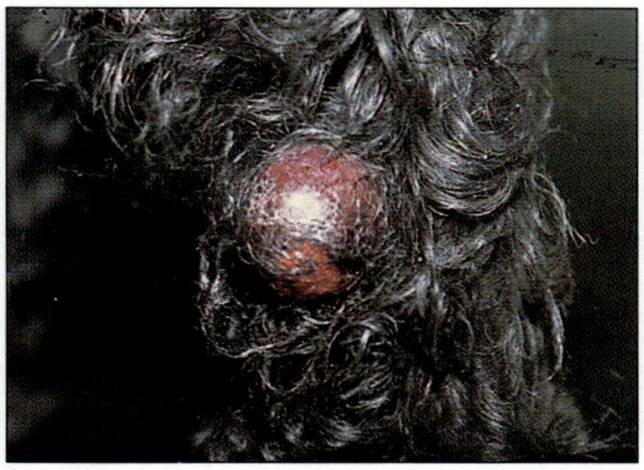
VIII-1

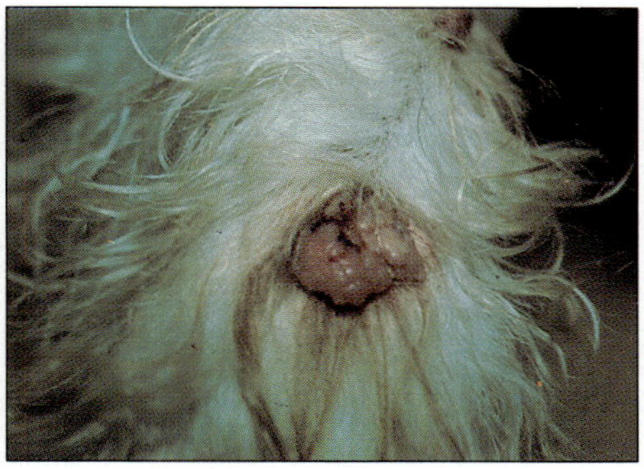
VIII-2

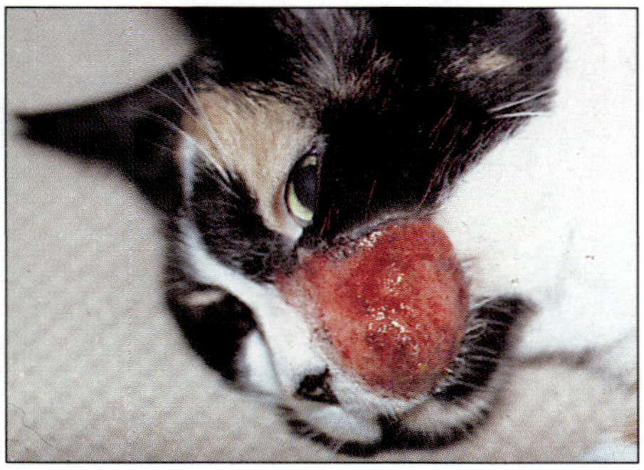
VIII-3

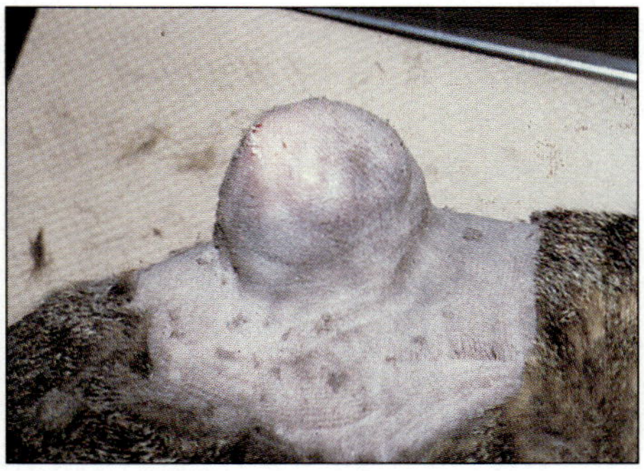
VIII-4

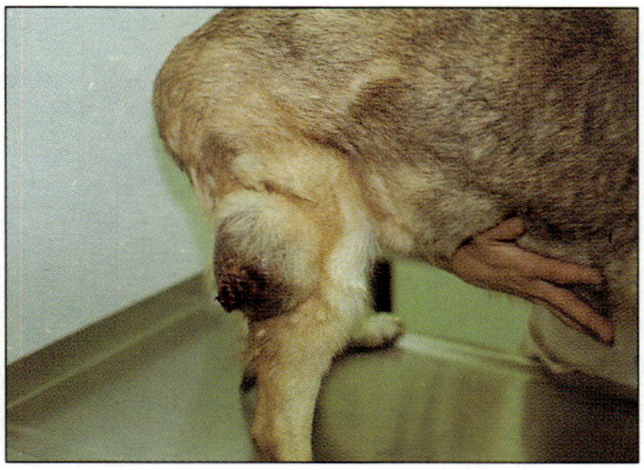
VIII-5

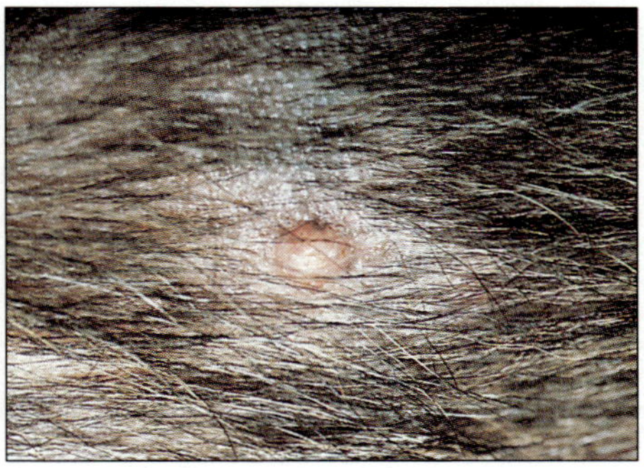
VIII-6

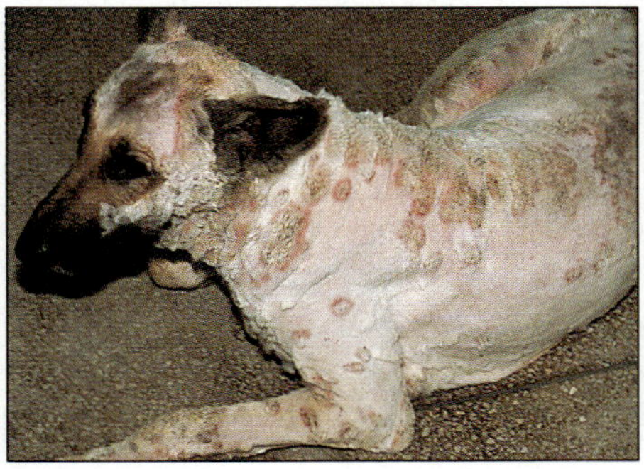
VIII-7

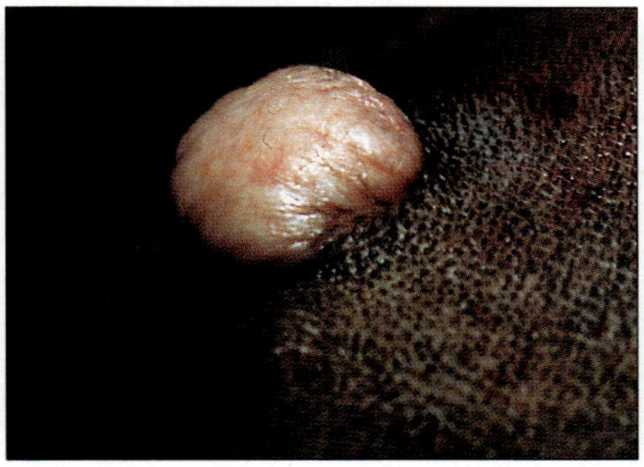
VIII-8

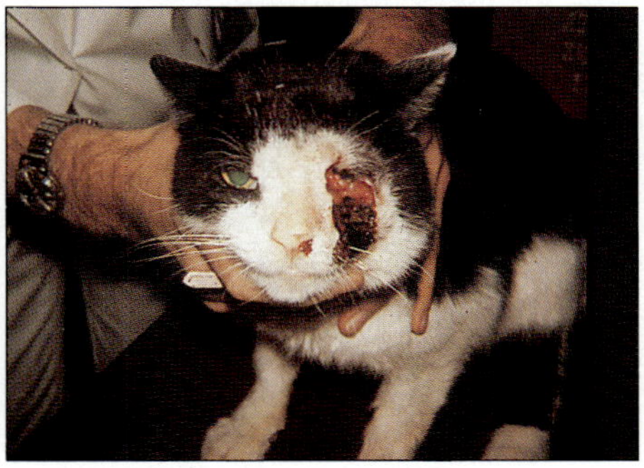
VIII-9

PLATE IX

IX-1. Irritant contact dermatitis: Diffuse erythema and erosion on the ventral abdomen of a dog caused by an ammoniated floor cleaner.

IX-2. Nasal solar dermatitis: Erythema and erosion on the anterior dorsal muzzle.

IX-3. Cutaneous asthenia: Boxer with marked hyperextensibility of the skin. (Courtesy of Anthony Stannard, School of Veterinary Medicine, University of California, Davis)

IX-4. Cutaneous asthenia: A 1-year-old Siamese cat with marked hyperextensibility of the skin.

IX-5. Dermatomyositis: Facial scaling, hair loss, and scarring in a young affected dog.

IX-6. Acanthosis nigricans: Axillary hyperpigmentation in a dachshund.

IX-7. Acral lick dermatitis: Ulceration and induration on a limb.

IX-8. Nodular panniculitis: Multiple, ulcerative, draining subcutaneous nodules and associated crusting in the lateral flank and thigh regions of a dog.

IX-9. Anal sac abscess: Taut abscess in the perineal region of a dog.

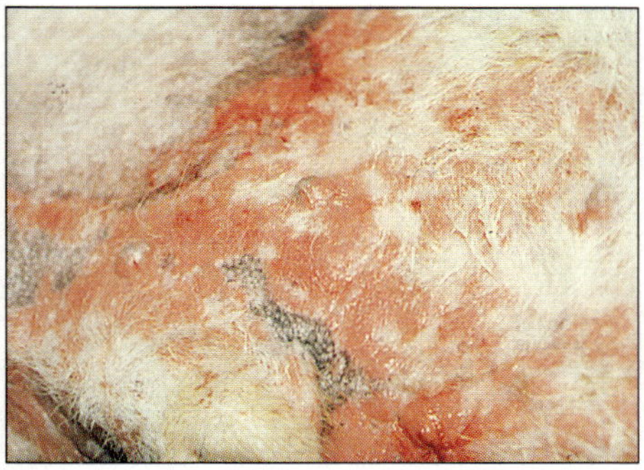

IX-1

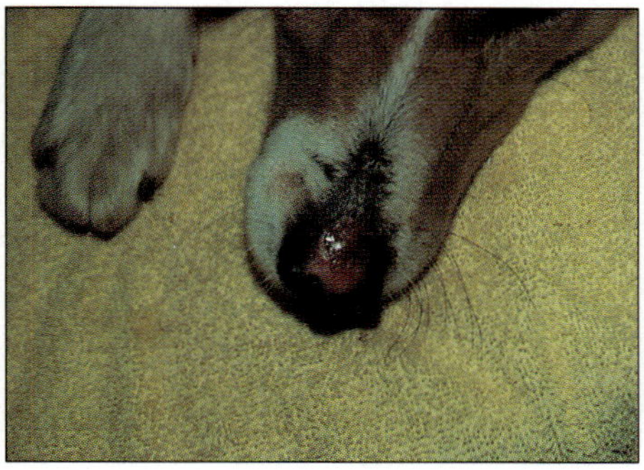

IX-2

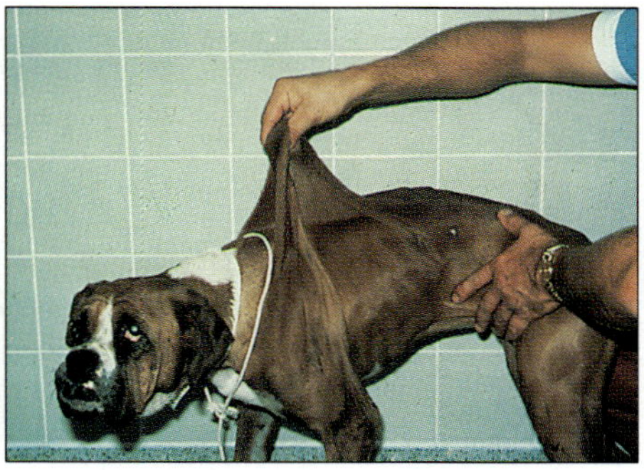

IX-3

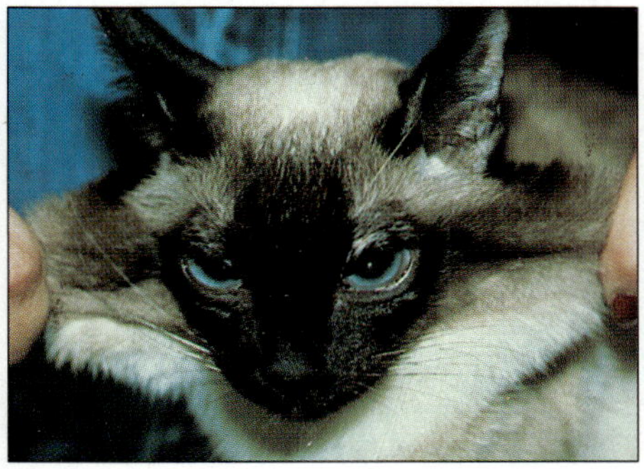

IX-4

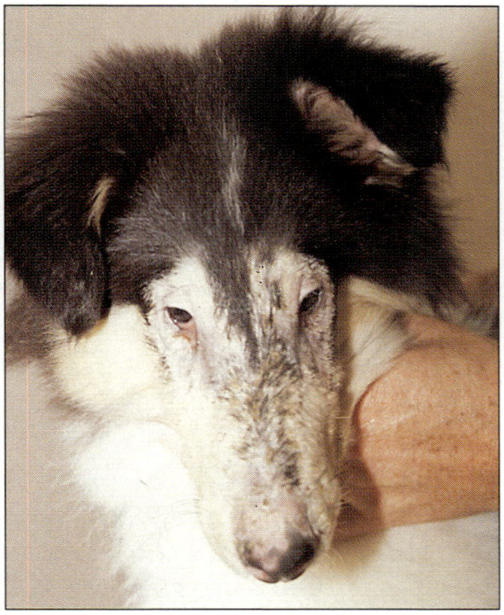

IX-5

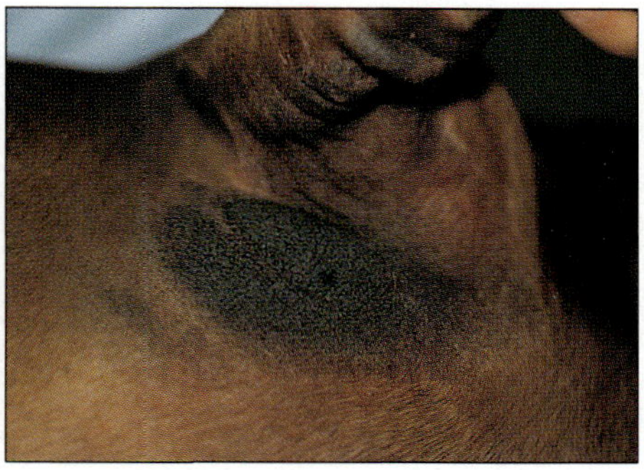

IX-6

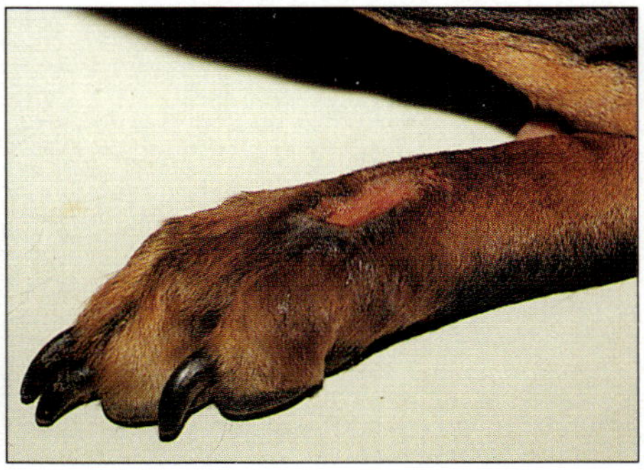

IX-7

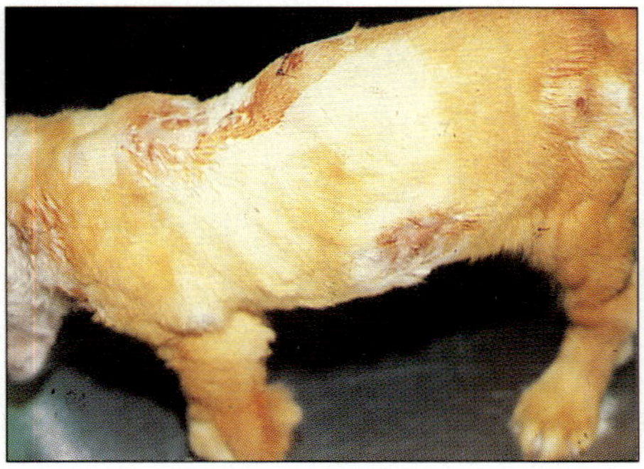

IX-8

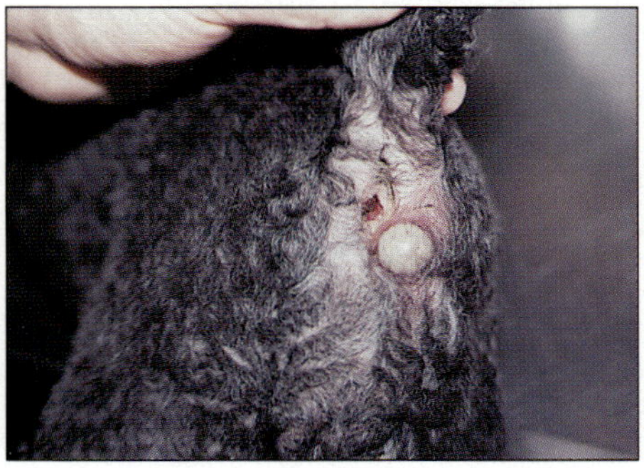

IX-9

PLATE X

X-1. Indolent ulcer: Ulceration on the margins of the lips in a cat.

X-2. Indolent ulcer: Ulceration and thickening of the upper anterior lip of a cat. Note the eosinophilic granuloma on the hard palate (*arrow*).

X-3. Eosinophilic plaque: Focal plaque with a moist, erythematous, ulcerative surface on the abdomen of a cat.

X-4. Linear granuloma: Linear pattern of multiple, raised, dry, granulomatous lesions on the posterior thigh of a cat. (Courtesy of Paul Caciolo, St. Louis, Missouri)

X-5. Miliary dermatitis: Multiple erythematous papules on the lateral thorax of a cat. (Courtesy of Gail Kunkle, College of Veterinary Medicine, University of Florida, Gainesville)

X-6. Feline endocrine alopecia: Diffuse alopecia with soft, noninflamed skin on the ventrum and medial thighs.

X-7. Psychogenic alopecia: Noninflamed hair loss on the lateral aspects of a cat in a bilaterally symmetric pattern.

X-8. Feline immunodeficiency virus infection (FIV): Nocardiosis in a cat immunosuppressed by FIV.

X-9. Plasma cell pododermatitis: Swollen, erythematous footpads on a cat.

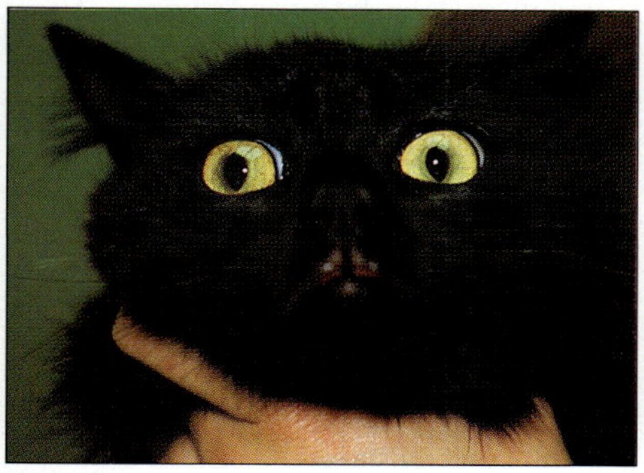
X-1

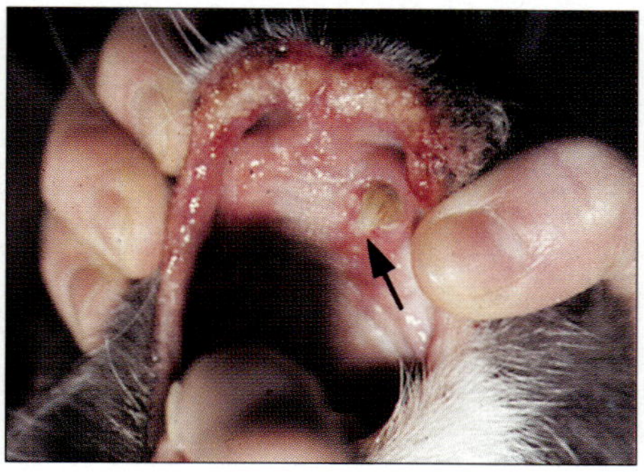
X-2

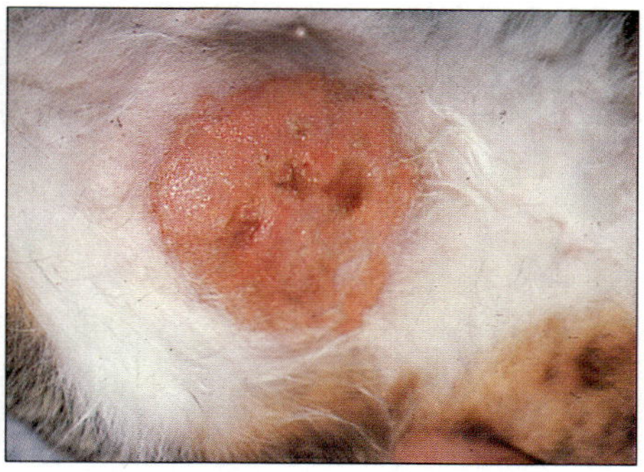
X-3

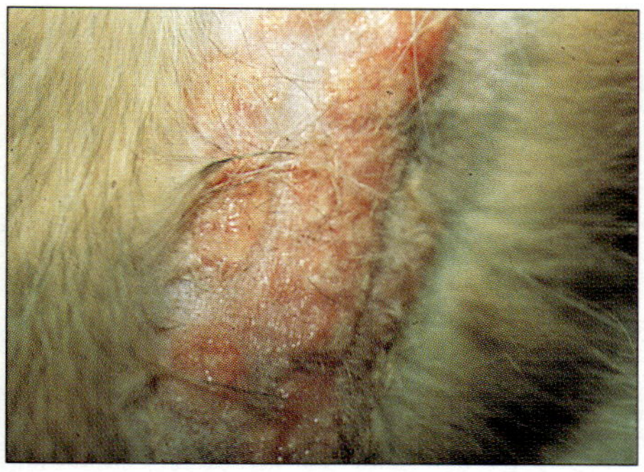
X-4

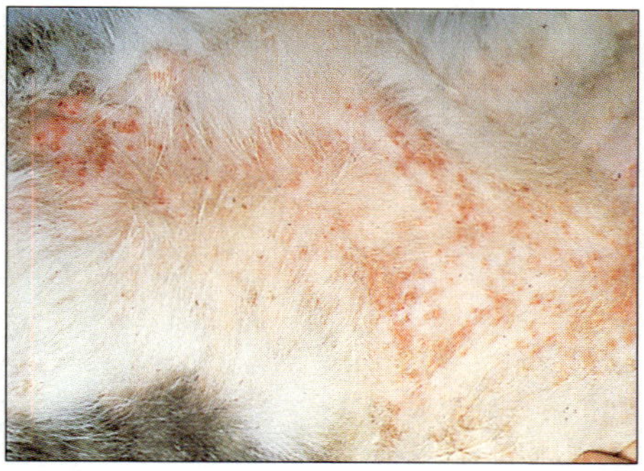
X-5

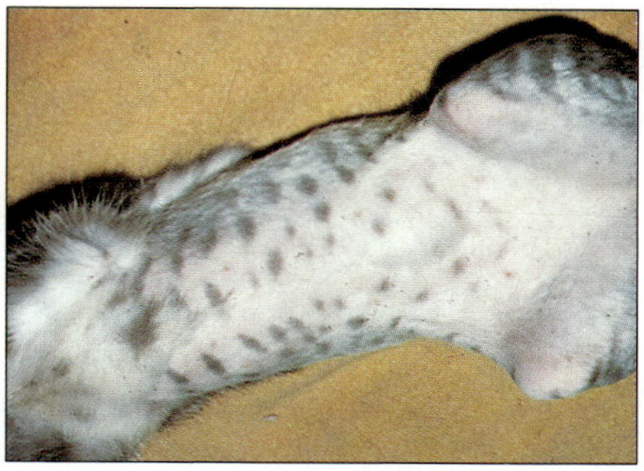
X-6

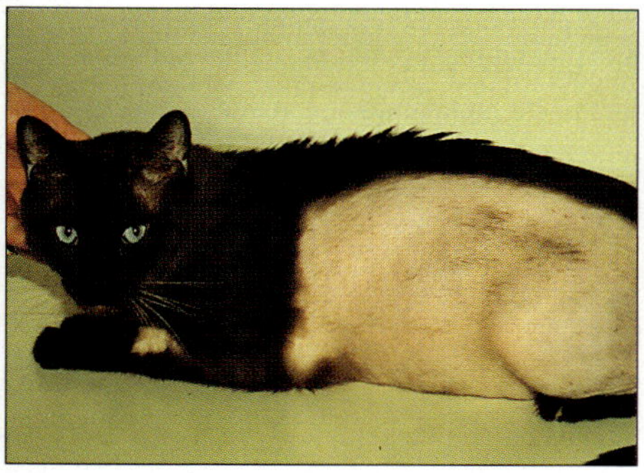
X-7

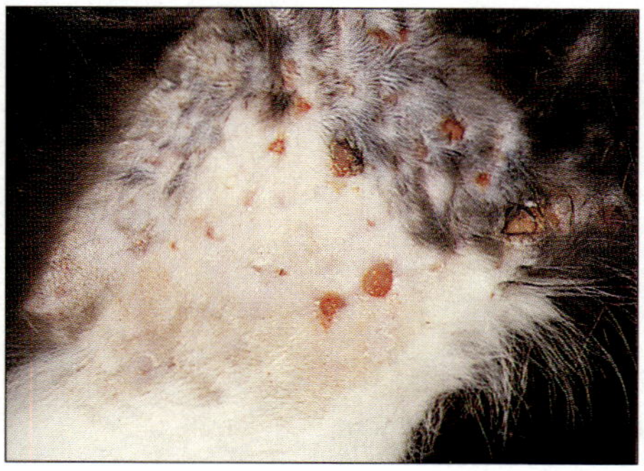
X-8

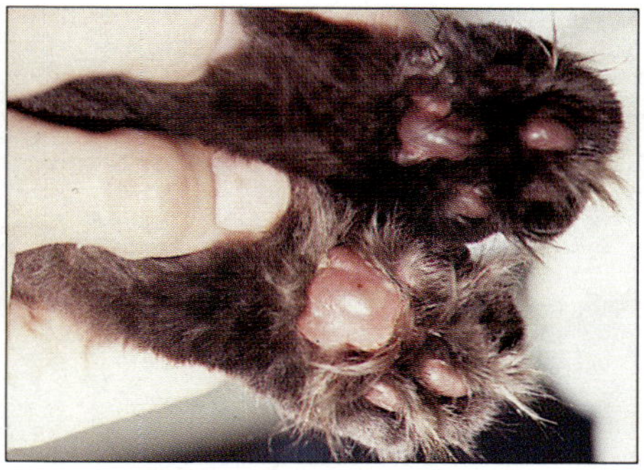
X-9

PLATE XI

XI-1. *Knemikodoptes* infestation on the face and feet of a buderigar.

XI-2. Amazon parrot recovering from parrot pox.

XI-3. Cockatoo with beak deformed by psittacine beak and feather disease syndrome.

XI-4. A young budgerigar with French molt.

XI-5. Cockatiel with a large abscess below the right eye.

XI-6. Yellow-billed Jamaican Amazon parrot with an erosive abscess of the right nares.

XI-7. Cloacal papilloma.

XI-8. Fibrosarcoma on the wing of a lovebird.

XI-9. Large feather cysts on a canary's wing.

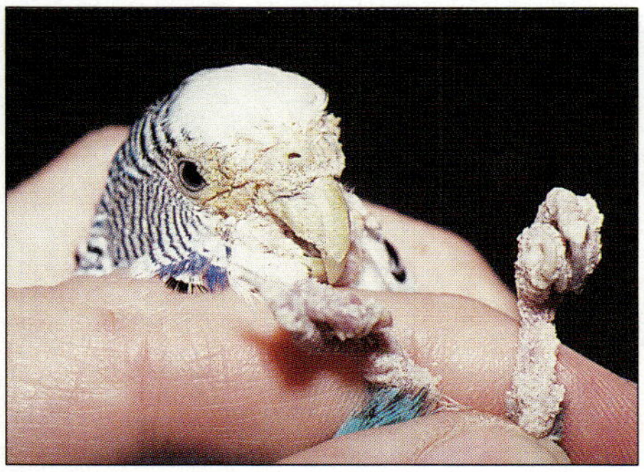
XI-1

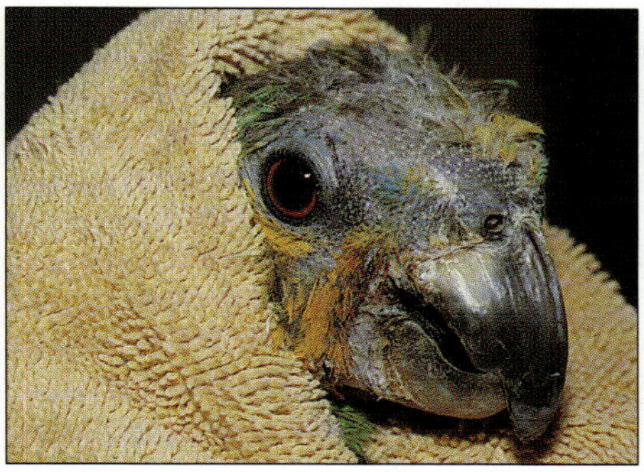
XI-2

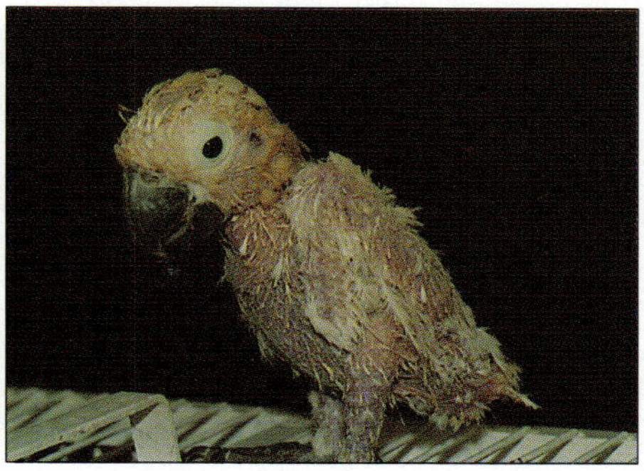
XI-3

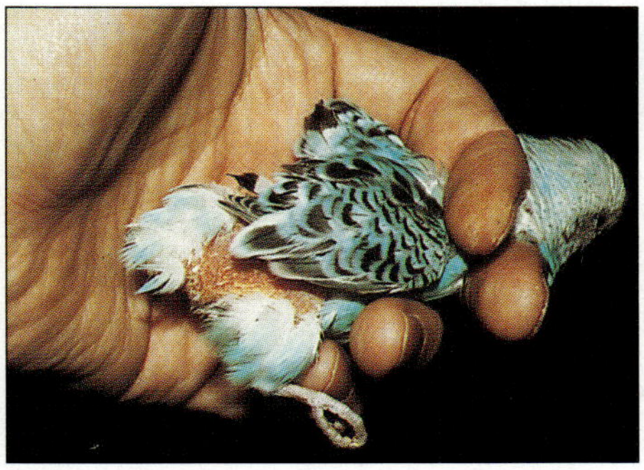
XI-4

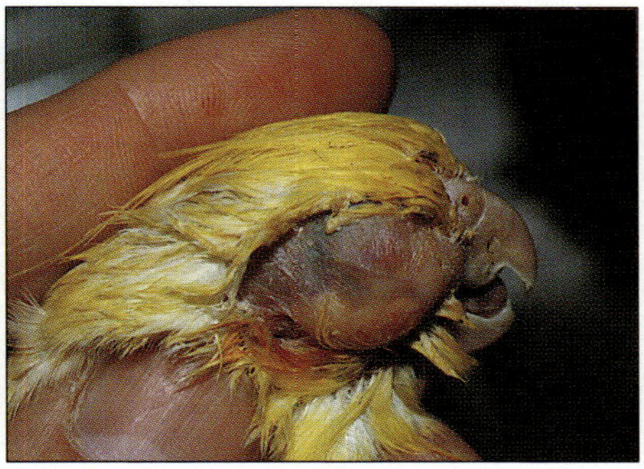
XI-5

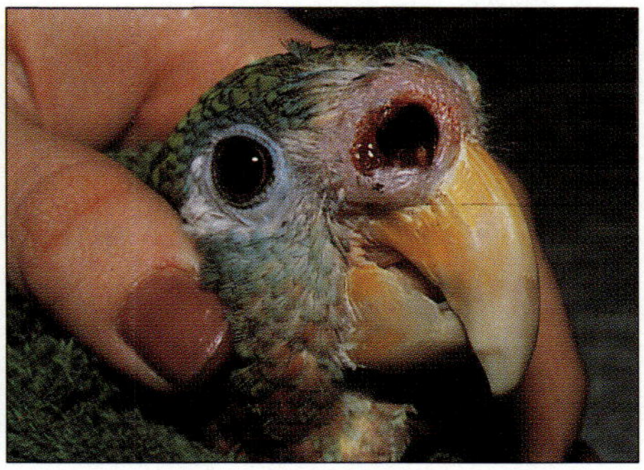
XI-6

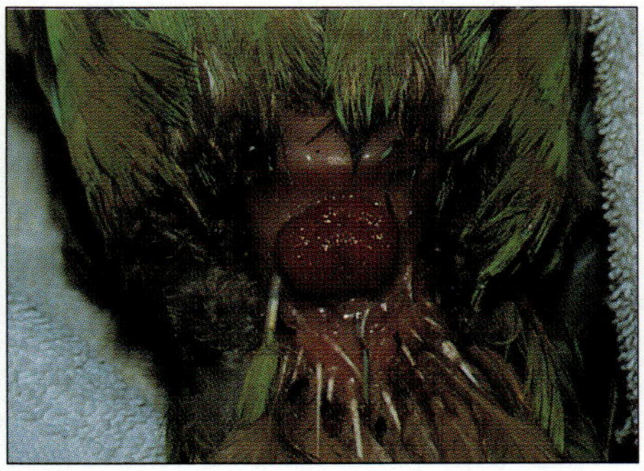
XI-7

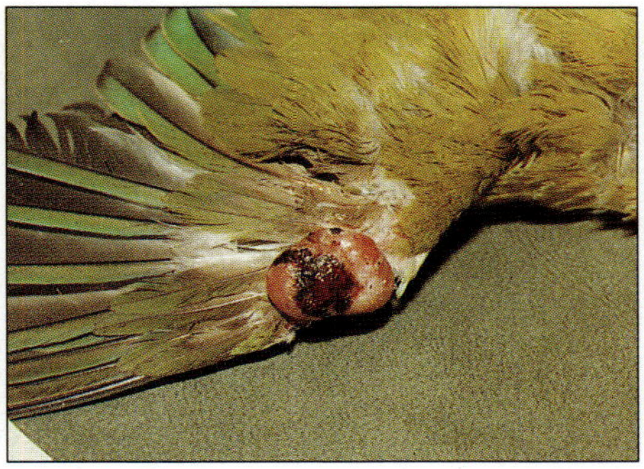
XI-8

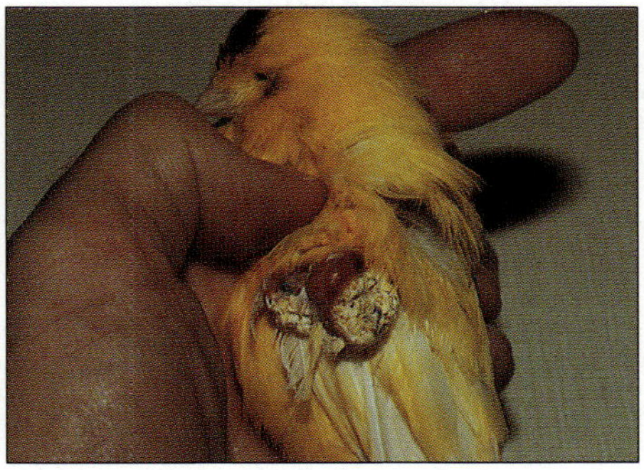
XI-9

PLATE XI (continued)

XI-10. Uric acid deposits or *tophi* on a budgerigar's foot caused by gout.

XI-11. Hyperkeratosis of the feet on a canary.

XI-12. Pododermatitis in a ring-necked dove.

XI-13. A "bald" canary.

XI-14. A self-mutilated cockatiel.

XI-15. A hypothyroid African Grey parrot that had a low thyroxine (T_4) level and responded to thyroid therapy.

XI-16. Xanthomatosis on a budgerigar's wing.

XI-17. Brown hypertrophy of the cere.

XI-18. An overgrown beak resulting from a tumor on the dorsal surface near the cere of a budgerigar.

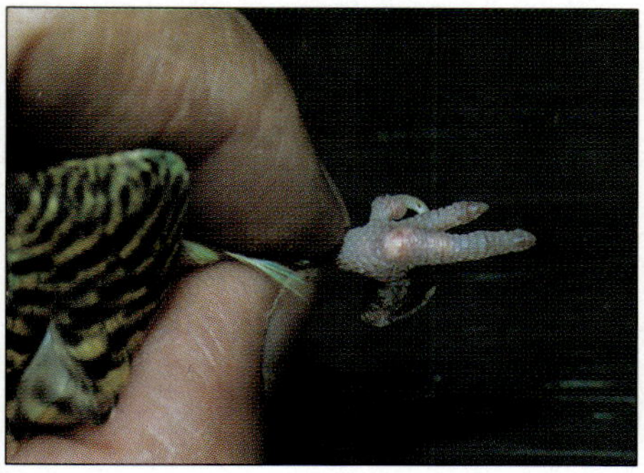
XI-10

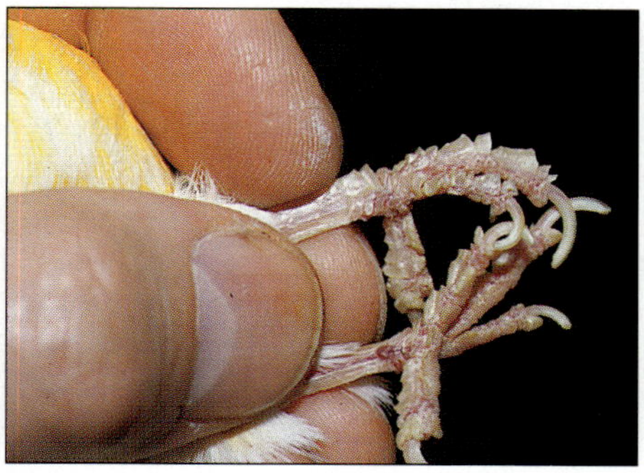
XI-11

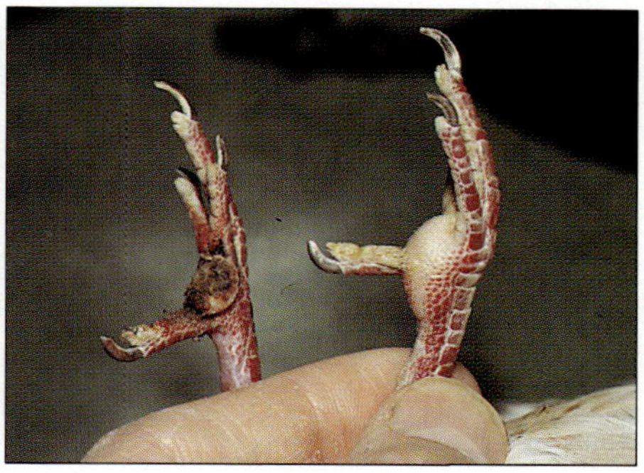
XI-12

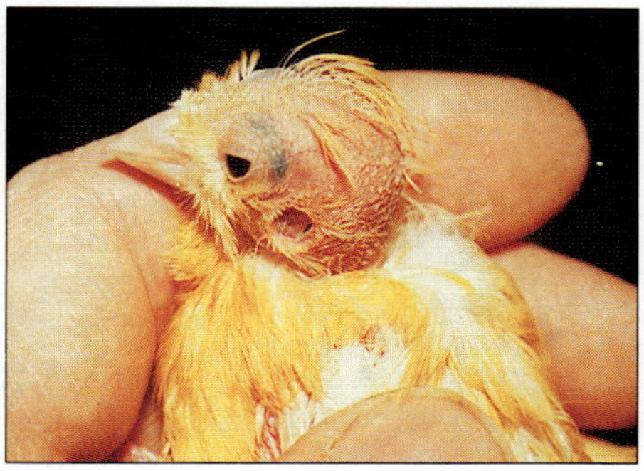
XI-13

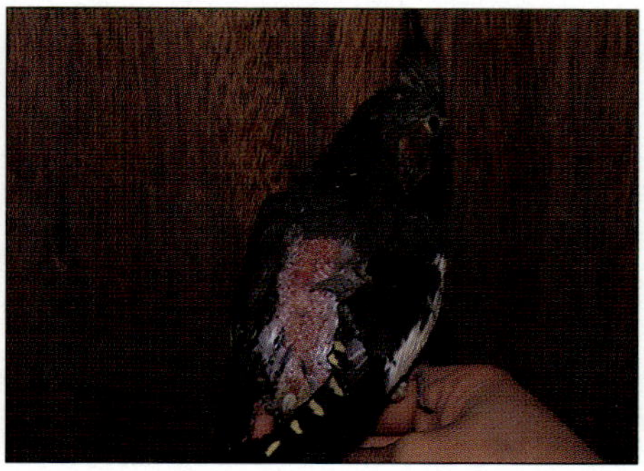
XI-14

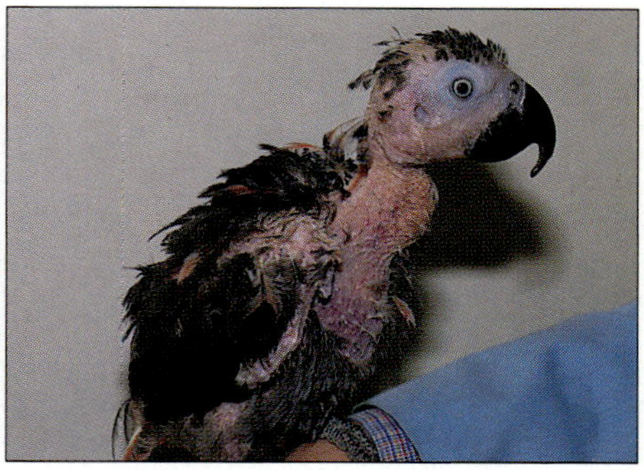
XI-15

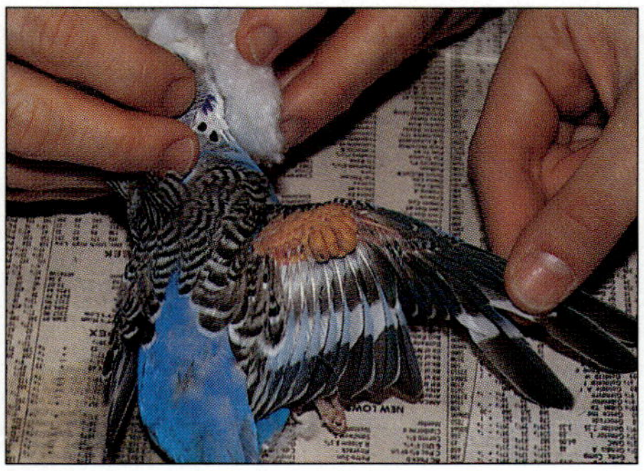
XI-16

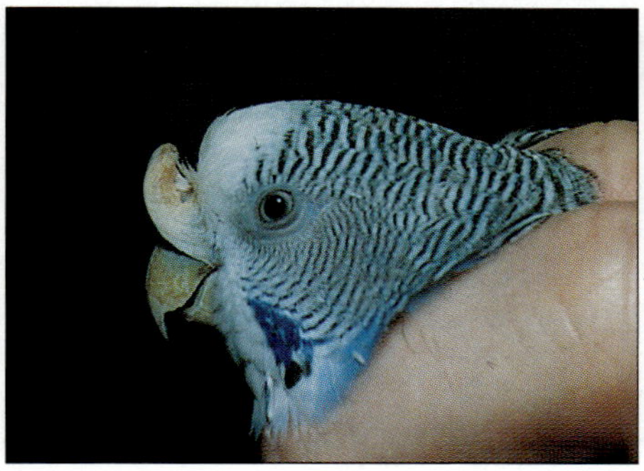
XI-17

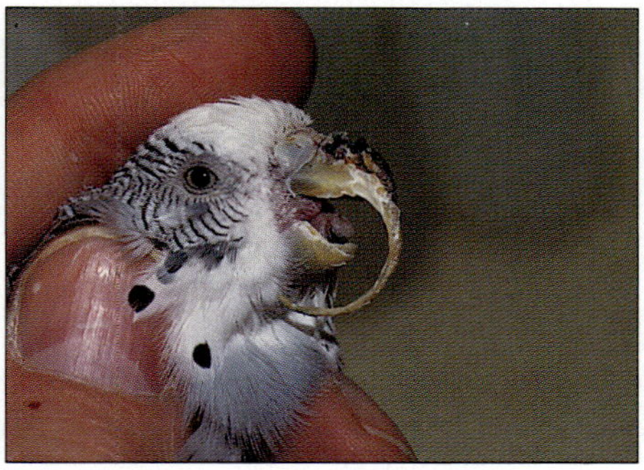
XI-18

PLATE XII

XII-1. Clinical lesions of *Myobia musculi* infestation on the head and flank.

XII-2. *Myobia musculi*. (Courtesy of S.W. Barthold, Yale University, New Haven, Connecticut)

XII-3. Barbering in a mouse. (Courtesy of D.H. Percy, Ontario Veterinary College, Guelph, Ontario, Canada)

XII-4. Ringtail in a rat. (Courtesy of D.H. Percy, Ontario Veterinary College, Guelph, Ontario, Canada)

XII-5. Normal pigmented "hip" or "flank" gland in a male hamster.

XII-6. Jaw abscess in a hamster.

XII-7. Demodicosis in a hamster.

XII-8. Cutaneous T-cell lymphoma in a hamster. (Courtesy of L.J. Ackerman, Mesa, Arizona)

XII-9. Normal sebaceous "scent" gland in a gerbil.

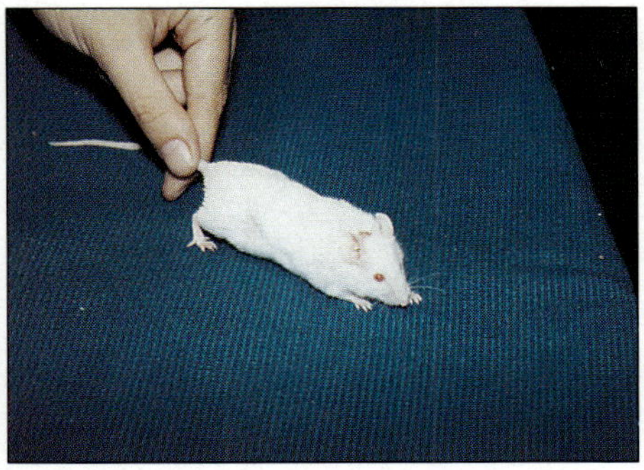
XII-1

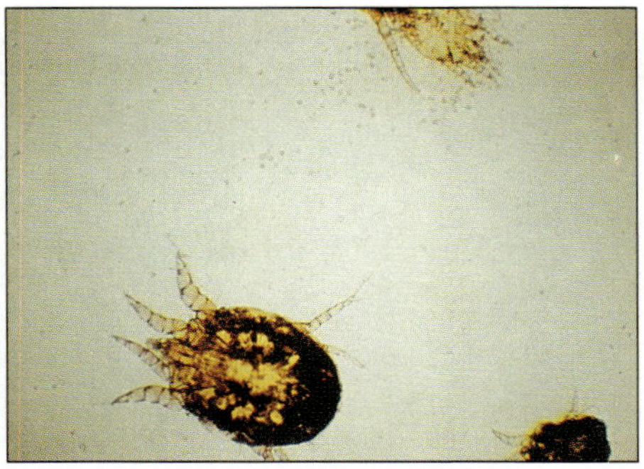
XII-2

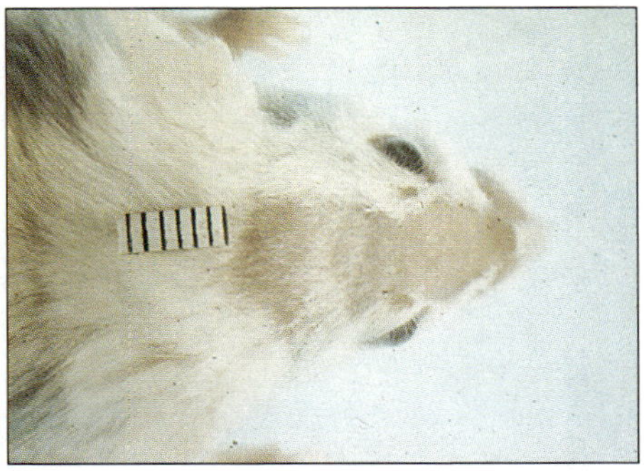
XII-3

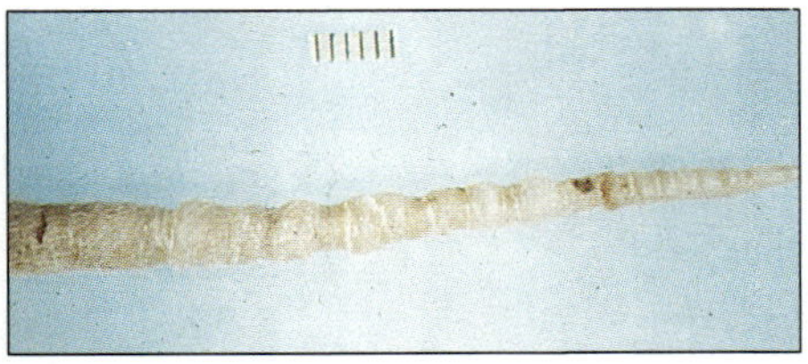
XII-4

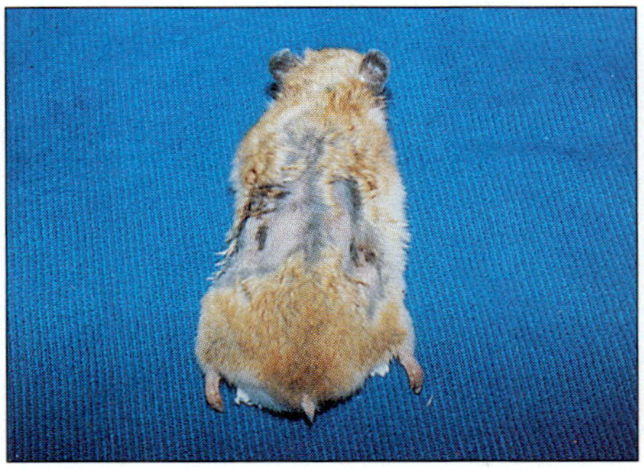
XII-5

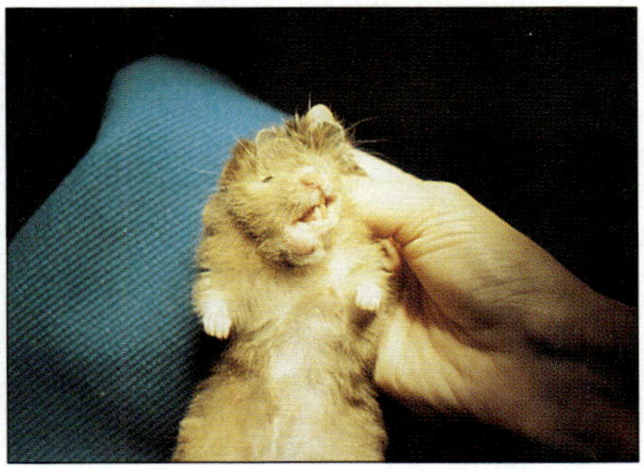
XII-6

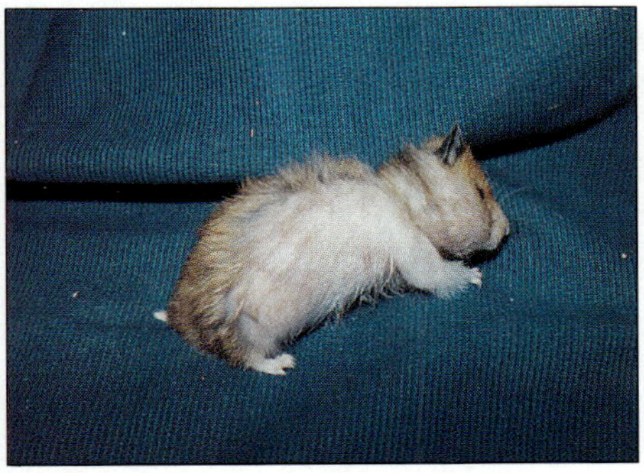
XII-7

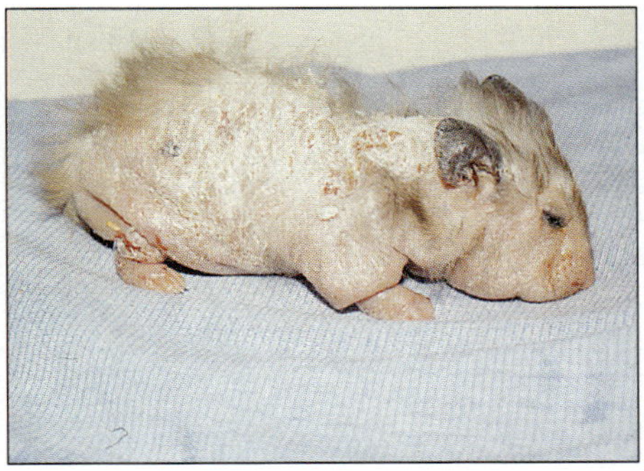
XII-8

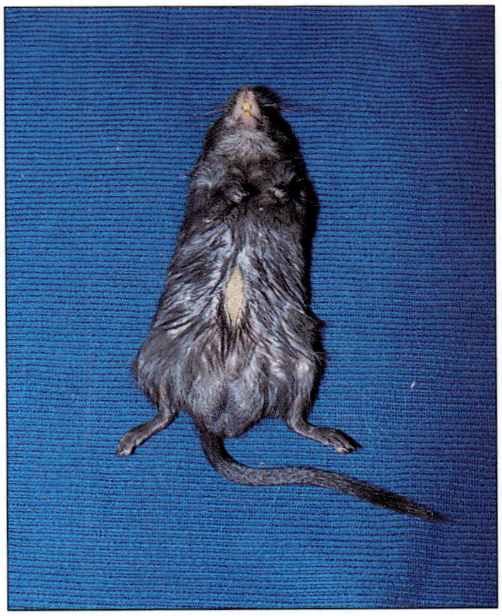
XII-9

PLATE XII (continued)

XII-10. Nasal dermatitis in a gerbil. (Courtesy of R.D. Axelson, Willowdale, Ontario, Canada)

XII-11. *Gliricola porcelli* in a guinea pig. (Courtesy of P. Lautenslauger, Ontario Veterinary College, Guelph, Ontario, Canada)

XII-12. *Trixacarus caviae* infestation in a guinea pig. (Courtesy of L.J. Ackerman, Mesa, Arizona)

XII-13. Dermatitis and jaw abscess caused by *Pasteurella multocida* infection in a rabbit. (Courtesy of R.D. Axelson, Willowdale, Ontario, Canada)

XII-14. *Trichophyton mentagrophytes* infection in a rabbit.

XII-15. *Psoroptes cuniculi*. (Courtesy of D.H. Percy, Ontario Veterinary College, Guelph, Ontario, Canada)

XII-16. *Psoroptes cuniculi* infestation in a rabbit. (Courtesy of R.D. Axelson, Willowdale, Ontario, Canada)

XII-17. Hutchburn in a rabbit.

XII-18. Hyperadrenocorticism caused by an adrenal adenoma in a ferret.

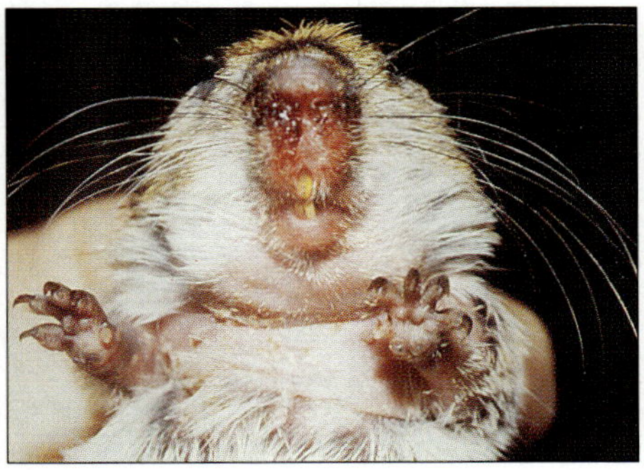

XII-10

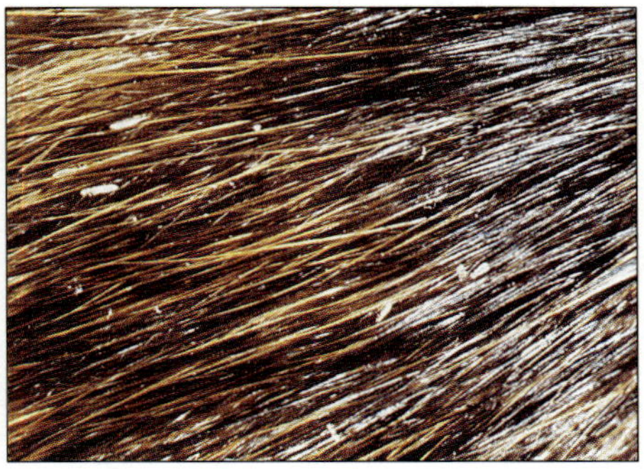

XII-11

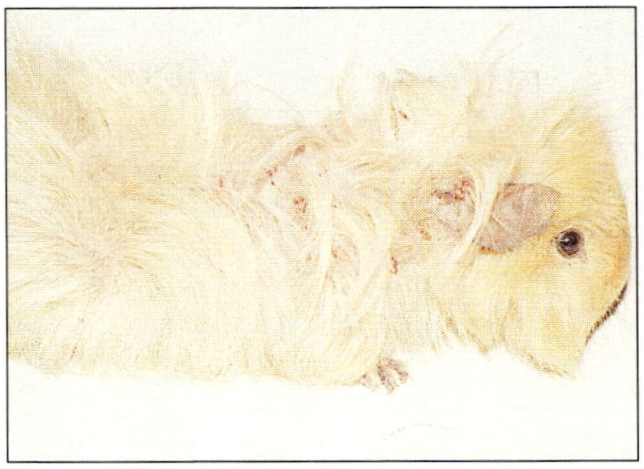

XII-12

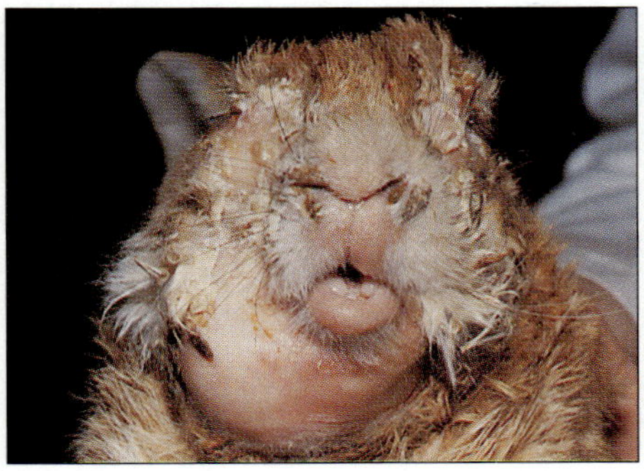

XII-13

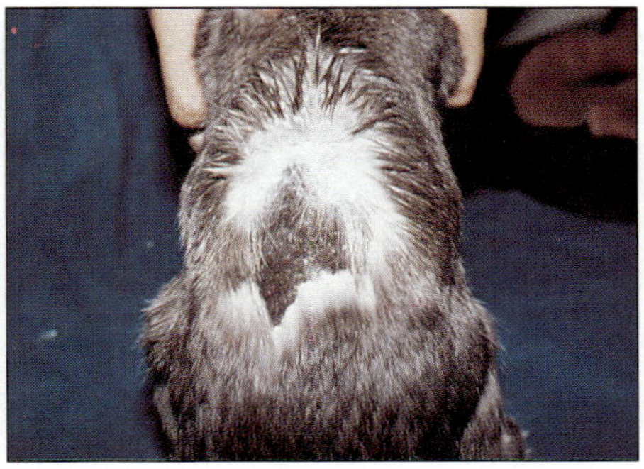

XII-14

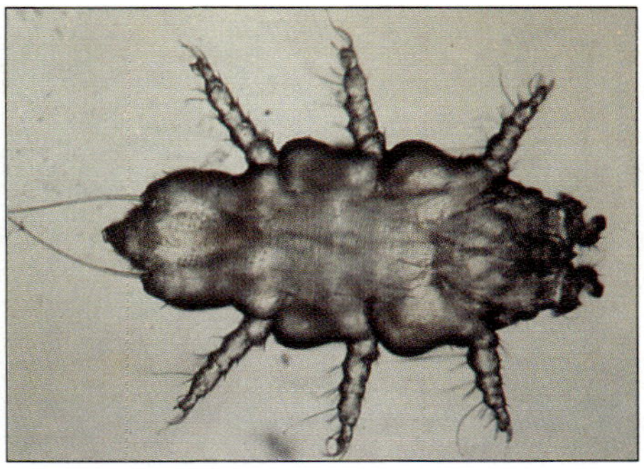

XII-15

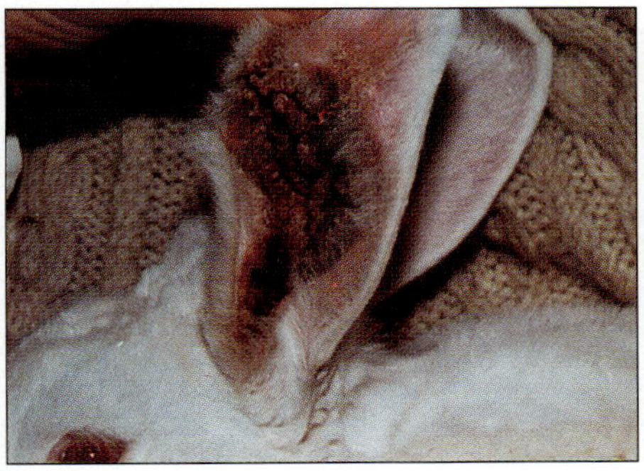

XII-16

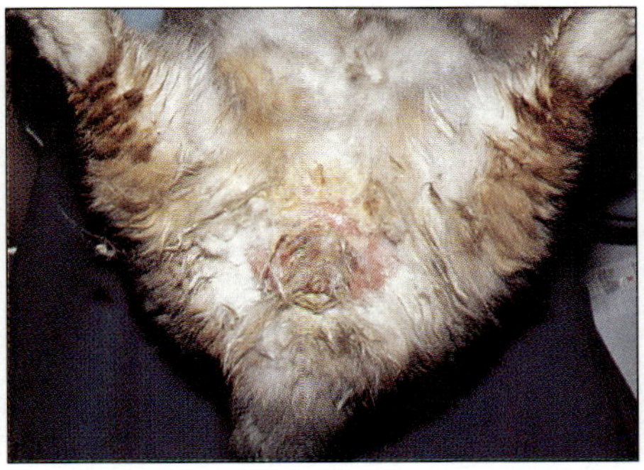

XII-17

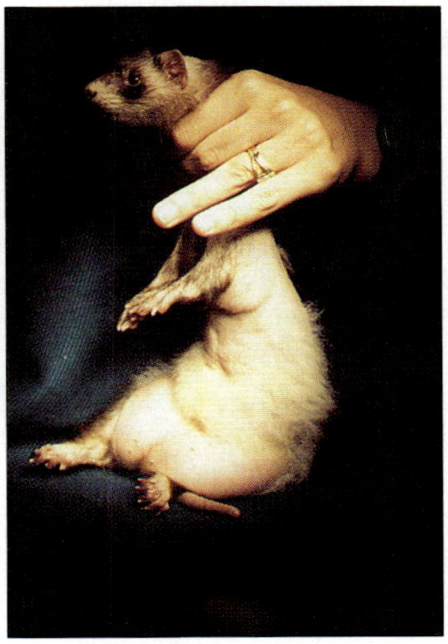

XII-18

PLATE XIII

XIII-1. Plastron of a leopard tortoise. Lightly pigmented areas of new growth are seen at suture lines (*s*), equidistant between embryonic shields (*e*).

XIII-2. A painted turtle shedding its scutes.

XIII-3. Histologic section of the skin of an American anole. Melanophores (*m*) and iridophores (*i*) are seen in the dermis. (H&E, x160)

XIII-4. Gray patch disease in a juvenile green turtle. Note the prominent lesions on the head and cervical region. (From Jacobson ER: Diseases of reptiles. Part I. Noninfectious diseases. *Compend Contin Educ Pract Vet* 3:122–126, 1981, with permission)

XIII-5. Poxvirus infection of a caiman. Multiple white patches are seen on the body surface.

XIII-6. Bolivian side-neck turtle with confluent white skin lesions caudal to the right eye. (From Jacobson ER, Gaskin JM, Clubb SL: Papilloma-like virus infection in Bolivian side-neck turtles. *JAVMA* 181:1325–1328, 1982, with permission)

XIII-7. Papillomas on a European emerald lizard are seen as darkly pigmented proliferative lesions.

XIII-8. Middle ear infection in a juvenile eastern box turtle. (From Jacobson ER: Diseases of reptiles. Part I. Noninfectious diseases. *Compend Contin Educ Pract Vet* 3:122–126, 1981, with permission)

XIII-9. A subcutaneous abscess being surgically removed from a boa constrictor. The abscess was the result of a bite wound from a rodent.

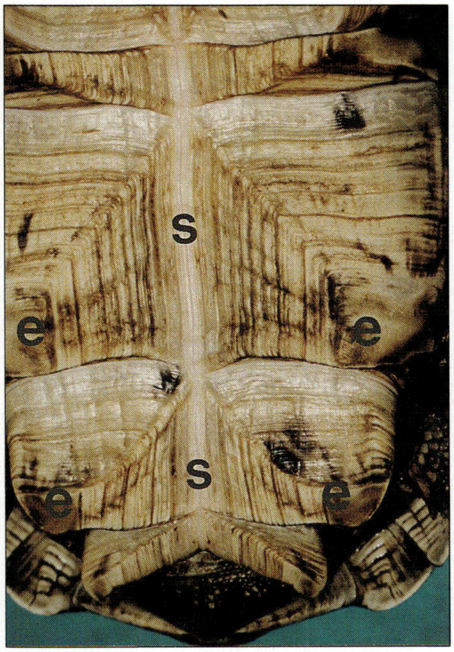

XIII-1

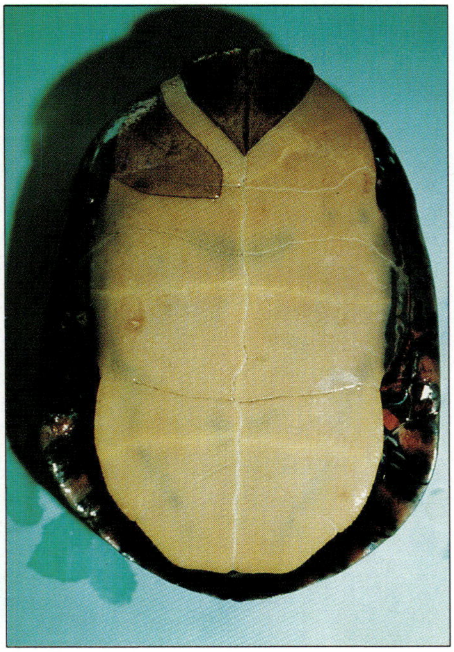

XIII-2

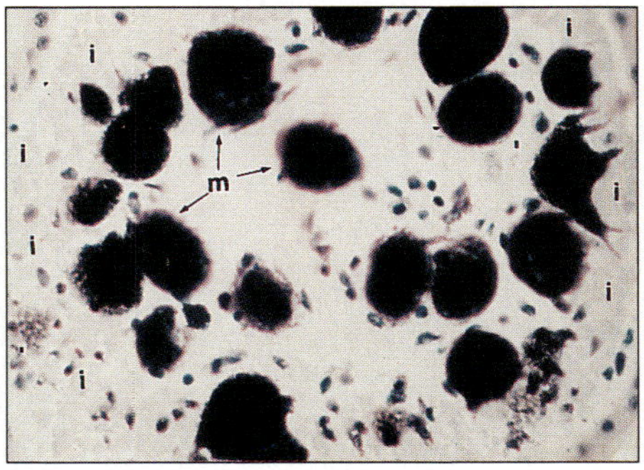

XIII-3

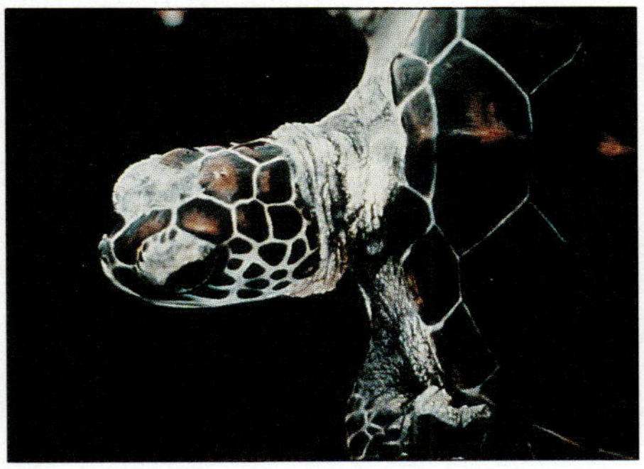

XIII-4

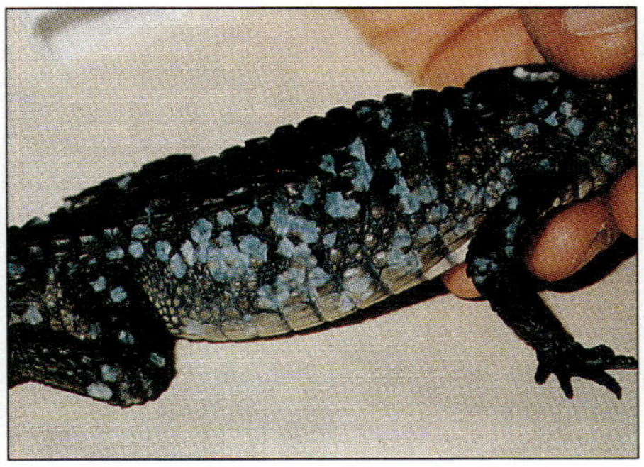

XIII-5

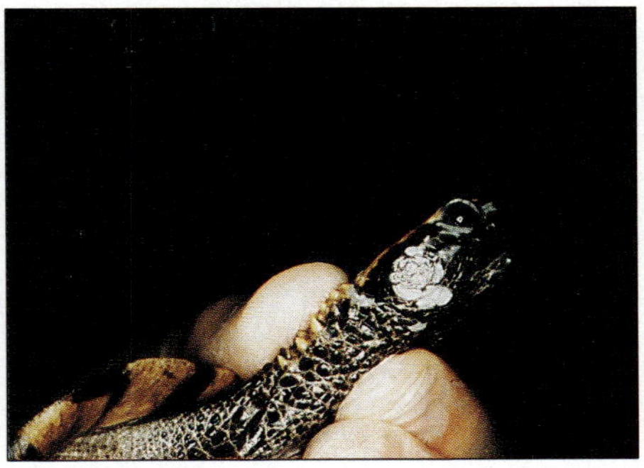

XIII-6

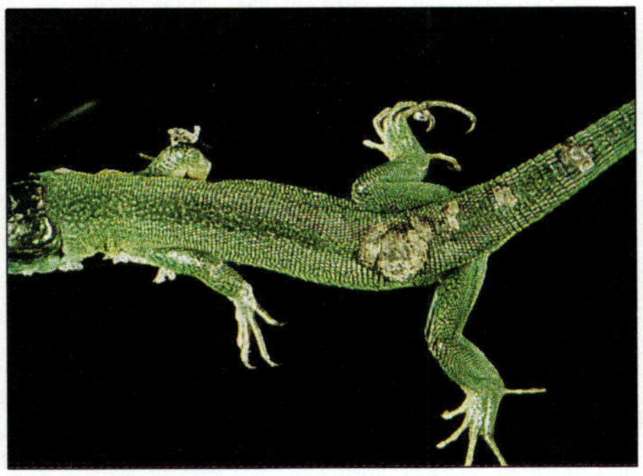

XIII-7

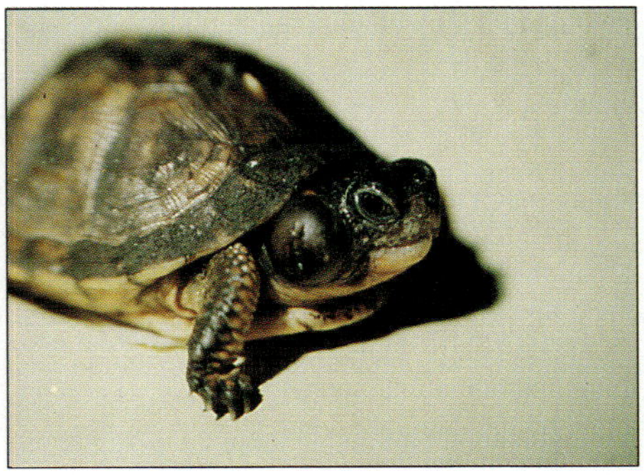

XIII-8

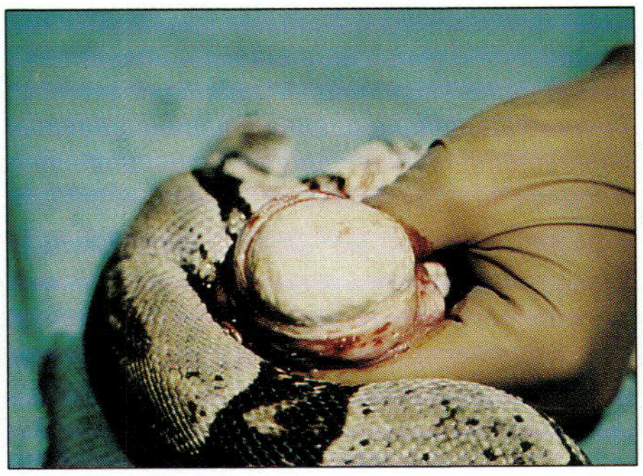

XIII-9

PLATE XIII (continued)

XIII-10. *Corynebacterium pyogenes* abscess in a green iguana.

XIII-11. Burn wound colonized by *Pseudomonas aeruginosa* in a Burmese python.

XIII-12. Loss of stratum corneum of body scales in a taipan that had a severe enteritis.

XIII-13. Necrotizing shell and skin lesions in a juvenile Florida softshell turtle. (From Jacobson ER, Calderwood MB, Clubb SL: Mucormycosis in hatchling Florida softshell turtles. *JAVMA* 177:838–841, 1980, with permission)

XIII-14. Histologic section of a shell lesion in a juvenile Florida softshell turtle showing a branching nonseptate fungus. (GMS stain, x1000) (From Jacobson ER, Calderwood MB, Clubb SL: Mucormycosis in hatchling Florida softshell turtles. *JAVMA* 177:838–841, 1980, with permission)

XIII-15. Subcutaneous hematomas in an American anole. *Trichosporon beigelii* was cultured from this lesion.

XIII-16. Mycotic dermatitis in an eastern king snake.

XIII-17. Large fibropapillomas covering the right eye of a juvenile green turtle.

XIII-18. An albino hatchling green turtle.

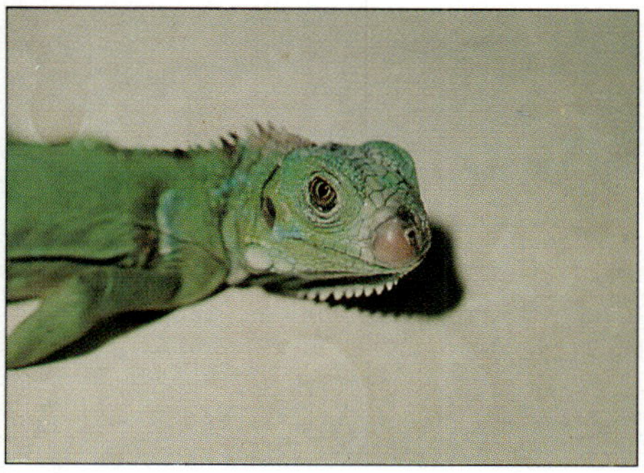

XIII-10

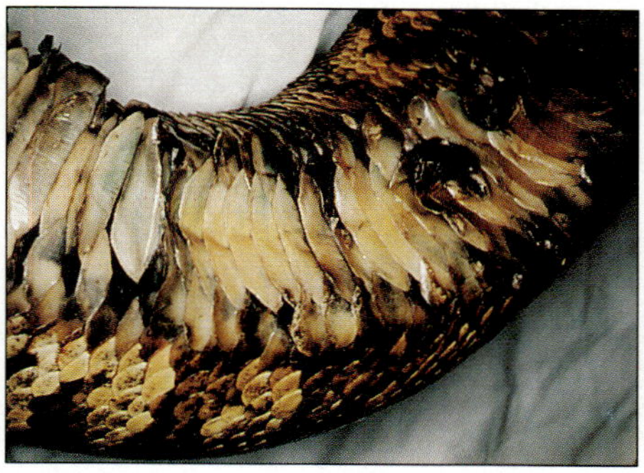

XIII-11

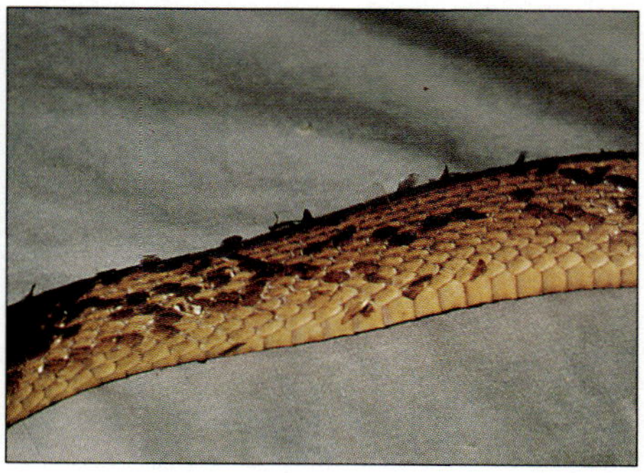

XIII-12

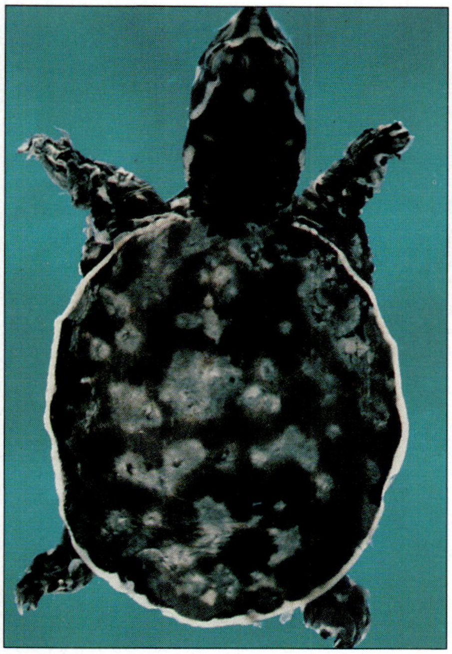

XIII-13

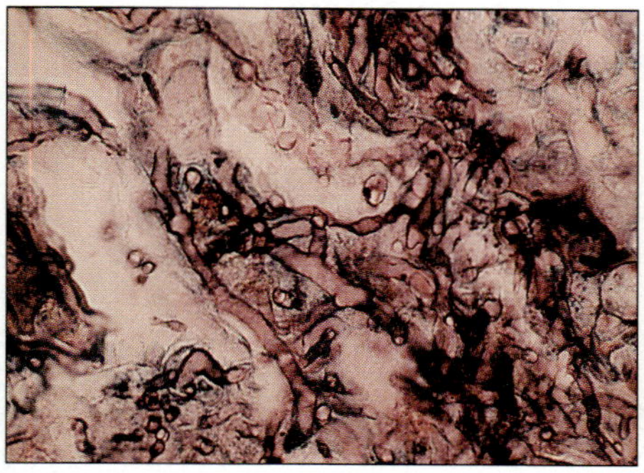

XIII-14

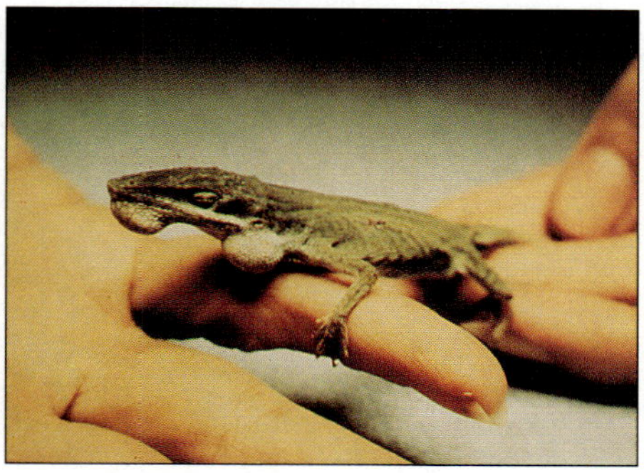

XIII-15

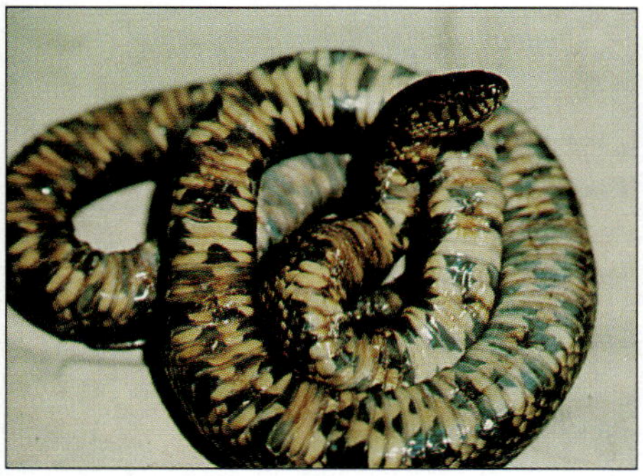

XIII-16

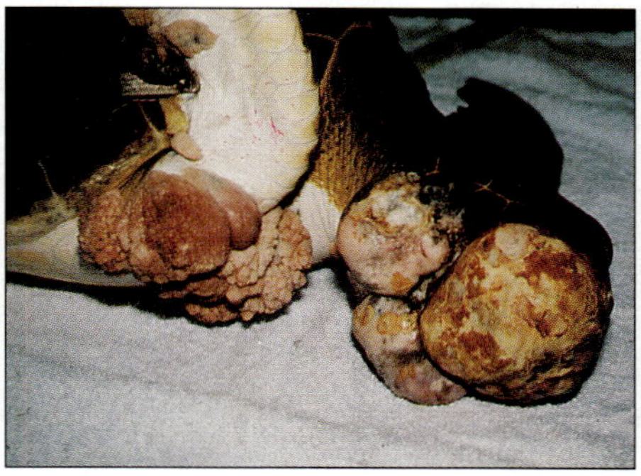

XIII-17

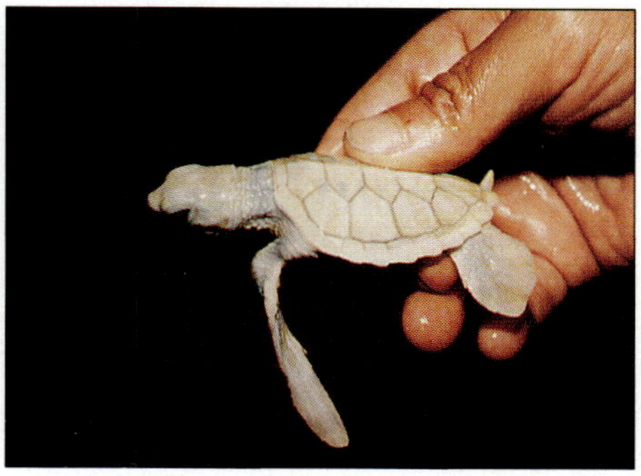

XIII-18

Chapter 9

ENDOCRINE SKIN DISEASES

Lowell Ackerman, DVM
Gene H. Nesbitt, DVM, MS

Endocrine disorders are relatively common in dogs and, although uncommon, are being reported more frequently in cats. Diagnostic Key 8 (see end of Chapter 2) lists the most pertinent historical and clinical findings and diagnostic tests necessary to differentiate the common canine and feline endocrine dermatoses.

HYPOTHYROIDISM

Canine hypothyroidism is characterized by a decreased level of circulating thyroid hormones. Clinical feline hypothyroidism has been reported only rarely.

Etiologic Factors

Several pathophysiologic mechanisms can lead to hypothyroidism. The most common cause of primary hypothyroidism in dogs is atrophy of the thyroid gland, usually associated with lymphocytic thyroiditis. Antibodies to thyroglobulin, microsomal antigen, and a second colloid antigen have been identified in dogs with lymphocytic thyroiditis. Other causes are classified as idiopathic follicular atrophy. Congenital thyroid agenesis is rare. Secondary hypothyroidism is caused by a lack of thyroid-stimulating hormone (TSH), which can result from either congenital hypopituitarism or an acquired disorder associated with pituitary neoplasia. Other potential causes of hypothyroidism include iodine deficiency, dyshormonogenesis (an intrinsic defect in synthesis of thyroid hormone), a defect in the transport of thyroid hormone, a peripheral defect in the conversion of thyroxine (T_4) to triiodothyronine (T_3), and inappropriate deiodination of T_4 associated with an excess of reverse T_3. All of these conditions are uncommon. Dietary insufficiency of iodine leading to atrophy of the thyroid gland has been reported in cats.

Thyroid Physiology

The canine thyroid gland secretes two hormones, T_4 and T_3, in a ratio of 20:1. The large majority of both hormones are bound to plasma proteins. The unbound or free thyroid hormones are those available for the tissues. The binding affinity of plasma proteins for T_4 is lower in dogs than in humans; thus, the total T_4 is lower, the unbound or free T_4 is higher, and the hormone turnover is more rapid in dogs than in humans. Approximately 40% of the extrathyroidal T_4 is in the plasma; the majority of the remaining portion is taken up by the liver where conversion to T_3 occurs. Although there is controversy concerning the biologic activity of T_4 and T_3, it is generally agreed that T_3 is the most biologically active. Some evidence does indicate, however, that T_4 also has intrinsic biologic activity.

Extrathyroidal T_4 is metabolized in two ways, 45% by deiodination and 55% by fecal excretion. Approximately 70% of T_3 is metabolized by deiodination and 30% by fecal excretion. Fecal excretion contributes to the inefficiency of hormone utilization and raises the level of tolerance to exogenous thyroid hormone.

The half-life of T_4 is 24 hours; the peak plasma or serum level occurs 4 to 12 hours after thyroid replacement. The half-life of T_3 is approximately 3 to 4 hours, with a peak blood level occurring approximately 3 hours after administration of the hormone.

Serum or plasma thyroid hormone levels are lowered by the administration of several drugs including glucocorticoids, phenytoin, phenobarbital, and phenylbutazone. Levels of T_3 are more susceptible to the influence of corticosteroids than T_4; thus, stress conditions can result in a rather sudden and sustained decrease in T_3 concentration. Long-term corticosteroid influence, either endogenous or exogenous in origin, results in a marked decrease of both T_3 and T_4.

Several important actions of thyroid hormones correlate with the clinical signs observed in a hypothyroid animal. The most pronounced action of both T_3 and T_4 is the stimulation of metabolism in the tissues resulting in an increased oxygen consumption. These thyroid hormones activate the enzyme systems which are responsible for oxidation processes. These hormones also promote growth and development of tissue, regulate lipid metabolism, increase the absorption of carbohydrates from the intestine, and influence function of the central nervous system.

The major modulator of thyroid-hormone production is thought to be TSH, which is secreted by the anterior pituitary gland. TSH is regulated at the level of the anterior pituitary by the antagonistic effects of thyroid hormone and TSH-releasing hormone (TRH), which is released by the hypothalamus.

History

The historical findings in dogs with hypothyroidism are variable. An overrepresentation of akitas, chow chows, Great Danes, Irish wolfhounds, boxers, English bulldogs, dachshunds, Afghans, Newfoundlands, Malamutes, Doberman pinschers, basenjis, Brittany spaniels, poodles, golden retrievers, Irish setters, shar peis, and schnauzers has been observed.

The age of onset of clinical signs associated with hypothyroidism is usually 2 to 5 years, although the disease has been reported in younger dogs. The two most common owner observations are diminished physical activity denoted by fatigue, lethargy, and increased sleeping time, and haircoat changes. Slow regrowth of hair after clipping for a routine procedure may be the primary complaint. A history of sensitivity or intolerance to cold manifested by the avoidance of cold areas and the seeking out of warm areas, such as heat vents or radiators, may be reported.

Clinical Signs

Clinical signs are variable. In an untreated dog, they tend to increase in number and severity with age. The primary problem in one dog, however, may remain a minor problem or be nonexistent in another dog. Owners may not recognize the signs of hypothyroidism if there is minimal opportunity for the dog to exercise, and the signs are generally characterized by subtle changes over a prolonged period of time. In the clinically most extreme form of hypothyroidism, animals may become comatose. Other affected animals may appear clinically normal.

Haircoat changes include dryness, dullness, coarseness, and sparseness. Hair loss can occur on the trunk in a bilaterally symmetrical pattern, in a multifocal pattern (Plate VI-1), or on pressure points or wear areas, such as the posterior thighs and the neck beneath a collar. In large-breed dogs, hair loss may be more prevalent on the extremities than the trunk (Plate VI-2). Skin changes can include hyperpigmentation, thickened skin, scaling, and swelling. Edema of the facial folds and periorbital skin may cause a tragic expression but this is less commonly seen in practice than reported in the veterinary literature. Superficial pyoderma is commonly associated with hypothyroidism.

The incidence of obesity in hypothyroid dogs is likely overestimated and is more often a consequence of diet than hormonal status. Subtle changes in cardiac function may be manifested by a slow heart rate, weak apex beat and pulse, and low voltage on an electrocardiogram. Abnormal sexual activity may be noted in intact animals; females may have a shortened estrus or prolonged anestrus and infertility, and males may show a lack of libido.

Cats with congenital hypothyroidism have signs of disproportionate dwarfism with an enlarged, broad head but short neck and limbs. Additional signs include lethargy, constipation, bradycardia, and radiographic evidence of nearly complete absence of ossification centers in long bones.

Clinically, hypothyroidism in cats is typified by lethargy and a nonpruritic exfoliative dermatosis. Alopecia and crusting of the pinnae has been reported in radiothyrectomized cats. Bilateral symmetrical alopecia has been associated with iodine deficiencies. Cases of hypothyroidism have also resulted from surgical removal of the thyroid glands in hyperthyroid cats.

Diagnosis

The diagnosis of canine hypothyroidism is based on history, clinical signs, quantitation of baseline serum or plasma thyroid hormone levels, thyroid stimulation testing, free levels of thyroid hormones, K values, and therapeutic trials. Biopsies and blood profiles (complete blood count [CBC], creatinine phosphokinase [CPK], cholesterol) are supportive but never diagnostic. Nonspecific findings include anemia in about a fourth of cases, high circulating levels of cholesterol in about a third of cases, and elevated levels of the enzyme creatine phosphokinase in about half of cases. Biopsies for histopathology are often consistent for an endocrinopathy (Fig. 9-1) but are rarely diagnostic.

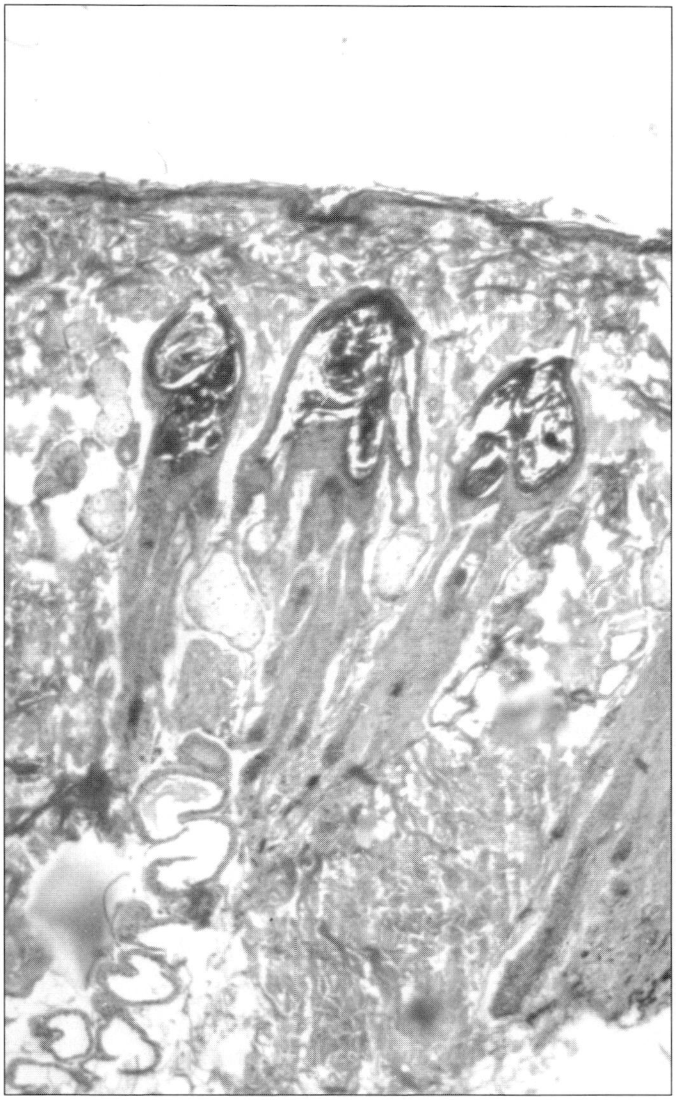

Figure 9-1. Hypothyroidism: Microscopic section with follicular plugging and atrophy of the pilosebaceous units as seen with most endocrinopathies (scan power).

A test measuring simply T_3 and T_4 levels is easy to perform and inexpensive but quite unreliable because thyroid hormone levels fluctuate greatly throughout the day. The finding of low baseline levels is an easy screening test for hypothyroidism, although it is not possible to distinguish among primary, secondary, tertiary, or drug-induced disease. Human reference laboratories must make adjustment to their techniques if they are to accurately detect the low T_4 and T_3 values of canine blood.

The classic diagnostic test for primary hypothyroidism has been the TSH stimulation test, in which a baseline blood level is determined, 0.5 IU of TSH/kg body weight (or 1.0 to 5.0 IU TSH empirically) are injected intravenously, and a second blood sample is obtained in 4 to 6 hours. The remaining reconstituted TSH can be separated into aliquots of 1.0 to 2.5 IU, frozen, and thawed as needed over a period of perhaps 3 months. In primary hypothyroidism there is minimal response after TSH stimulation.

A TSH assay measuring endogenous blood TSH levels has potential value but the assay apparently does not significantly increase the predictive value for hypothyroidism using current methodologies.

The TRH stimulation test is performed by giving TRH intravenously at 0.1 mg/kg and serum is collected 4 to 6 hours later. An increase of 1.5 times over basal T_4 levels is considered normal. Potential transient side effects of TRH administration reported include salivation, vomiting, tachycardia, tachypnea, pupillary dilatation, urination, and defecation.

Free (non–protein bound) thyroxine and triiodothyronine levels also can be obtained but their ultimate value in assisting diagnosis of hypothyroidism has yet to be determined. Accurate measurement of free hormones is believed to correlate closely with the true functional status of the thyroid gland.

Predictive formulas (K values) have also been proposed to enhance accuracy in the diagnosis of primary hypothyroidism. The K value is obtained using the linear discriminant formula $K = 0.5 \times$ basal T_4 (in nmol/L) plus the increase in T_4 after TSH stimulation. It is proposed that those animals with K values less than 15 are hypothyroid, while those with K values greater than 30 are normal or nonresponsive to treatment. Another formula, $K = 0.7 \times$ free T_4 (in pmol/L) – cholesterol (in mmol/L), has also been proposed. Dogs with K values less than –4 are considered hypothyroid while those with K values greater than 1 are considered normal or nonresponsive to treatment. Those with K values between –4 and 1 should be reevaluated using the TSH stimulation test. Large clinical trials are warranted.

Thyroid autoantibodies to both T_4 and T_3 can be determined by some laboratories (Michigan State University Endocrine Diagnostic Laboratory, East Lansing, MI).

Thyroglobulin autoantibodies occur with greater frequency in dogs with clinical hypothyroidism or other endocrine diseases than in normal dogs. In some dogs autoantibody levels may be predictive of impending thyroid failure. Approximately 50% of canine hypothyroid cases have demonstrable circulating antithyroglobulin antibodies. Continued research is needed.

Many dogs evaluated for thyroid function have values considered only borderline for normal. Some of these dogs are actually hypothyroid, but probably many more have nonthyroidal illness. Many medications, especially corticosteroids, profoundly influence the levels of thyroid hormones in circulation and in addition marked decreases may be seen with any disease that results in anorexia for more than 2 days.

A therapeutic trial has in the past been considered a practical and economical diagnostic test for hypothyroidism but it must be cautioned that beneficial effects do not confirm the diagnosis. The danger also exists of creating a hyperthyroid state, even if this is rare in dogs. Because of the tendency toward hyperthyroidism in cats, thyroid supplementation should never be considered a substitute for laboratory assessment.

Cutaneous biopsies are helpful in ruling out nonendocrine differential diagnoses. The microscopic findings of hypothyroidism usually are consistent with an endocrinopathy. Epidermal atrophy, orthokeratosis, hyperkeratosis, follicular atrophy and dilatation, and sebaceous gland atrophy are common nonspecific findings (Fig. 9-1). Microscopic changes most consistent with hypothyroidism include hypertrophy of the arrector pili muscles, increased dermal mucin, and thickened dermis.

Treatment

Several satisfactory treatment protocols have been used for canine hypothyroidism (see Table 3-14). L-Thyroxine is the most widely used replacement hormone; it is given once or twice daily at at a dosage of 0.02 mg/kg. Triiodothyronine and combination T_3-T_4 products have been used with good clinical results but are seldom warranted. The dosage for supplementation with T_3 is 4.4 μg/kg two to three times daily. Treatment should be continued for a minimum of 3 to 4 months because treatment response time is variable. An increase in activity usually is seen within 1 to 2 weeks if lethargy has been a problem. Haircoat and skin changes may require treatment for 1 to 4 months before a satisfactory clinical response is obtained. Lifelong therapy usually is required, although the dosage may be decreased in some dogs.

Monitoring

All animals prescribed thyroid hormones should be reevaluated approximately 6 weeks after initiating therapy, allowing for modification of the regimen if needed. The blood sample is collected 4 to 6 hours after the morning dose was administered. If levels are well into the normal range, dosing may be lessened to once daily for T_4 and twice daily for T_3. Indications for continued therapeutic monitoring include either an exaggerated or inadequate response to the standard recommended dosage of thyroid hormone replacement, a change in the type or dosage of thyroid hormone replacement, or the development of thyrotoxicosis. Several factors must be considered when using posttreatment serum or plasma T_4 or T_3 values to monitor therapeutic response or to decide on changes in therapy.

The best time to monitor T_4 and T_3 concentrations after treatment is dependent on the half-life of these hormones in the circulation. The maximal increase from baseline values occurs in approximately 4 to 12 hours for T_4 and 3 hours for T_3 after treatment with L-thyroxine. Peak blood levels for T_3 after triiodothyronine replacement are more variable and have not been determined accurately. If the dog is on T_3 replacement, the T_4 values will be depressed and of no interpretive value because of a negative feedback effect; thus, the monitoring of T_4 levels would not be indicated. The single most important criterion for therapeutic monitoring is the response to thyroid hormone replacement based on physical examination and history.

HYPERADRENOCORTICISM (CUSHING'S SYNDROME)

The terms *hyperadrenocorticism*, *hypercortisolism*, and *Cushing's syndrome* all refer to a general disease state resulting from a chronic excess of plasma cortisol. Hyperadrenocorticism is the second most common endocrine dermatosis in dogs but is rare in cats.

Etiologic Factors

The most common cause of excessive cortisol levels (85%) is bilateral adrenocortical hyperplasia, which results from an excessive secretion of adrenocorticotropic hormone (ACTH) by the pituitary gland; this is classified as pituitary-dependent hyperadrenocorticism. Functional neoplasms of the adrenal cortex are found in 10 to 15% of dogs with Cushing's syndrome. These neoplasms secrete cortisol independent of pituitary control. Long-term exogenous administration of corticosteroids can cause iatrogenic Cushing's syndrome. In cats, most cases are caused by pituitary adenomas, although pituitary carcinomas, adrenocortical adenomas, and adrenocortical carcinomas have been reported. Females appear to be predisposed to developing hyperadrenocorticism.

Pathogenesis

Cortisol influences the function of most body systems. An excess of cortisol causes atrophy of the hair follicles and sebaceous glands, which leads to the development of alopecia. Inhibition of fibroblast activity results in atrophy of the collagen and fibroelastic tissue in the dermis. This leads to loss of the primary support of the skin, which results in thin skin and a pendulous abdomen.

Excess glycogen is accumulated within hepatocytes leading to impaired liver function and hepatomegaly. The catabolic action of cortisol causes rearrangement of the molecular structure of collagen and elastic tissue, leading to the dystrophic binding of calcium to the altered protein matrix and subsequent calcinosis cutis. The antiinflammatory and immunosuppressive effects of cortisol excess result in secondary superficial pyoderma and systemic infection. Cortisol excess causes a collagen defect in vessel walls, which predisposes to an abnormal hemostatic reaction between collagen, platelets, and coagulation factors, leading to bruising and ecchymoses.

Anestrus and testicular atrophy are believed to result from the inhibition of gonadotropin release by cortisol. The mechanisms of action of cortisol that lead to polydipsia, polyuria, polyphagia, and hyperpigmentation are not completely known.

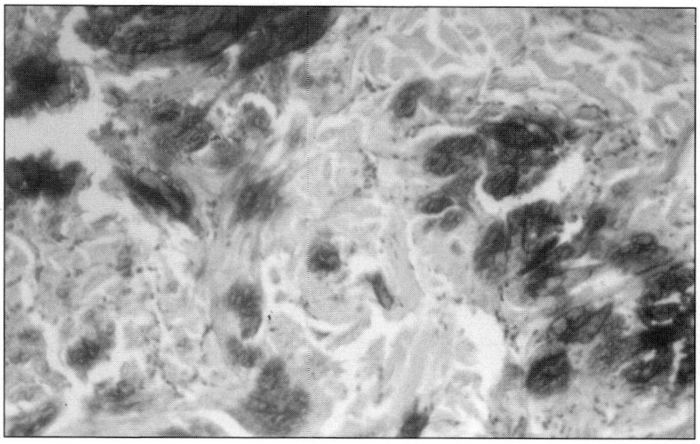

Figure 9-2. Calcinosis cutis: Microscopic section of dermis with multifocal areas of calcium deposition among disrupted collagen fibers.

History

The history associated with hyperadrenocorticism typically (in about two thirds of cases) includes the signs of polydipsia, polyuria, and polyphagia in a middle-aged animal. There is a breed predilection for the poodle, dachshund, boxer, and terrier breeds. Often there is a gradual, progressive, truncal thinning of hair with the legs and head spared. A drug history of chronic corticosteroid administration may suggest an exogenous cause. Prolonged anestrus may be seen in females or lack of libido and infertility in males. A history of pruritus and excoriation associated with focal proliferative lesions also may be reported.

Clinical Findings

The clinical signs of cortisol excess often include polydipsia, polyuria, polyphagia, and a noninflammatory hair loss equally distributed along both sides of the back (bilaterally symmetric alopecia). It should be cautioned, however, that these signs may be apparent in about two thirds of cases and therefore a third of dogs will not manifest them.

Physical examination of the dog with hyperadrenocorticism usually reveals hepatomegaly, some distention of the abdomen, and various degrees of truncal alopecia (Plate VI-3). These signs often are slowly progressive over a 6- to 12-month period from the time the haircoat starts thinning. A thin skin, often with comedone formation and prominent veins, is commonly found together with a distended abdomen. Mild to moderate hyperpigmentation may be observed in the alopecic areas. Hyperpigmentation occurs noticeably less in dogs with hyperadrenocorticism than in most dogs with hypothyroidism or sex hormone–related dermatosis. Testicular and temporal muscle atrophy are observed with longstanding disease.

Superficial pyoderma and urinary and respiratory tract infections are relatively common findings. Evidence may be seen of ecchymoses, especially following venipuncture. In a small percentage (10%) of dogs, calcinosis cutis (Plate VI-4 and Fig. 9-2) is present manifested by focal areas of proliferation of silver-white to red, firm plaques, often found over the dorsal shoulder area and/or ventral abdomen. Tissue reaction to dermal calcium deposits varies from none to marked.

In addition, animals may have neurologic signs (such as rotary nystagmus, seizures, symmetric tetraparesis) as a result of large, compressive pituitary tumors. Hypertension is seen in a considerable number of cases (perhaps 60%).

Dermatologic signs of Cushing's disease usually are absent in cats although thinning of the haircoat may be noted. The most common signs in cats include a pot-bellied appearance, concurrent diabetes mellitus, and organomegaly.

Diagnosis

Screening clinical laboratory tests include hemogram, biochemical profile, urinalysis, and thoracic and abdominal radiography. The hemogram usually reveals mild to moderate leukocytosis, with neutrophilia, lymphopenia, and eosinopenia. An elevated serum alkaline phosphatase concentration is seen in most dogs; this elevation is the result of isoenzyme production by the biliary epithelium in response to excessive levels of glucocorticoids. Some of the increase may also result from hepatocyte swelling and bile stasis. This elevation is not seen in cats because they have the ability to rapidly clear the serum of excess alkaline phosphatase. In general, if over 80% of the serum alkaline phosphatase is attributable to a corticosteroid-induced isoenzyme, a diagnosis of hyperadrenocorticism (natural or iatrogenic) is usually warranted. Mild to marked elevation of alanine aminotransferase (ALT, SGPT) can occur, especially in disease of long duration.

Elevated blood glucose and associated glucosuria are seen in about 15% of cases of canine hyperadrenocorticism and concurrent urinary tract infection and hyposthenuria is commonly recognized. Thyroid hormone levels also are often depressed, yet stimulate normally after administration of TSH depending on the duration of the condition and sustained level of endogenous or exogenous corticosteroid.

Radiographs of the thorax and abdomen may reveal mineralization of the skin, tracheobronchial tree, vasculature, skeletal muscles, kidneys, and occasionally the adrenal gland (Fig. 9-3). Hepatomegaly is the most common radiographic finding and osteoporosis may also be seen. Mineral deposits occur frequently in the adrenal

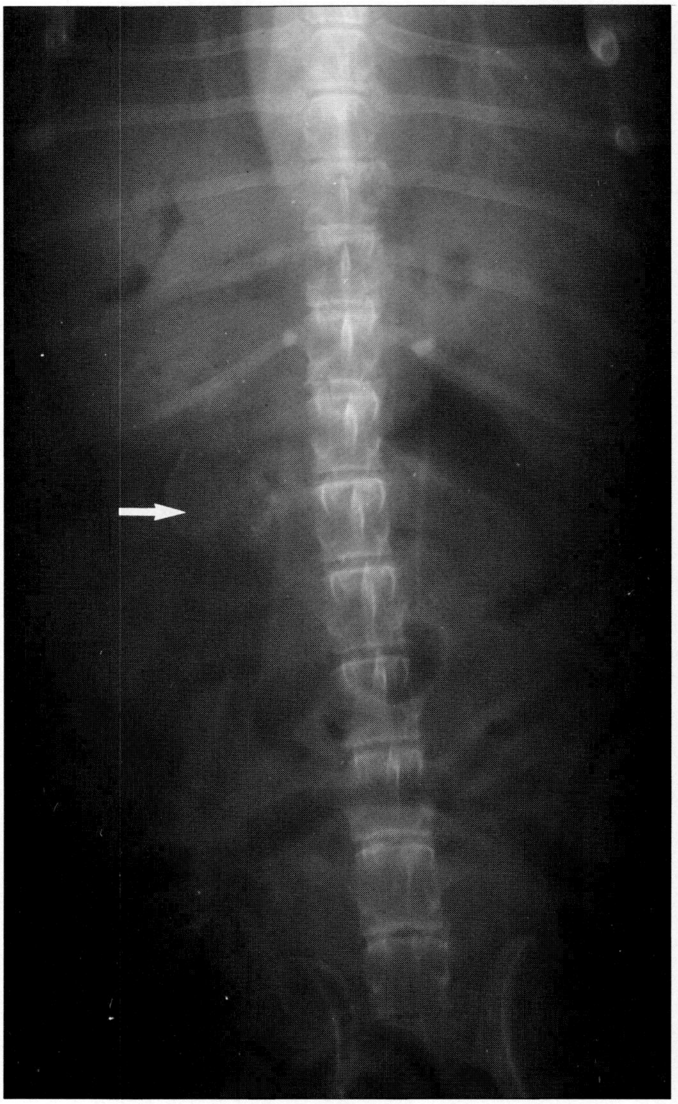

Figure 9-3. Hyperadrenocorticism: Abdominal radiograph with calcification of the left adrenal gland (*arrow*). (Courtesy of Robert Sikes, Glendora, California)

glands of cats and usually are not associated with clinical signs.

Cutaneous biopsy may reveal epidermal and pilosebaceous atrophy and occasionally, dystrophic mineralization.

Cortisol is released from the adrenal glands in episodic fashion and therefore baseline levels of cortisols are rarely of benefit in confirming a diagnosis of hyperadrenocorticism.

The ACTH stimulation test measures cortisol levels in the blood before and 2 hours after (1 hour after in cats) administration of ACTH gel (2.2 IU/kg intramuscularly). In most cushingoid dogs and some cushingoid cats, the poststimulation cortisol values range well above those considered normal. Dogs with iatrogenic hyperadrenocorticism usually have low to normal resting cortisol values and none to minimal response after ACTH administration. An additional drawback is that up to half of dogs with adrenal tumors fail to hyperrespond. The ACTH response test does not differentiate between pituitary-dependent and adrenal-dependent disease.

The low-dose dexamethasone suppression test is accomplished by taking a blood sample for a baseline cortisol value, injecting dexamethasone intravenously at 0.015 mg/kg, and measuring cortisol levels at intervals over an 8-hour period. The most important time interval is 6 to 8 hours, but a sample taken at 3 to 4 hours sometimes also is helpful. The test is considered about 90% diagnostic, and normal dogs show postinjection cortisol levels less than 30 nmol/L (1.0 μg/dl) by 8 hours. Most dogs with Cushing's disease caused by either pituitary or adrenal disease fail to respond at all, have values not less than 30 nmol/L (1.0 μg/dl), or do not have suppressed levels by 8 hours. The low-dose dexamethasone suppression test does not distinguish between adrenal-dependent and pituitary-dependent Cushing's disease. Cats with nonadrenal illnesses, such as diabetes mellitus, chronic renal disease, and congestive heart failure, may have inadequate suppression of cortisols with the low-dose dexamethasone suppression test.

Combinations of the dexamethasone suppression test and the ACTH stimulation test have been evaluated but these tests are often ambiguous and offer no real advantage over the individual tests. The combined test also does not suitably differentiate between adrenal- and pituitary-related disease.

A high-dose dexamethasone suppression test is used to differentiate between pituitary-dependent adrenal hyperplasia and adrenal tumor. In dogs with functional adrenal tumors, a high dose of dexamethasone (1.0 mg/kg) should not suppress the plasma cortisol level because it is only acting by suppressing ACTH secretion. With pituitary-dependent hyperadrenocorticism there will be suppression of the plasma cortisol compared with the baseline. The test should only be used cautiously in diabetic animals because ketoacidosis can result from the high doses of corticosteroids being administered. At this time, the high-dose dexamethasone suppression test may be the preferred screening test for feline hyperadrenocorticism.

Plasma ACTH assays currently available that measure the actual plasma concentration of ACTH are being evaluated to discriminate between pituitary- and adrenal-related disease. Optimal sample handling includes prompt cooling of blood after collection in plastic tubes and shipment on dry ice or with a freeze pack via overnight delivery service. Further controlled studies need to be completed on this assay before it becomes widely available.

Treatment

Both medical and surgical treatment have been advocated for pituitary-dependent hyperadrenocorticism in dogs. The medical treatment of choice is o,p′-DDD, a chlorinated hydrocarbon that causes selective necrosis of the adrenal zona reticularis and fasciculata while sparing the mineralocorticoid-producing zona glomerulosa. A loading dose of 15 to 50 mg/kg is given daily for a week, then maintained on a weekly basis. Glucocorticoids are commonly given concurrently in low doses to help offset the side effects of o,p′-DDD administration initially. Toxicity from o,p′-DDD is common and might include vomiting, diarrhea, anorexia, weakness, lethargy, and depression.

An ACTH response test should be performed 3 to 4 days after the week of daily administration to allow monitoring of plasma cortisols and allow dosage adjustments as necessary. If warranted, daily therapy can be continued until the cortisols remain in the normal range. ACTH stimulation tests should be performed after 3 months initially (earlier if warranted) and then every 6 to 12 months to monitor the condition.

Ketoconazole offers an alternative to o,p′-DDD and administration results in rapid but transient reduction in plasma cortisol concentration and the clinical signs of hyperadrenocorticism. Ketoconazole is administered orally with food (10 mg/kg twice daily) for 7 to 10 days at which time an ACTH stimulation test is done and the dosage adjusted as necessary. Once adequate control has been achieved, the maintenance dosage is administered twice daily and the patient is monitored by ACTH stimulation testing every 3 to 6 months. Although ketoconazole offers some advantages over o,p′-DDD, it is more cumbersome to administer (daily versus weekly) and a much more expensive option in the long term.

Adrenal tumors account for less than 15% of cases. Unilateral adrenalectomy is the treatment of choice for an adrenal tumor in dogs and cats but requires much intraoperative and postoperative care because shock is a common sequel to rebounding low cortisol levels once the gland is removed. Glucocorticoid supplementation is necessary until the opposite adrenal gland regains its normal function.

About half of all dogs surviving surgery will succumb to postoperative complications, such as acute renal failure, pneumonia, and thromboembolism. If the diagnosis was adrenal carcinoma, hyperadrenocorticism will likely recur at some point, despite surgery. With an adrenal carcinoma and liver metastasis, o,p′-DDD at 50 to 150 mg/kg daily may postpone the inevitable.

Therapy of naturally occurring hyperadrenocorticism in cats requires adrenalectomy (bilateral for pituitary diseases, unilateral for adrenal tumor). Animals in which both adrenals have been removed need to be supplemented with both corticosteroids and mineralocorticoids on a lifelong basis.

GROWTH HORMONE–RESPONSIVE DERMATOSIS

Growth hormone–responsive dermatosis of adult onset is a disorder that is presumed to be the result of decreased growth hormone levels in the blood, yet there is much evidence to suggest that this may not be the ultimate cause of the problem. Additional causes might include adrenocortical hyperprogestinism and/or hyperandrogenism. Growth hormone deficiency from birth results in dwarfism (Plate VI-5).

History

There appears to be a breed predilection in the keeshond, chow chow, Pomeranian, poodle, Airedale terrier, Samoyed, and American water spaniel. A sex predilection for males is reported. The owner observes initial alopecic lesions at 1 to 2 years of age in the absence of systemic problems. Hemograms and biochemical, thyroid, and adrenal profiles are invariably within normal ranges.

Clinical Signs

Regional alopecia sparing the legs and head is commonly seen along with hyperpigmentation of affected areas (Plate VI-6). Tufts of hair growth may be associated with areas of trauma, such as previous biopsy sites.

Diagnosis

Blood tests measuring growth hormone, or somatomedin, levels are the only way to confirm a diagnosis. These tests are expensive and performed by few laboratories and may be difficult to interpret. A growth hormone stimulation test can be performed by taking blood samples for growth hormone levels before and 15, 30, 45, and 60 minutes after injection of a measured amount of xylazine (100 to 300 μg/kg IV). Blood levels of somatomedin C, a growth hormone intermediary, are supposedly reduced in growth hormone–responsive dermatosis but this has not been convincingly demonstrated.

Biopsies taken from dogs with growth hormone–responsive dermatosis cannot be readily differentiated from those from dogs with other endocrinopathies. Changes include orthokeratotic hyperkeratosis, pilosebaceous atrophy, follicular plugging, and perhaps fewer elastin fibers than normal.

Treatment

The ultimate therapy of growth hormone–responsive dermatosis remains the subject of great debate. Because the condition is essentially cosmetic, management must not offer undue health risks to the animal. Intact animals should be neutered, a percentage of which will improve within 3 to 6 months from this measure alone.

Growth hormone is in short supply, seldom available commercially, and relatively expensive. It can be dosed at 0.1 IU/kg three times weekly for 4 to 6 weeks. A side effect is the development of transient or permanent diabetes mellitus; therefore, blood glucose levels should be monitored. Animals initially well controlled may relapse several months after discontinuation of therapy.

HYPERESTROGENISM

Pathogenesis

Hyperestrogenism, formerly known as *ovarian imbalance type I*, is a rare disorder caused mainly by formation of cysts on the ovaries or occasionally by development of ovarian tumors. A similar syndrome can be induced by administration of estrogens used to treat such conditions as urinary incontinence, mismating, and male aggression.

History

A middle-aged to older intact female dog is usually examined for a history of pseudocyesis or anestrus. Chronic, slowly progressive skin changes are observed in the ventral caudal abdomen, flank, and perineal regions.

Clinical Findings

The initial lesions are alopecia, hyperpigmentation, and scaling on the flanks and perineal region (Plate VI-7). Lichenification is prominent in the advanced stages. The axillae may also become involved with similar lesions. Other common findings include vulvar hyperplasia, crusting, and enlargement of the nipples. In the advancing stages of the syndrome, generalized scaling, greasiness, and ceruminous otitis are observed. Pruritus is variable.

Diagnosis

Diagnosis is made on the basis of the history, physical examination, and response to ovariohysterectomy.

Treatment

Ovariohysterectomy results in near-total reversal of clinical signs in most dogs several months after surgery. If greasiness is present, antiseborrheic shampoos are helpful.

ESTROGEN-RESPONSIVE DERMATOSIS

Pathogenesis

Estrogen-responsive dermatosis, presumably caused by low circulating levels of estrogens in the blood, was formerly known as *ovarian imbalance type II*. It has never been documented that these animals are actually deficient in estrogen.

History

A middle-aged to older female dog that has had an ovariohysterectomy at a young age is examined for a history of immature coat and progressive alopecia around the perineum, ventral abdomen, neck, and ears (Plate VI-8). Occasionally urinary incontinence is present.

Clinical Findings

The skin is soft, pliable, and smooth. Alopecia is noted on the perineum, ventral abdomen, neck, and head. The haircoat is fine and silky. The vulva and nipples often appear juvenile. All biochemical and hematologic parameters are normal.

Diagnosis

The history and clinical findings are suggestive. Normal thyroid serum levels and adrenal function tests further support the diagnosis. The most definitive diagnostic test is a therapeutic trial with estrogen replacement.

Treatment

Replacement therapy with 1 mg diethylstilbestrol, two to three times weekly, usually results in reversal of clinical signs within 2 to 4 months. In most dogs this therapy must be continued on a weekly basis for a lifetime because relapses often occur. If long-term maintenance therapy is required, potential bone marrow suppression and platelet dysfunction can occur; monitoring is critical.

TESTICULAR TUMORS

Pathogenesis

Testicular tumors, usually Sertoli cell tumors but occasionally interstitial cell tumors and seminomas, can secrete female sex hormones and result in hyperestrogenism in male dogs. The incidence is much higher in dogs whose testicles have not descended completely from the abdominal cavity into the scrotum.

History

Breeds reported to have a high incidence of Sertoli cell tumor include the Chihuahua, Pomeranian, miniature schnauzer, miniature and standard poodle, Shetland sheepdog, Siberian husky, boxer, and Yorkshire terrier. The age of onset is usually more than 7 years.

Most owners are unaware of the presence of a testicular tumor in their dog until it is revealed by physical examination or becomes so large as to be visibly evident. There may be a history of progressive symmetric alopecia and hyperpigmentation of the perineal and periscrotal regions. Attraction of male dogs and decreased libido may be reported. Systemic illness may result from long-standing testicular tumors secreting estrogens because of bone marrow suppression.

Clinical Findings

Palpation of the testes reveals one enlarged testis, either scrotal or, more commonly, abdominal or inguinal. The other testis, if descended, is usually smaller and softer.

Cutaneous changes consist of alopecia of the perineal area and posterolateral thighs, and often marked hyperpigmentation of the affected areas (Plate VI-9). Lichenification is evident in long-standing cases. Palpable prostatic hyperplasia is frequently observed as is a pendulous and edematous prepuce. Perianal gland tumors and perineal hernia may be seen with seminomas.

Diagnosis

The history and clinical findings are suggestive but diagnosis is confirmed by testicular biopsy, usually performed at the time of neutering. Estrogen and testosterone levels are indicated but results vary and interpretation is not standardized.

Treatment

Removal of the testes is required and the prognosis is usually good if metastasis has not occurred and if any bone marrow suppression present is reversible. Chest radiographs and blood counts (including platelet counts) should be considered before surgery.

SELECTED READINGS

Arnold U, Opitz M, Grosser I, et al: Goitrous hypothyroidism and dwarfism in a kitten. *JAAHA* 20:753–758, 1984.

Beale KM, Halliwell REW, Chen CL: Prevalence of antithyroglobulin antibodies detected by enzyme-linked immunosorbent assay of canine serum. *JAVMA* 196:745–748, 1990.

Bruyette DS, Feldman EC: Ketoconazole and its use in the management of canine Cushing's disease. *Compend Contin Educ Pract Vet* 10:1379–1386, 1988.

Dorn AS, Craig JA, Van Ee RT: Sex hormone–related diseases treated surgically in bitches. *Mod Vet Pract* 66:621– 625, 1985.

Dorn AS, Bone DL, Bellah JR: Sex hormone–related diseases treated surgically in male dogs. *Mod Vet Pract* 66:727–733, 1985.

Emms SG, Johnston DE, Eigenmann JE, Goldschmidt MH: Adrenalectomy in the management of canine hyperadrenocorticism. *JAAHA* 23:557–564, 1987.

Feldman EC: Comparison of ACTH response and dexamethasone suppression as screening tests in canine hyperadrenocorticism. *JAVMA* 182:506–510, 1983.

Feldman EC: Distinguishing dogs with functioning adrenocortical tumors from dogs with pituitary-dependent hyperadrenocorticism. *JAVMA* 182:195–199, 1983.

Feldman EC, Bruyette DS, Nelson RW, Farver TB: Plasma cortisol reponse to ketoconazole administration in dogs with hyperadrenocorticism. *JAVMA* 197:71–78, 1990.

Ferguson DC: Thyroid function tests in the dog: Recent concepts. *Vet Clin North Am [Small Anim Pract]* 14:783–808, 1984.

Ferguson DC: The effect of nonthyroidal factors on thyroid function tests in dogs. *Compend Contin Educ Pract Vet* 10:1365–1377, 1988.

Haines DM, Lording PM, Penhale WJ: Survey of thyroglobulin autoantibodies in dogs. *Am J Vet Res* 45:1493–1497, 1984.

Kemppainen RJ, Sartin JL: Evidence for episodic but not circadian activity in plasma concentrations of adrenocorticotrophin, cortisol and thyroxine in dogs. *Endocrinology* 103: 219–226, 1984.

Kemppainen RJ, Mansield PD, Sartin JL: Endocrine responses of normal cats to TSH and synthetic ACTH administration. *JAAHA* 20:737–740, 1984.

Larsson MG: Determination of free thyroxine and cholesterol as a new screening test for canine hypothyroidism. *JAAHA* 24:209–217, 1988.

Lothrop CD Jr: Pathophysiology of canine growth hormone–responsive alopecia. *Compend Contin Educ Pract Vet* 10:1346–1352, 1988.

Lothrop CD Jr, Tamas PM, Fadok VA: Canine and feline thyroid function assessment with the thyrotropin-releasing hormone response test. *Am J Vet Res* 45:2310–2313, 1984.

Medleau L: Sex hormone-associated endocrine alopecias in dogs. *JAAHA* 25:689–694, 1989.

Nelson RW, Feldman EC, Smith MC,: Hyperadrenocorticism in cats: Seven cases (1978–1987). *JAVMA* 193:245–250, 1988.

Nesbitt GH, Izzo J, Wilkins RJ, et al: Canine hypothyroidism: A retrospective study of 108 cases. *JAVMA* 177:1117–1122, 1980.

Panciera DL: Canine hypothyroidism. Part I. Clinical findings and control of thyroid hormone secretion and metabolism. *Compend Contin Educ Pract Vet* 12(5):689–701, 1990.

Peterson ME: Hyperadrenocorticism. *Vet Clin North Am [Small Anim Pract]* 14:731–750,1984.

Peterson ME, et al: Endocrine disorders in cats: Four emerging diseases. *Compend Contin Educ Pract Vet* 10:1353–1363, 1988.

Reimers TJ, Lawler DF, Sutaria PM, et al: Effect of age, sex, and body size on serum concentrations of thyroid and adrenocortrical hormones in dogs. *Am J Vet Res* 51:454–457, 1990.

Schmeitzel L, Lothrop CD Jr: Hormonal abnormalities in Pomeranians with normal coat and in Pomeranians with growth hormone–responsive dermatosis. *JAVMA* 197(10):1333–1341, 1990.

Scott DW, Walton DK: Hyposomatotropism in the mature dog: A discussion of 22 cases. *JAAHA* 22:467–473, 1986.

Voorhout G, Stolp R, Lubberink AAME, Van Waes PFGM, et al: Computed tomography in the diagnosis of canine hyperadrenocorticism not suppressible with dexamethasone. *JAVMA* 192:641–646, 1988.

Chapter 10

KERATINIZATION DISORDERS (SEBORRHEA)

Lowell Ackerman, DVM
Gene H. Nesbitt, DVM, MS

Disorders of keratinization (seborrhea, erythroderma, exfoliative dermatitis) refers to a broad classification of clinical entities ranging from simple dandruff to severe red, crusting, and scaly skin. The normal process of epidermal renewal involves the orderly turnover of epidermal cells, progressing from the basal cell layer to the shingle-like stratum corneum in about 21 to 23 days. In keratinization disorders, there is an increased turnover rate. The entire epidermis may be replaced in as little as 2 to 4 days, leaving scale on the skin surface.

The term *seborrhea* is a poor one because it literally means "flow of sebum" and most keratinization disorders have little or nothing to do with sebum production. Dozens of different disorders with different causes and different treatments have been lumped together under the heading "seborrhea" in the past. It is hoped that most conditions now are better diagnosed and specific therapy rendered.

Diagnostic Key 9 (see end of Chapter 2) lists the most pertinent historical and clinical findings and diagnostic tests necessary to differentiate the common keratinization disorders.

SECONDARY KERATINIZATION DEFECTS

Pathogenesis

Some animals undoubtedly are born with a defect in their keratinization process. By far most keratinization disorders occur secondary to underlying problems. Thus, it is always best to identify a specific cause so that a specific treatment can be applied.

Some common conditions that can result in secondary keratinization disorders include allergies, ectoparasites, dermatophytes, endocrinopathies, nutritional disorders, immune-mediated conditions, environmental conditions, and even some neoplasias.

Clinical Signs

Scaling, crusting, greasiness, and hair loss are the primary clinical signs of keratinization disorders. Secondarily, variable degrees of inflammation, scratching, self-trauma, and bacterial dermatitis are evidenced in some cases. The normal cutaneous bacterial flora of 100 to 200 colonies/cm^2 increases to an average of 16,000 colonies/cm^2 on skin with a keratinization defect. Ceruminous otitis externa and hyperplasia of the tail gland are also commonly noted. Lesions on dogs can vary from dry to greasy but most dogs have "combination skin" in which some areas are greasy and others dry.

The most common clinical signs associated with feline keratinization disorders are generalized dry skin and haircoat with excessive scaling. Signs of excessive oiliness are rare in cats, but when present usually are associated with systemic signs of feline leukemia, liver disease, neoplasia, or immune-mediated disorders.

Diagnosis

Multiple skin scrapings are always indicated to rule out external parasites. Therapeutic trials with parasiticides also help with the diagnosis. Fungal cultures also should be performed because dermatophytes routinely cause scaling and are sometimes associated with crusting. If allergies are suspected, hypoallergenic diet trials and intradermal allergy testing are indicated. Thyroid function tests and biochemical profiles should be performed if an endocrine-related or metabolic disorder is suspected, and therapeutic trials with fatty acid supplements are recommended if fatty acid deficiencies are suspected. All cats should be evaluated with a viral profile (feline immunodeficiency virus [FIV], feline leukemia virus [FeLV]) in addition to a complete blood count and biochemical profile.

Cutaneous biopsy is often useful and might demonstrate microscopic findings of crusts, orthokeratotic and/or parakeratotic and/or follicular hyperkeratosis, epidermal hyperplasia, a superficial perivascular dermatitis, and intercellular edema (Fig. 10-1). More specific findings, such as tissue eosinophilia, presence of fungal elements, dystrophic mineralization, acantholysis, and marked follicular hyperkeratosis, may allow a more definitive diagnosis.

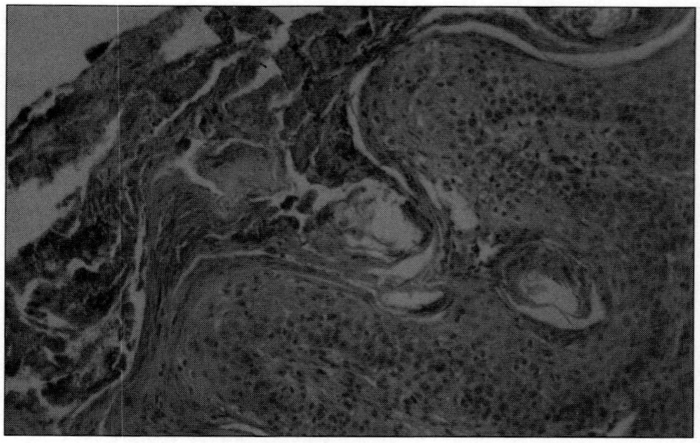

Figure 10-1. Seborrheic syndrome: Microscopic section with crusts, hyperkeratosis, parakeratotic hyperkeratosis, acanthosis, and a cellular infiltrate at the dermoepidermal junction (low power).

Treatment

Treatment usually is successful when the underlying provoking factors have been identified and corrected. For disorders in which the underlying condition has not been identified, treatment must be vigorous and intensive, although in most cases the animal's overall health status is not compromised. Frequent bathing and topical treatment of the skin, and perhaps dietary supplementation as well, may make the condition more tolerable. This usually means bathing from twice weekly to once every few weeks with an antiseborrheic shampoo (see Table 3-6). To maximize the effect of all antiseborrheic shampoos, they should be left on the animal's skin (not just the haircoat) for 5 to 15 minutes after thorough lathering, or as recommended by the manufacturer. Proper rinsing is essential, and animals should be air-dried or towel-dried rather than blown dry. Emollients and humectants (see Table 3-2) permit moisturizing of the skin in the intervals between baths.

PRIMARY IDIOPATHIC "SEBORRHEA"

Pathogenesis

The epidermal and follicular turnover times are more rapid in affected animals and their keratinization process is considered hyperproliferative. Cocker spaniels, springer spaniels, Irish setters, basset hounds, West Highland white terriers, Doberman pinschers, shar peis, and Labrador retrievers are most commonly affected. A primary epidermal cell defect is suspected.

Clinical Signs

Clinical signs vary from a dry scaling coat to greasiness and associated inflammatory reactions. A secondary pyoderma is often apparent as is ceruminous otitis externa. Commonly involved areas include the periocular region, interdigital spaces, axillae, and perineum.

Diagnosis

A diagnosis can be suspected by ruling out the other causes of keratinization defects. Biopsy specimens often demonstrate orthokeratotic, parakeratotic, and follicular hyperkeratosis, dyskeratosis, and a superficial perivascular dermatitis.

Treatment

Idiopathic seborrhea can be controlled but not cured. Treatment must be intensive and includes frequent antiseborrheic shampooing, systemic and topical corticosteroids, antibiotics for concurrent pyoderma, and dietary supplementation. Use of synthetic retinoids may also be beneficial but they are expensive, have side effects, and are not approved for use in dogs and cats.

EPIDERMAL DYSPLASIA

Pathogenesis

Epidermal dysplasia is a congenitohereditary keratinization defect seen most commonly in the West Highland white terrier. There is no apparent sex predilection.

Clinical Signs

Epidermal dysplasia starts at an early age and is a pruritic, scaling disorder seen most commonly on the extremities, axillae, inguinal area, and perineum. Erythema, hair loss, hyperpigmentation, and lichenification are often pronounced (Plate VII-1).

Diagnosis

Biopsy specimens from affected tissue often reveal epidermal hyperplasia, dyskeratosis, epidermal disorientation, epidermal budding, parakeratotic mounding, and a superficial perivascular dermatitis.

Treatment

There is no satisfactory treatment for epidermal dysplasia and the condition usually becomes progressively worse despite treatment. Drugs affecting the keratinization process, such as corticosteroids and retinoids, may offer temporary benefit.

ICHTHYOSIS

Pathogenesis

Canine ichthyosis is a hereditary disease characterized by extreme hyperkeratosis and exaggerated thickening of the digital, carpal, and tarsal pads. The actual causes are unknown and it is uncertain if all of the cases reported actually represent the same defect.

History and Clinical Signs

The incidence of canine ichthyosis is rare. Typically, a young dog (less than 6 months) is examined for excessive scaling, usually generalized, which progresses with age (Plate VII-2). There are tightly adhering tannish-gray scales and feathered keratinous projections. The digital pads are thickened with large accumulations of keratin at the margins of the pads; pain may also be associated with this disease.

Diagnosis

History and clinical appearance are diagnostic. Cutaneous biopsy rules out other etiologic factors and also supports the diagnosis with findings of orthokeratotic hyperkeratosis and hypergranulosis.

Treatment

Palliative treatment with warm water soaks and antiseborrheic and keratolytic shampoos are sometimes helpful. Emollient rinses may help prevent dryness of the skin. Some of the newer retinoids, especially etretinate, may have an important role in the management of patients with ichthyosis. Even intense treatment, however, will only mask the disorder. As with all hereditary defects, a cure is impossible.

FATTY ACID DEFICIENCY

Pathogenesis

Fats usually make up 5 to 20% of the dry matter of dog foods and may provide 25 to 50% of the daily caloric needs of the animal. Essential fatty acids should constitute at least 1% of the diet, or 2% of the caloric intake. Poor-quality dog foods may be deficient in fatty acids. Dry foods especially are limited in the amount of fats that can be incorporated without causing rancidity. Antioxidants normally are added to foods to delay this process, but foods stored for long periods at high temperatures can lose their fatty acid content. Medical conditions that limit the body's ability to absorb or metabolize ingested fats can also result in fatty acid deficiency.

Clinical Signs

Animals must normally be fed a fatty acid–deficient diet for many months before they begin to show signs. A dry, lusterless coat and prominent dandruff are often the first signs evident. Bacterial infections can further affect the skin and haircoat.

Diagnosis

Diagnosis is often based on history and clinical signs and can be supported but not confirmed by biopsy.

Treatment

Therapy involves feeding a good-quality food with adequate fat content and supplementing the diet with a suitable fatty acid compound. Topical applications of essential fatty acids also result in some absorption directly through the skin. Antiseborrheic shampoos remove the scales and oiliness from the skin.

ZINC-RELATED DERMATOSES

Pathogenesis

Zinc-related dermatoses include the clinical skin conditions characterized by focal scaling and crusting lesions that are either associated with zinc or respond to zinc supplementation. Three syndromes have been recognized, one in rapidly growing puppies, one with a predisposition for the sled dog breeds, and one associated with the feeding of generic dog foods.

Anything that interferes with the absorption of zinc, affects its longevity or function in the body, enhances its excretion, or causes general body wasting and catabolism also reduces the body stores of zinc.

Clinical Signs

Some Siberian huskies, malamutes, Samoyeds, and perhaps Great Danes and Doberman pinschers may have a genetic defect that results in a decreased ability to absorb zinc from the intestine. The clinical presentation is usually one of tenacious crusts, redness, and a variable degree of itchiness. The most commonly affected areas include the face, footpads (Plate VII-3), elbows, and hocks. Hyperpigmentation may be seen in chronic lesions.

In young rapidly growing dogs, the primary skin lesions are focal hyperkeratotic plaques and crusts over the head, trunk, and extremities. Thickening and fissuring of the footpads and planum nasale are common signs as is a moderate lymphadenomegaly.

Clinical signs of generic dog food disease usually develop in dogs between 2 and 4 weeks after being given the generic diet as the sole food source. Affected animals are often normal on physical examination but lethargic and depressed. Extensive crusting and scaling is noted, and the predominant sites of involvement include the distal extremities, face, pressure points, mucocutaneous junctions, and trunk. Pruritus, hyperpigmentation, erythema, alopecia, and lichenification are variable but enlarged lymph nodes are common.

Diagnosis

History and clinical signs are usually suggestive and biopsies are supportive but nonconfirmatory. Response to therapy is the most definitive test.

Treatment

Dietary management consists of first putting the animal on a good plane of nutrition, removing any and all dietary supplements, and ensuring the animal is fed a brand name dog food. These animals should get better within 6 to 8 weeks. Animals requiring zinc supplementation usually benefit from administration of zinc sulfate, zinc gluconate, or zinc methionine at a dose of 1.1 mg elemental zinc/kg twice daily. Symptomatic treatment with antiseborrheic shampoos, emollient rinses, and antibiotics usually is indicated.

VITAMIN A–RESPONSIVE DERMATOSIS

Pathogenesis

This is not a deficiency syndrome but rather a skin condition that responds to large doses of vitamin A supplementation. The principal breed affected is the cocker spaniel, but other breeds, such as the Labrador retriever and cairn terrier, have also been affected. Anything that interferes with the absorption of vitamin A or enhances its excretion can result in a relative deficiency.

Clinical Signs

The condition is characterized by scaling, hair loss, and marked crusting, especially on the back and head. The center of the problem is the hair follicle, from which the scaling and crusting (follicular keratosis) originates.

Diagnosis

Diagnosis is based on the history, clinical signs, and biopsies for histopathologic evaluation. Biopsies reveal dyskeratosis (abnormal keratinization) and marked follicular hyperkeratosis.

Treatment

Therapy includes megadose vitamin A administration on a daily basis (10,000–100,000 IU/day), usually for life. Most cocker spaniels benefit from doses approximating 10,000 IU daily. Because vitamin A is stored in the liver, liver function evaluation should be an important component of any monitoring program.

PERIAPPENDAGEAL DERMATITIS (SEBACEOUS ADENITIS)

Pathogenesis

Periappendageal dermatitis describes a condition in which the hair follicles and adnexa are involved in an inflammatory process that results clinically in a keratinization disorder. It is most commonly reported in standard poodles, but Samoyeds, Irish setters, golden retrievers, yellow Labrador retrievers, and collies have also been affected. These disorders are grouped collectively because of our current limited knowledge of their etiology.

Clinical Signs

Most dogs are initially affected at 1 to 5 years of age. Symmetric nonpruritic scaling and hair loss begin on the dorsal midline and progress (Plate VII-4). Secondary bacterial infection is common and may cause pruritus.

Diagnosis

The diagnosis is based on the history, clinical signs, and histopathologic examination of biopsies, which shows inflammatory destruction of the follicle and/or associated adnexa.

Treatment

Treatment is only palliative and corticosteroids may halt progression of the disease. Later, frequent antiseborrheic shampooing and application of emollients, such as propylene glycol, urea, or lactic acid, may be beneficial. Treatment with isotretinoin (Accutane®—Roche) at 1 mg/kg daily may also be beneficial but animals must be carefully monitored for adverse effects. This product is not licensed for use in dogs or cats.

FOOTPAD HYPERKERATOSIS

Pathogenesis

Footpad hyperkeratosis (hyperkeratotic footpads) describes conditions in which the pads tend to become thickened, cracked, and scaly when diseased.

Footpad diseases have various causes. In the past, many cases were undoubtedly the result of infection with distemper virus (hard pad disease). With today's more sophisticated methods of diagnosis, many different conditions have been implicated in footpad disorders, including parasitism, bacterial infections, fungal infections, contact allergy, autoimmune diseases (lupus erythematosus, pemphigus foliaceus), nutritional skin diseases (zinc-responsive dermatosis, generic dog food disease), congenitohereditary diseases, neoplasms (squamous cell carcinoma), contact irritation, cutaneous horns, and nasodigital hyperkeratosis.

Clinical Signs

As described above, footpad hyperkeratosis is reflected by pads that are thickened, cracked, and scaly (Plate VII-5). Accompanying clinical signs may be helpful in distinguishing the underlying cause.

Diagnosis

Because footpad hyperkeratosis can result from so many different causes, it is important that a thorough search for underlying disorders be initiated. A minimum data base should include skin scrapings, complete blood count, and fungal culture. Biopsies are often warranted. In cats, viral profiles (especially for feline leukemia virus) should be considered mandatory.

Treatment

Treatment should always be directed at the underlying cause if it can be determined. Symptomatic treatment is attempted by shaving away the excess dead tissue and applying hydrating ointments and keratolytics to increase shedding of the accumulated material.

LICHENOID-PSORIASIFORM DERMATOSIS

Pathogenesis

Clinical lichenoid dermatoses are uncommon in dogs and include idiopathic lichenoid dermatosis, lichenoid keratosis, and lichenoid-psoriasiform dermatitis of springer spaniels.

Lichenoid-psoriasiform dermatosis connotes a pathologic description (psoriasiform dermatitis with a lichenoid tissue reaction) in a specific breed. To date, no other breeds have been affected, suggesting that inheritance has a role in the etiology.

Clinical Signs

The dermatitis usually is manifested as plaques on the skin of the pinnae and ventral abdominal skin (Plate VII-6). Affected dogs are often under 3 years of age. The condition is more of a cosmetic defect than a health concern.

Diagnosis

Diagnosis is easily accomplished by biopsies for histopathology in which the characteristic changes (irregular epidermal hyperplasia with a lichenoid band of mononuclear cells at the dermoepidermal junction) are seen.

Treatment

No treatment is necessary as the condition poses no health concern.

LARGE PLAQUE PARAPSORIASIS

Pathogenesis

Large plaque parapsoriasis has only recently been described in dogs and cats. It refers to a focal exfoliative dermatosis with certain historical, clinical, and histopathologic consistencies. In humans, large plaque parapsoriasis is sometimes a precancerous state of cutaneous

T-cell lymphoma. No pathogenesis has been proposed in animals.

Clinical Signs

Lesions consist of exfoliative dermatitis in which papules, plaques, and crusts are noted. Hyperpigmentation and associated alopecia may be recognized. The condition does not appear to be either pruritic or painful.

Diagnosis

A diagnosis can be suspected on the basis of clinical signs and histopathologic findings but there are no confirmatory tests. Skin biopsies often reveal orthokeratotic and parakeratotic hyperkeratosis, superficial perivascular dermatitis, lymphocytic exocytosis, and accumulation of lymphocytes at the stratum basale.

Treatment

Treatment consists of antiseborrheic shampooing regimens, emollients, and corticosteroids. Initial doses of 2.2 mg/kg/day usually result in remission, and maintenance doses of 1.1 mg/kg on alternate days usually are sufficient.

FOLLICULAR DYSPLASIA/DYSTROPHY

Follicular dysplasia and dystrophies consist of color-mutant alopecia and black hair follicular dysplasia.

Color-mutant alopecia describes the patchy poor haircoat that develops in these abnormally colored animals. They are born with normal coats but later suffer from hair loss, dry skin, and cutaneous bacterial infections (Plate VII-7). The principal breeds involved include blue Doberman pinschers, Great Danes, dachshunds, whippets, Italian greyhounds, and standard poodles. Red Doberman pinschers and fawn Irish setters may have milder forms of the disorder.

Black hair follicular dysplasia is a tardive hereditary alopecia in black and white spotted dogs. It has been observed in mongrels, papillons, and dachshunds. Dysplasia of the follicle in the alopecic areas of black skin occurs with resulting abnormal hair development, shedding, and scaling. The white skin is not affected.

Diagnosis

Diagnosis is based on clinical signs, direct examination of hair shafts (large clumps of free melanin with color-mutant alopecia), and biopsies for histopathology. Biopsies often reveal profound follicular hyperkeratosis and cystic dilatation of affected hair follicles.

Treatment

Treatment is symptomatic and lifelong because the abnormal hair follicles cannot be replaced. Antiseborrheic shampoos (see Table 3-6) normally are prescribed to remove the prominent scale that forms on the skin surface. Therapy should be considered lifelong and animals should not be used for breeding.

ACNE

Pathogenesis

Acne is a follicular keratinization disorder frequently resulting in secondary bacterial involvement. Certain breeds, such as the Great Dane, Doberman pinscher, bulldog, and bull terrier, are particularly at risk, but any animal can be afflicted with acne. With chronic bacterial involvement, lesions can develop into furunculosis and have draining tracts. Feline acne has no age, sex, or breed predilection.

Clinical Signs

The condition often begins as comedones associated with plugging of the hair follicles. Papules, pustules, nodules and furuncles frequently result (Plate VII-8). The most common areas for involvement are the chin, muzzle, and lip margins.

In cats, acne lesions are characterized by comedones on the chin and lower lips that only occasionally are painful or pruritic (Plate VII-9).

Diagnosis

The diagnosis normally is based on clinical presentation but can be confirmed by biopsy. Chronic lesions often are associated with granulomas. Canine lesions are often contaminated with staphylococci while cultures from cats usually reveal *Pasteurella multocida* or β-hemolytic streptococci.

Treatment

Treatment is aimed at cleansing the hair follicle and therefore benzoyl peroxide cleansers frequently are used. Systemic antibiotics are palliative but will not cure the condition. Intralesional or systemic corticosteroids are sometimes used to reduce inflammation. Retinoids, such as isotretinoin, may be helpful in troublesome cases but are not licensed for use in dogs or cats.

SCHNAUZER COMEDO SYNDROME

Pathogenesis

Schnauzer comedo syndrome is a congenitohereditary disorder characterized by abnormal follicular keratinization. The actual cause is unknown.

History and Clinical Signs

The owner observes small crusts on the back, often at the time of grooming, which initially cause little or no discomfort to the dog. Pain and pruritus normally accompany the condition once folliculitis results. The lesions are well-demarcated crusted papules associated with the individual hair follicles on the entire dorsum of the back from the shoulder to the tail. Soft, waxy comedones rather than crusting may also be observed.

Diagnosis

The history, breed predilection, and distribution of clinical signs are normally sufficient to permit diagnosis but biopsies (gross distention of hair follicles with keratin) are confirmatory. Hypothyroidism is found as a concurrent problem in approximately 25% of cases.

Treatment

Schnauzer comedo syndrome is treated with antiseborrheic shampoos. Bathing every 2 to 4 weeks helps prevent recurrence. Antibiotics may contribute to a faster clinical response. Thyroid replacement should be instituted if warranted (see Table 3-14). Alcohol rubs twice weekly are helpful in preventing a recurrence of lesions.

KERATOSES

Pathogenesis

Keratoses are accumulations of large amounts of keratin; they can be seborrheic, actinic, or proliferative (cutaneous "horns"). Actinic keratosis may be a premalignant lesion that can develop into squamous cell carcinoma.

Clinical Signs

Seborrheic keratoses are nodular to plaque-like growths that often are hyperpigmented and have a greasy texture. Actinic keratoses are caused by excessive exposure of skin to ultraviolet light. They form on lightly haired or lightly pigmented skin, which receives a comparatively large amount of ultraviolet irradiation from sunlight. Proliferative keratoses (cutaneous horns) form from compacted scale.

Diagnosis

Keratoses are suspected on the basis of history and clinical signs and are confirmed by characteristic biopsy findings. Seborrheic keratoses have extreme orthokeratotic hyperkeratosis and papillomatous epidermal hyperplasia. Actinic keratoses show dysplastic epidermal cells and hyperkeratosis. Proliferative keratoses form from accumulations of compact lamellated orthokeratotic hyperkeratosis that may overlay tumors, virus-induced lesions, or other keratoses.

CALLUS

Pathogenesis

Calluses develop over pressure points subjected to repeated trauma. They are most commonly seen on the elbows and hocks of large breeds of dogs, and occasionally on the sternum of others (for example, dachshunds). They are formed by the repeated impact of these body parts on hard surfaces, such as concrete, wood, or tile.

Clinical Signs

Calluses are hyperkeratotic plaques most commonly found on the elbows, hocks or sternum. They initially are scaly but may become infected when chronic. Furunculosis and draining tracts are an eventuality. Persistent exudate, erosions, and crusting result from constant irritation and friction.

Diagnosis

Calluses are suspected on the basis of clinical appearance as well as breed and site predilection. Biopsies are confirmatory.

Treatment

Most calluses are harmless and require no treatment. For minor problems, application of skin softeners, emollients, and keratolytics is sufficient. For large calluses and callous pyoderma, the use of antibiotics and protective padding is warranted. Surgery is often an unsatisfactory option because of the sites involved.

SELECTED READINGS

Ackerman LJ: Lichenoid-psoriasiform dermatosis in a springer spaniel. *Mod Vet Pract* 69:32–33, 1988.

Anderson RK: Exfoliative dermatitis in the dog. *Compend Contin Educ Pract Vet* 3:885–890, 1981.

Austin VH: A clinical approach to abnormal keratinization diseases of the dog. *Compend Contin Educ Pract Vet* 5:890–897, 1983.

Baker BB, Maibach HI: Epidermal cell renewal in seborrheic skin of dogs. *Am J Vet Res* 48:716–718, 1987.

Briggs OM, Botha WS: Color mutant alopecia in a blue Italian greyhound. *JAAHA* 22:611–614, 1986.

Carpenter JL, Thornton GW, Moore FM, King NW Jr: Idiopathic periadnexal multinodular granulomatous dermatitis in 22 dogs. *Vet Pathol* 24:5–10, 1987.

Degryse AD, Fransen J, Van Cutsem J, Ooms L: Recurrent zinc-responsive dermatosis in a Siberian husky. *J Small Anim Pract* 28:721–726, 1987.

Fadok VA: Treatment of canine idiopathic seborrhea with isotretinoin. *Am J Vet Res* 47:1730, 1986.

Ihrke PJ, Goldschmidt MH: Vitamin A–responsive dermatosis in the dog. *JAVMA* 182:687–690, 1983.

Kwochka KW, Rademakers AM: Cell proliferation of epidermis, hair follicles, and sebaceous glands of beagles and cocker spaniels with healthy skin. *Am J Vet Res* 50:587–591, 1989.

Kwochka KW, Rademakers AM: Cell proliferation kinetics of epidermis, hair follicles, and sebaceous glands of cocker spaniels with idiopathic seborrhea. *Am J Vet Res* 50:1918–1922, 1989.

Mason KV, Halliwell REW, McDougal BJ: Characterization of lichenoid-psoriasiform dermatosis of springer spaniels. *JAVMA* 189:897–901, 1986.

Miller WH Jr, Scott DW, Buerger RG, et al: Necrolytic migratory erythema in dogs: A hepatocutaneous syndrome. *JAAHA* 26:573–581, 1990.

Muller GH: Ichthyosis in two dogs. *JAVMA* 169:1313–1316, 1976.

Rosser EJ, Dunstan RW, Breen PT, Johnson GR: Sebaceous adenitis with hyperkeratosis in the standard poodle: A discussion of 10 cases. *JAAHA* 23:341–345, 1987.
Scott DW: Lichenoid reactions in the skin of dogs: Clinicopathologic correlations. *JAAHA* 20:305–317, 1984.
Scott DW: Granulomatous sebaceous adenitis in dogs. *JAAHA* 22:631–634, 1986.
Scott DW: Vitamin A–responsive dermatosis in the cocker spaniel. *JAAHA* 22: 125–129, 1986.
Scott DW: Exfoliative dermatoses in a dog and a cat resembling large plaque parapsoriasis in humans. *Compan Anim Pract* 2(4):22–29, 1988.
Sousa CA, Stannard AA, Ihrke PJ, et al: Dermatosis associated with feeding generic dog food: 13 cases (1981–1982). *JAVMA* 192:676–680, 1988.
Van den Broek A, Thoday KL: Skin disease in dogs associated with zinc deficiency: A report of 5 cases. *J Small Anim Pract* 27:313–323, 1986.
Williams ML, Elias PM: Ichthyosis. *Arch Dermatol* 122:529–531, 1986.

Chapter 11

CUTANEOUS NEOPLASTIC AND CYSTIC DISEASES

Gene H. Nesbitt, DVM, MS
Lowell Ackerman, DVM

Cutaneous neoplasms are the most frequently recognized neoplasms and represent more than 30% of all tumors in dogs and 20% of all tumors in cats. The relative incidence of cysts generally is not reported but they are common in dogs and uncommon in cats.

Diagnostic Keys 10 and 11 (see end of Chapter 2) outline the pertinent historical and clinical findings and screening and definitive diagnostic tests that help to differentiate the most commonly encountered neoplasms and cysts in dogs and cats.

ETIOLOGIC FACTORS

Specific etiologic factors of most cutaneous tumors are unknown. Both intrinsic and extrinsic factors have been implicated. Solar and ionizing radiation, as well as viral, chemical, hormonal, genetic, and immunologic factors, all potentially play a role in the cause or origin of cutaneous tumors.

PATHOGENESIS

The pathogenesis of most cutaneous tumors is unknown. An irritant factor may act as an initiator, setting the stage for cell transformation. When the skin is exposed to another factor, called a promoter, overt clinical or histologic signs of cancer result.

HISTORY

Several breeds of dogs have a predilection for cutaneous tumors, including the boxer, Scottish terrier, Kerry blue terrier, Norwegian elkhound, basset hound, and weimaraner. No breed predilection has been reported in cats. A lower incidence of skin tumors in Siamese cats than in other breeds has been reported.

CLASSIFICATION AND INCIDENCE

Cutaneous neoplasms are often classified according to their origin, that is, as epithelial tumors, mesenchymal tumors, or tumors of melanin-producing cells. Multiple histologic types of skin tumors often occur simultaneously in the same animal.

Knowledge of the relative frequency and biologic behavior of skin tumors is important. The origin, relative incidence, and biologic behavior of canine cutaneous neoplasms are presented in Table 11-1. Similar data for feline cutaneous tumors are found in Table 11-2.

Differentiating benign from malignant lesions is not always easy based on the gross appearance and history. Guidelines for differentiation of biologic activity are presented in Table 11-3. Cats have a higher proportion of malignant skin tumors than dogs. Only three of the ten most common canine cutaneous tumors are considered to be malignant. The malignant tumors are mast cell tumor, squamous cell carcinoma, and melanoma. The more benign form of the mast cell tumor predominates in dogs. Squamous cell carcinoma is often highly invasive at the primary site, but is seldom metastatic. Only the oral and digital forms of melanoma are highly metastatic.

Of the four feline cutaneous tumors of highest incidence, three are usually malignant: fibrosarcoma, mast cell tumor, and squamous cell carcinoma.

Incidence of skin tumor types varies with geographic location. Squamous cell carcinoma has a higher incidence in areas where animals are exposed to excessive amounts of sunlight. The incidence of skin cancer increases with age in both dogs and cats.

NEOPLASMS AND CYSTS OF EPITHELIAL ORIGIN

Basal Cell Tumors

Basal cell tumors are frequently seen in both dogs and cats over 6 years of age. They grow slowly and often are observed for years as asymptomatic, solitary tumors. Basal cell tumors are seen most commonly in cocker spaniels and poodles.

Basal cell tumors are most often found near the commissures of the mouth, eyes, pinnae, cheeks, and jaw. The trunk is less frequently affected. Tumors of this type are usually small, often less than 2.5 cm in diameter, circumscribed, encapsulated, and hairless with a pinkish-white glistening surface (Plate VIII-1). These tumors also can have a large central cyst. A large tumor may ulcerate. Feline basal tumors often are pigmented. Surgical excision is the treatment of choice.

Epidermoid, Sebaceous, and Epidermal Inclusion Cysts

Epidermoid, sebaceous, and epidermal inclusion cysts occur commonly in dogs and rarely in cats. These non-neoplastic lesions are observed most frequently in middle-aged and older dogs, but may be present when the dog is 1 to 2 years of age. The cysts are dermal or subcutaneous masses 0.2 to 5 cm in diameter. They may remain relatively static or may slowly increase in size. There is usually no discomfort or inflammation unless the cyst ruptures. The sebaceous cyst is filled with a doughy or semifluid gray to brownish material that is easily expressed from most larger cysts with gentle pressure. This procedure is not recommended, however, because a rupture of the cyst wall and release of the keratin can cause an inflammatory response in the adjacent dermis and subcutis.

Milia (also known as follicular cysts) develop when the os of a hair follicle is lost or obstructed, resulting in the accumulation of keratin and possibly sebaceous and apocrine gland material. No age, sex, or breed predisposition has been noted. Milia generally are thought to be asymptomatic and are white or yellow, small (less than 5 mm) papules that resemble pustules because of their color. Careful examination will reveal that milia do not have an erythematous base.

Diagnosis is supported by finding only keratinous debris on cytology, but definitive diagnosis requires histopathology. Topical benzoyl peroxide is the treatment of choice, but vitamin A or potentially even retinoids could be considered in severe cases.

Intracutaneous Cornifying Epithelioma (Keratinization)

Intracutaneous cornifying epithelioma is most common in young male dogs, many under 5 years of age. A breed predilection for the multicentric form of the tumor is seen in the Norwegian elkhound and keeshond. German shepherds, Old English sheepdogs, and collies also have the generalized form. Although many of these

TABLE 11-1

The Origin, Relative Incidence, and Biologic Behavior of Canine Cutaneous Neoplasms

Tumor or Cyst	*Origin*	*Relative Incidence (%)*[a]	*Biologic Behavior*		
			Always Benign	*Occasionally Locally Invasive or Metastatic*	*Malignant*
Lipoma	Mesenchymal	24.2	yes	no	no
Perineal gland adenoma	Epithelial	12.0	no	yes	no
Mast cell tumor	Mesenchymal	10.5	no	yes	yes
Squamous cell carcinoma	Epithelial	8.7	no	no	yes
Sebaceous gland adenoma	Epithelial	7.3	yes	no	no
Hemangiopericytoma	Mesenchymal	7.1	no	yes	no
Papilloma	Epithelial	4.4	yes	no	no
Melanoma	Melanin-producing cell	4.4	no	yes	yes
Basal cell tumor	Epithelial	4.1	no	yes	no
Histiocytoma	Mesenchymal	4.0	yes	no	no
Hemangioma	Mesenchymal	2.8	yes	no	no
Trichoepithelioma	Epithelial	2.1	no	yes	no
Sebaceous gland adenocarcinoma	Epithelial	1.9	no	no	yes
Fibroma	Mesenchymal	1.6	yes	no	no
Fibrosarcoma	Mesenchymal	1.3	no	no	yes
Cutaneous lymphosarcoma	Mesenchymal	1.2	no	yes	yes
Hemangiosarcoma	Mesenchymal	1.2	no	no	yes
Intracutaneous cornifying epithelioma	Epithelial	1.0	yes	no	no
Hair matrix tumor	Epithelial	0.9	yes	no	no
Neurofibroma	Mesenchymal	0.4	no	yes	no
Leiomyoma	Mesenchymal	0.3	yes	no	no
Myxosarcoma	Mesenchymal	0.3	no	no	yes
Sweat gland adenoma	Epithelial	0.25	yes	no	no
Sweat gland adenocarcinoma	Epithelial	0.2	no	no	yes
Liposarcoma	Mesenchymal	0.1	no	no	yes
Leiomyosarcoma	Mesenchymal	0.1	no	no	yes
Myxoma	Mesenchymal	0.1	yes	no	no
Mammary gland tumor	Epithelial	NR[b]	no	yes	yes

[a]Relative incidence is based on the averaging of data from Priester WA: *J Natl Cancer Inst* 50:457, 1973, and Theilen GH, Madewell BR: *Veterinary Cancer Medicine*. Philadelphia, Lea & Febiger, 1979, p 126.
[b]NR, not reported.

tumors are asymptomatic, there may be a history of biting at the site of the larger ones. Most tumors occur on the back, neck, thorax, and shoulders.

The gross appearance of intracutaneous cornifying epithelioma is variable. A dermal mass, usually from 1 to 4 cm in diameter, has a small central pore opening onto the skin surface from which a cheesy-like material can be expressed. At times a larger pore opening is observed that contains a hard mass of keratin. A third type of epithelioma consists of multiple, small dermal masses within a large, protruding keratinized structure that emerges from the central pore. Surgical excision is the treatment of choice.

Papilloma (Warts)

Viral papillomas (canine viral papillomatosis) most commonly occur in the oral cavity and on the lips of dogs under 1 year of age. Such growths are occasionally seen on the medial aspect of the thighs. The growths may be observed by the owner before any other signs are

TABLE 11-2

The Origin, Relative Incidence, and Biologic Behavior of Feline Cutaneous Neoplasms

Tumor or Cyst	Origin	Relative Incidence (%)[a]	Biologic Behavior: Always Benign	Biologic Behavior: Occasionally Locally Invasive or Metastatic	Biologic Behavior: Malignant
Squamous cell carcinoma	Epithelial	26.2[b]	no	yes	yes
Fibrosarcoma	Mesenchymal	18.2	no	yes	yes
Basal cell tumor	Epithelial	15.7	yes	no	no
Mast cell tumor	Mesenchymal	10.4	no	yes	yes
Fibroma	Mesenchymal	4.1	yes	no	no
Trichoepithelioma	Epithelial	2.8	yes	no	no
Hemangioma	Mesenchymal	2.5	yes	no	no
Melanoma	Melanin-producing cell	2.1	no	yes	yes
Sebaceous gland adenoma	Epithelial	1.8	yes	no	no
Lipoma	Mesenchymal	1.8	yes	no	no
Sebaceous gland adenocarcinoma	Epithelial	1.0	yes	no	no
Hemangiopericytoma	Mesenchymal	1.0	yes	no	no
Papilloma	Epithelial	1.0	yes	no	no
Leiomyoma	Mesenchymal	1.0	yes	no	no

[a]Relative incidence is based on the averaging of data from Priester WA: *J Natl Cancer Inst* 50:457, 1973; and Theilen GH, Madewell BR: *Veterinary Cancer Medicine*. Philadelphia, Lea & Febiger, 1979, p 126.
[b]The incidence of feline squamous cell carcinoma is reported to be from 9 to 25% in other published reports.

noted. Hemorrhage from the lips and oral cavity may be noted as well as a reluctance to eat. Viral papillomas have not been reported in cats.

Viral papillomas are initially smooth, white growths located around the lips that develop into roughened cauliflower-like surfaces. As the number of papillomas increases, more are observed on the tongue, hard palate, and medial cheek.

Cutaneous papillomas of nonviral origin occur in old dogs and cats. Male cocker spaniel and Kerry blue terriers have a higher incidence. These lesions usually are small, up to 5 mm, and of variable shape from pedunculated to smooth, are firm or soft, and usually are found on the head, eyelids, or feet.

Viral papillomas are often self-limiting within a period of 3 months. The growths can be surgically excised if traumatized or for cosmetic reasons.

TABLE 11-3

Differentiation of Benign and Malignant Tumors on the Basis of History and Physical Examination

Historical and Clinical Findings: Benign	Historical and Clinical Findings: Malignant
Slow growth	Rapid growth
Well circumscribed	Poorly circumscribed
Nonulcerated	Often ulcerated
Not attached to surrounding structures	Fixation to overlying skin or underlying fascia
No local invasion	Local invasion
No regional lymphadenopathy	Regional lymphadenopathy
Long clinical course (weeks to years)	Rapid clinical course

Perianal Gland Adenoma

Perianal gland adenoma is a common tumor of older male and occasionally female dogs. The most common age of occurrence is 8 to 12 years. There is a predilection in the dachshund, cocker spaniel, English bulldog, Samoyed, Afghan hound, and beagle.

Perianal gland tumors are located primarily around the anus; occasionally they extend to the prepuce, the base of the tail, and along the sacral and lumbar regions of the back. They may be solitary or multiple nodules of variable size. Pruritus is common, and the subsequent scooting and licking of the tumor results in ulceration, hemorrhage, and sometimes secondary infection.

Although the majority of perianal gland tumors are benign, metastasis can occur to regional lymph nodes, especially in female dogs. Castration is the treatment of choice in males. Surgical excision is recommended for perianal tumors of females and ulcerative nodules in males.

Pilomatrixoma

Pilomatrixomas are likely derived from the pilar portion of the hair matrix and usually present as solitary masses. Kerry blue terriers and poodles appear to be predisposed. The average age of onset is 6 years. The tumors are firm, well-circumscribed, elevated, and often alopecic masses.

Diagnosis is confirmed by biopsies for histopathology that demonstrate a connective tissue capsule surrounding a zone of basophilic cells which undergo abrupt transition to "shadow cells." Focal calcification is often apparent in the shadow cells.

Pilomatrixomas rarely recur or metastasize although malignant variants have been reported.

Sebaceous Gland Tumors

Sebaceous gland tumors are divided into the following categories based on the level of maturation of the cells: nodular hyperplasia, sebaceous adenoma, sebaceous epithelioma, and sebaceous adenocarcinoma. These tumors are common in the cocker spaniel, poodle, Kerry blue terrier, Boston terrier, beagle, dachshund, Norwegian elkhound, and basset hound. Sebaceous gland tumors are uncommon in cats.

Most of these tumors are observed incidentally by the owner and are asymptomatic. They often remain static in size and shape for years. Adenocarcinoma, which is uncommon in dogs and rare in cats, is the exception with rapid growth observed.

Distribution is usually on the dorsal and lateral aspects of the trunk, legs, head, and neck. Sebaceous gland tumors can be solitary or multiple.

The most common type of sebaceous gland tumor is nodular hyperplasia, which is characterized as a discrete, lobulated, yellow mass, 2 to 10 mm in diameter (Plate VIII-2). Sebaceous adenoma is wider in diameter (up to 2 cm), and less lobulated than a hyperplastic lesion. Sebaceous epithelioma is a firm, well-circumscribed, dermal mass that is frequently ulcerated and alopecic, and moves freely over underlying tissue. Sebaceous adenocarcinoma is characterized by rapid growth, ill-defined borders, and ulceration. Greasy sebaceous material can be forced from most sebaceous gland tumors. Histologic features assist in the characterization of the sebaceous gland tumor.

Most sebaceous gland tumors do not require treatment. Surgical excision is performed for cosmetic reasons, or in cases of traumatized or infected growths or those that are growing rapidly.

Squamous Cell Carcinoma

Squamous cell carcinoma is one of the most common cutaneous tumors in dogs and cats. It is most prevalent in animals that are exposed to excessive sunlight. Dogs and cats at highest risk are at least 5 years old (average of 9 years) and lack melanin pigment (for example, white cats). Scottish terriers, Pekingese, boxers, poodles, and Norwegian elkhounds are reported to have a higher incidence of squamous cell carcinomas.

There may be a history of a previous solar dermatitis. In dogs, concurrent papillomas may also be observed in the same lesion. Often, there is a history of poor response to previous conservative treatment with antibiotics and corticosteroids.

Squamous cell carcinoma has a predilection for mucocutaneous areas. In dogs, the oral cavity is the primary site with associated tumors of the lips and nose. The ventral abdomen of the dog is also a common site, and digital tumors occur rarely. The ears are the most common site for squamous cell carcinoma in cats (Plate VIII-3); nostrils and mammary glands are other sites of moderate to high incidence.

Clinical signs associated with squamous cell carcinoma vary depending on predisposing factors and duration and degree of malignancy of the tumor. The early, precancerous lesion is erythematous and scaly. A thickened, infiltrative, frequently ulcerated lesion then develops. If the tumor becomes aggressive, erosion and ulceration of the tissue and rapid local invasion as well as regional lymph node involvement may be seen. Squamous cell tumors of the digits usually are malignant with involvement of the footpads and underlying bone. A proliferative form of squamous cell carcinoma with a cauliflower appearance may be seen.

Radiation and surgical excision are the most common forms of treatment. Hyperthermia is also effective, but chemotherapy is ineffective.

Trichoepithelioma

Trichoepithelioma represents a small percentage of cutaneous skin tumors of dogs and cats. These tumors range in diameter from 1 to 10 cm and are found in the subcutaneous tissue, usually on the back. Ulceration may be observed. They are usually solitary tumors with a predilection for the back and head. Treatment is surgical excision.

NEOPLASMS OF MESENCHYMAL ORIGIN

Fibroma

Fibromas occur in both older dogs and cats, although a higher incidence is reported in cats. No breed or sex predilection has been reported for feline fibroma. Boxers, Boston terriers, and fox terriers most commonly have canine fibromas. There is a predilection for females.

Solitary or multiple lesions are observed in canine fibromas, although feline fibromas usually are solitary. Fibromas usually are asymptomatic unless traumatized. Canine fibroma has a predilection for areas lined by mucous membranes, such as the gingiva, vagina, and rectum, and also for the limbs and flank. There is no site predilection for feline fibroma.

Fibromas are characterized as firm or soft discrete masses of varying size located in the dermis and subcutis. The surface may be alopecic and the tumor may be pedunculated.

Fibrosarcoma

Fibrosarcomas are the most frequently observed mesenchymal tumors and the second most common skin tumor in cats; they occur infrequently in dogs. Tumors may appear benign for a variable period of time before growing rapidly and metastasizing to regional lymph nodes and lungs. They respond poorly to symptomatic treatment.

Solitary non–viral-induced feline fibrosarcomas occur most commonly in older cats, with an average age of 11 years. Multicentric, feline sarcoma virus (FeSV)–induced tumors occur in kittens under 4 months of age. These kittens test positive for feline leukemia virus (FeLV).

Fibrosarcomas are firm, poorly circumscribed dermal or subcutaneous masses of irregular size and shape (Plate VIII-4). They usually are found on the limbs and trunk. Ulceration, infection, and edema are common in advanced fibrosarcoma.

Recurrence and metastasis is relatively common with fibrosarcomas. Wide surgical excision is recommended.

Nodular Dermatofibrosis

Generalized nodular dermatofibrosis has been observed in German shepherds with internal malignancy (renal cystadenocarcinoma).

The condition is characterized by a papulonodular eruption usually involving the head, trunk, and back legs of adult dogs.

The diagnosis is based on history, appearance of the lesions, and biopsies. Treatment is usually not attempted unless the nodules interfere with movement. The prognosis remains guarded even if the neoplastic kidney is removed.

Cutaneous Hemangioma

The incidence of hemangioma is low in both dogs and cats. It occurs most frequently in middle-aged or older dogs and cats, although occurrences have been noted in younger dogs. Boxers are reported to be at increased risk for developing hemangioma.

Hemangiomas usually are solitary and located on the extremities, neck, and face. They are characterized as soft or spongy, circumscribed, spherical to ovoid, dermal or subcutaneous masses, 0.5 to 3.0 cm in diameter. The overlying skin often has a dark red or bluish discoloration and may be alopecic. Some large tumors have an ulcerated surface and bleed easily.

Cutaneous Hemangiosarcoma

Hemangiosarcomas occur occasionally in dogs and rarely in cats. Male German shepherd dogs, Bernese mountain dogs, and boxers have a higher incidence than other breeds. Occurrence is most common in middle-aged to older dogs.

Hemangiosarcoma is usually a solitary, large, firm, poorly circumscribed tumor located in the subcutis or deep dermal layers of the skin. Necrosis and ulceration are common. The tumors are rapidly growing and highly invasive.

Canine Hemangiopericytoma (Dermatofibroma, Spindle Cell Tumor, Perithelioma)

Hemangiopericytoma occurs commonly in older dogs (average age of 10 years). There is a predilection for the boxer, German shepherd, cocker spaniel, springer spaniel, and fox terrier. Females are more commonly affected. Tumor growth is slow and progressive.

The majority of hemangiopericytomas are located on the extremities. They range in size from 0.5 to 25 cm in diameter. Small tumors are smooth or lobulated, well circumscribed, and move freely (Plate VIII-5). Large tumors infiltrate the surrounding tissues, have indistinct borders, and frequently ulcerate. Secondary infection may follow.

Surgical excision is recommended. A relatively high recurrence rate is experienced.

Canine Cutaneous Histiocytoma

Histiocytomas are common benign tumors that occur in young dogs. The average age is 2 years although immature dogs can be affected. The highest incidence is seen in boxers and dachshunds; cocker spaniels, Great Danes, and Shetland sheepdogs are also predisposed. Tumors usually grow rapidly. Solitary tumors predominate but multiple histiocytomas have been reported.

Histiocytomas usually are located on the head, especially the pinnae; the neck; trunk; and legs. They are firm, well circumscribed, dome or button shaped, and range in size from 0.3 to 3 cm in diameter (Plate VIII-6). The surface usually is erythematous and may be ulcerated.

Many histiocytomas undergo spontaneous remission within a 3-month period. The specific treatment is surgical excision.

Malignant Histiocytosis

Malignant histiocytosis has been described in dogs and the Bernese mountain dog appears to be predisposed. It is a rapidly progressive and fatal disease characterized by a generalized nodular eruption. Concurrent disease in the lungs, lymph nodes, spleen, and liver is to be anticipated, and central nervous and respiratory systems also can be involved. The prognosis is poor and no satisfactory treatment has been reported.

Lipoma

Lipoma is the most common cutaneous neoplasm in dogs. It is uncommon in cats. Incidence is highest in older (7 or more years of age), overweight, female dogs. Breeds reported to have the highest incidence include the dachshund, weimaraner, cocker spaniel, and Labrador retriever.

Lipomas grow slowly and usually are asymptomatic, round to ovoid, solitary or multiple, well-circumscribed masses ranging in size from 0.5 to 30 cm in diameter. They usually are found in the subcutaneous tissue of the trunk and mammary gland areas. Lipomas occasionally are found between intraabdominal or intrathoracic muscle masses (infiltrative lipomas) and can be soft or firm. A large ventral tumor can occasionally become traumatized and ulcerate.

The majority of lipomas remain relatively small and asymptomatic. Most of these can be left untreated. Surgical excision is the most common treatment when the lipomas are removed for cosmetic reasons or if they are causing other clinical signs. A 10% solution of calcium chloride injected intratumorally has resulted in a high percentage of remission or reduction of tumor mass.

Liposarcoma

Liposarcomas are rare malignancies that are locally invasive and rarely metastatic. Incidence is highest in older animals, with an average age of 10 years. In dogs, male dachshunds and Brittany spaniels are reported to have the highest incidence.

Liposarcomas usually are solitary subcutaneous masses that are poorly circumscribed, firm, and of variable size. They are found most commonly on the ventral abdomen and thorax.

Wide surgical excision is the treatment of choice.

Cutaneous Lymphosarcoma

Primary cutaneous lymphosarcoma is uncommon in dogs and rare in cats. The highest rate of occurrence is in older dogs. A breed predilection for boxers, St. Bernards, basset hounds, cocker spaniels, beagles, German shepherds, golden retrievers and Scottish terriers has been reported. A sex predilection has not been reported. There is a history of poor response to systemic corticosteroids and antibiotics. The course of tumor growth may be weeks to years. Pruritus varies. Most cases of cutaneous lymphosarcoma are generalized although solitary lymphosarcoma has been reported.

Cutaneous lymphosarcoma is characterized by variable clinical signs. Multiple nodules are present in the majority of dogs and cats (Plate VIII-7). Alopecic, erythematous, scaly macules or patches are frequently observed in epitheliotropic lymphosarcoma (mycosis fungoides or cutaneous T cell–like lymphoma). Early lesions frequently are diagnosed as allergy, seborrhea, pyoderma, or bullous disease. In the epitheliotropic form, nodules may not be noted until the disease becomes more advanced. Involvement of the mucocutaneous junctions and skin with diffuse infiltration of the tissue, erythema, ulceration, and crusting may be confused with signs of a bullous disease. In advanced disease, peripheral lymphadenopathy may be noted.

Treatment of generalized cutaneous lymphosarcoma is seldom successful. Chemotherapy protocols that are efficacious for other forms of lymphosarcoma have failed with the primary cutaneous form. Nitrogen mustard has been reported to be of some benefit in the epitheliotropic lymphosarcoma.

Mastocytoma (Mast Cell Tumor)

Mastocytomas are frequently observed in both dogs and cats. The boxer, Boston terrier, English bulldog, English bull terrier, fox terrier, Staffordshire terrier, Labrador retriever, dachshund, and weimaraner have a predilection for mast cell tumors. The highest incidence is in dogs older than 6 years with the risk increasing with age (average age of 8.5 years). No sex predilection is found in dogs. Mast cell tumors in cats occur most frequently in older males with no breed predilection reported.

Benign mast cell tumors may grow slowly over a period of months to years. There may be a history of temporary clinical response to corticosteroids. In contrast, malignant mast cell tumors rapidly increase in size and usually show minimal if any response to corticosteroids.

Cutaneous canine mastocytoma is usually benign. It is characterized by dermal or subcutaneous masses that have a predilection for the upper posterior limbs and perineal and preputial regions. The tumors may be found on any part of the body. The tumors range in size from one to several centimeters in diameter and can be either solitary or multiple.

Benign tumors are firm, circumscribed, encapsulated, and are attached to the epidermis (Plate VIII-8). In contrast, malignant tumors are nonencapsulated and extend deep into subcutaneous tissue. Ulceration, erythema, edema, and inflammation are common in the surrounding tissue. Metastasis to regional lymph nodes usually occurs. Systemic signs of duodenal and gastric ulceration, dysproteinemia, coagulopathies, and inflammatory glomerular disease have been associated with malignant canine mastocytoma.

Feline mast cell tumors may be benign or malignant. Cutaneous tumors have variable clinical presentation. Most cats have multiple tumors in the region of the head and neck. Lesions usually are firm, raised, dermal masses of 0.5 to 5 cm in diameter (Plate VIII-9). The borders usually are well demarcated, although a few tumors are soft with nondiscrete borders; the color may be pink, yellow, or white. Lesions may be ulcerated, especially if they are large. Small papules and ulcerated plaques are other clinical presentations of mast cell tumors. Splenomegaly and sometimes hepatomegaly are frequently associated with mast cell tumors, as is metastasis to regional lymph nodes and lungs.

Treatment is variable depending upon the distribution and grade of mast cell tumor but includes surgical excision, cryosurgery, corticosteroids, radiation therapy, and immunotherapy (see Table 3-13).

TUMORS OF MELANIN-PRODUCING CELLS

Melanoma (Junctional or Dermal Melanocytoma, Malignant Melanoma)

Melanoma is seen commonly in dogs and infrequently in cats. Tumors usually occur in animals 7 years and older. The Scottish terrier, cocker spaniel, Airedale terrier, springer spaniel, boxer, Irish setter, Irish terrier, chow chow, Chihuahua, Doberman pinscher, and Boston terrier breeds have the highest incidence.

Benign melanoma usually is solitary and can persist for years with minimal growth. Malignant melanoma usually grows rapidly and often metastasizes early. The majority of feline melanomas are malignant.

Melanoma can occur on any part of the dog. The most common sites are the oral cavity, lips, eyelids, trunk, and digits. Digital and oral melanomas usually are highly malignant. The pinnae and head of cats are most commonly involved. Benign melanomas usually are brown to black growths, 0.5 to 2 cm in diameter, that can be round, ovoid, or pedunculated. Malignant melanomas are discrete, dome-shaped, or sessile masses with infiltration into the surrounding tissue. They usually are pigmented but can be amelanotic or nonpigmented. Necrosis, hemorrhage, and ulceration are common. Signs of metastasis to regional lymph nodes and lungs are frequently observed.

Because of the high potential for malignancy in many melanotic growths, radical excision is recommended. There is a relatively low rate of recurrence when benign tumors are excised and a high rate of recurrence with malignant tumors.

OTHER CUTANEOUS TUMORS

Nevi

Nevi are developmental defects (cutaneous hamartomas) that are well demarcated and reflect a hyperplastic response of one or more elements from the epidermis, dermis, or panniculus. Thus, there are collagenous nevi, epidermal nevi, melanocytic nevi, organoid nevi, sebaceous nevi, vascular nevi, and so forth. These growths are benign proliferations of cells that most often appear early in life but some (such as collagenous nevi) may not appear until the animal is many years old.

Transmissible Venereal Tumor

As the name suggests, transmissible venereal tumor is transmitted as a tissue allograft by exfoliation of cells onto traumatized vaginal, penile, or oral epithelium. Most of these abnormal cells have a chromosome number of 59 (with ranges of 57 to 64) compared with 78 in the normal canine cell. Transmission usually occurs during coitus but can occur with other behavior patterns, such as fighting, licking, or scratching. Affected dogs often are young, free roaming, and sexually active.

Lesions consist of nodules that can be small to extremely large (10 cm) and often are described as being cauliflower-like in appearance. They are gray to white to red in color. Edema, necrosis, and hemorrhage often are associated with the tumor. Affected areas include the penis and inner sheath, vagina, and oral cavity, but lesions can spread to the cervix and uterus, scrotum, eyes, nose, lymphatics, and even visceral organs.

Cytology of the transmissible venereal tumor reveals a round cell tumor with multiple clear cytoplasmic vacuoles that often are arranged in a chain. Histopathology is diagnostic.

Spontaneous regression is reported in experimental cases only, and treatment is always indicated in naturally occurring transmissible venereal tumors. Surgery is effective if all the tumors are accessible, but this usually is not the case. Chemotherapy is rewarding, with both vincristine (0.5 mg/m^2 weekly) and doxorubicin (30 mg/m^2 given intravenously every 3 weeks) being effective as singular agents. Metastasis may be difficult to control. Radiation therapy when available has also been reported effective in treating transmissible venereal tumors.

Many other cutaneous tumors have been described that are not discussed in this chapter. These include other tumors of epithelial origin, such as trichofolliculoma, dilated pore of Winer, warty dyskeratosis, sweat gland tumors, and epithelial sarcoma. Other tumors of mesenchymal origin include fibrovascular papilloma, myxoma and myxosarcoma, undifferentiated sarcoma, leiomyoma and leiomyosarcoma, nodular fasciitis, schwannoma, granular cell tumor, liposarcoma, angiokeratoma, lymphangioma, lymphangiosarcoma, and osteoma and osteosarcoma. Other tumors of lymphohistiocytic origin include systemic histiocytosis, cutaneous histiocytosis, fibrous histiocytoma, malignant fibrous histiocytoma, leukemia cutis, cutaneous plasmacytoma, and primary cutaneous neuroendocrine tumor.

The reader is referred to other texts for discussion of these very uncommon and rare cutaneous neoplasms.

DIAGNOSIS

Definitive diagnosis of a specific tumor or type of cyst is often difficult to determine on the basis of history and clinical signs. Aspiration, incisional, and excisional biopsies are the diagnostic tests of choice.

Aspiration biopsy is of diagnostic value in the following types of tumors or cysts: epidermoid or sebaceous cyst, lipoma, mast cell tumor, and perianal gland adenoma. Results of aspiration biopsy are often suggestive but not definitive for a specific diagnosis.

Tissue biopsy is the definitive diagnostic test for all cutaneous neoplasms and cysts. Size, location, and suspected biologic behavior of the growth should be considered when selecting incisional or excisional biopsy.

The reader is referred to dermatopathology references for microscopic differentiation of the cutaneous cysts and tumors.

TREATMENT

Indications for specific therapeutic protocols and suggested therapy are given in Chapter 3 (see Table 3-13).

The treatment of choice for most cutaneous tumors involves surgical excision. A few benign tumors and cysts may not require any treatment except for cosmetic reasons, including the epidermoid cyst, lipoma, sebaceous gland nodular hyperplasia and adenoma, papilloma, and intracutaneous cornifying epithelioma. Adjunct therapy in the form of chemotherapy or immunotherapy is only indicated for the most malignant tumors, usually after metastasis has occurred. Neoplasms in this group include mast cell tumor, perianal gland tumor, and sebaceous adenocarcinoma. Squamous cell carcinoma, mast cell tumor, and perianal gland tumor are all partially responsive to radiotherapy.

SELECTED READINGS

Ackerman LJ: Cutaneous T cell-like lymphoma in the dog. *Compend Contin Educ Pract Vet* 6:37–42, 1984.

Barton CL: Cytologic diagnosis of cutaneous neoplasia: An algorithmic approach. *Compend Contin Educ Pract Vet* 9:20–33, 1987.

Bevier DE, Goldschmidt MH: Skin tumors in the dog. Part I. Epithelial tumors and tumorlike lesions. *Compend Contin Educ Pract Vet* 3:389–400, 1981.

Bevier DE, Goldschmidt MH: Skin tumors in the dog. Part II. Tumors of the soft (mesenchymal) tissues. *Compend Contin Educ Pract Vet* 3:506–516, 1981.

Cosenza SF, Seely JC: Generalized nodular dermatofibrosis and renal cystadenocarcinomas in a German shepherd dog. *JAVMA* 189:1587–1590, 1986.

Gilbert PA, Griffin CE, Walder EJ: Nodular dermatofibrosis and renal cystadenoma in a German shepherd dog. *JAAHA* 26:253–256, 1990.

Goldschmidt MH, Bevier DE: Skin tumors in the dog. Part III. Lymphohistiocytic and melanocytic tumors. *Compend Contin Educ Pract Vet* 3:588–594, 1989.

Macy DW, Reynolds HA: The incidence, characteristics and clinical management of skin tumors of cats. *JAAHA* 17:1026, 1981.

O'Keefe DA, Couto CG, Burk-Schwartz C, Jacobs RM: Systemic mastocytosis in 16 dogs. *J Vet Intern Med* 1:75–80, 1987.

Richardson RC: Canine transmissible venereal tumor. *Compend Contin Educ Pract Vet* 11:951–956, 1981.

Scott DW, Yager-Johnson JA, Manning TO, et al: Nevi in the dog. *JAAHA* 20:505–512, 1984.

Vail DM, Withrow SJ, Schwarz PD, Powers BG: Perianal adenocarcinoma in the canine male: A retrospective study of 41 cases. *JAAHA* 26:329–334, 1990.

Wilcock BP, Yager JA: The behavior of epidermotropic lymphoma in twenty-five dogs. *Can Vet J* 30:754–756, 1989.

Chapter 12

MISCELLANEOUS SKIN DISEASES

Lowell Ackerman, DVM
Gene H. Nesbitt, DVM, MS

In the future, the etiologic factors of some of the canine and feline skin diseases discussed in this chapter will be better understood and the diseases then can be classified more specifically. Pertinent historical and clinical findings and diagnostic tests are summarized in Diagnostic Key 12 (see end of Chapter 2). More specific information on treatment modalities can be found in Chapter 3.

PHYSICAL AND CHEMICAL DISORDERS

Irritant Contact Dermatitis

Irritant contact dermatitis is not immune-mediated in contradistinction to allergic contact dermatitis (allergic contact dermatitis is discussed in Chapter 4).

Etiologic Factors

Irritant contact dermatitis can be caused by either chemical or physical agents. The specific etiologic agents are similar for irritant and allergic contact dermatitis (Table 12-1). Some chemical and physical agents are primary irritants on the first exposure and act as allergens on subsequent exposures. It is often difficult to distinguish between an irritant and allergic reaction on the basis of history and clinical signs.

Pathogenesis

The pathogenesis of irritant contact dermatitis is not as well understood as that of allergic contact dermatitis. Precise mechanisms by which chemicals cause irritation to skin are not known. These materials may not be toxic in themselves, but may be carried in a petroleum derivative that is toxic, or they may potentiate the toxicity of an otherwise mildly toxic material. Irritating qualities of petroleum distillate products are directly proportional to their fat solvent properties.

Substances that contact skin can cause varying degrees of damage to the epidermis. Heavy metals act as direct toxins to cells. Mildly irritant substances can dry the skin, which then becomes less resistant to further insults by the same or other materials. Severe or continued toxic damage by a contactant can result in the development of an acute edematous reaction, which leads to epidermal necrosis and ulceration. Milder acting toxicants can result in thickened skin with minimal erythema. The most mild toxicants used over extended periods of time may cause only hyperpigmentation and slight fissuring of the epidermis.

History

A classic history for irritant contact dermatitis is a sudden onset at any age of pruritus and dermatitis associated with recent exposure to a potentially irritating chemical or physical agent. The lesions can be severe within a period of a few days or may gradually progress over a period of several weeks. It is common to observe lesions that persist for a variable period of time after removal from or lack of contact with the suspected irritant because of the initial damage to the skin.

Pruritus and self-trauma vary, but are often severe. Distribution of lesions is usually more variable with irritant than with allergic contact dermatitis. Many irritant contact problems are caused by liquids that come in contact with any part of the body. Irritant reactions to the fibers of rugs or bedding result in a predominantly ventral and lateral distribution of lesions as is observed in the majority of allergic contact dermatitis reactions.

Clinical Signs

Physical examination reveals variable signs depending on many factors, such as specific cause, severity of the pruritus, location of the lesions, and degree of secondary skin changes. Acute irritant contact dermatitis is usually characterized by erythema and a moist, edematous lesion (Plate IX-1). The most common distribution is on the less-haired areas of the body (ventral abdomen, medial thighs, axillae, footpads, scrotum, and pinnae). A liquid irritant contactant also can cause lesions on the haired areas. With irritant reactions this often progresses rapidly to excoriation, ulceration, crusting, and alopecia. If there is a slower progression or less severe irritant reaction, excessive scaling and hyperpigmentation will be prominent. Lichenification may be observed and scarring may result from severe dermal inflammation.

TABLE 12-1

Etiologic Agents of Irritant Contact Dermatitis in Dogs and Cats

Chemicals and Ions	*Materials and Products*
Chrome	Wool
Nickel	Synthetic fibers
Iodine	Rubber
Formaldehyde	Plastic
Dyes	Cleaning materials
Finishes (floor, fibers)	Polishes
Oleoresins	Leather
Sterols	Vehicles for drugs
Antioxidants	Flea collars
	Fertilizer

Diagnosis

History of recent exposure to a potentially irritating chemical or physical agent supports a diagnosis of irritant contact dermatitis as does a history of improvement of clinical signs after isolation from the suspected irritant. Several screening diagnostic tests are indicated to rule out other primary and secondary causes; these include skin scraping, fungal culture, bacterial culture, diet testing, and biopsy.

The most definitive diagnostic test for contact irritant dermatitis is isolation from the suspected irritant, followed by provocative exposure; however, such exposure is frequently avoided because many irritant reactions are severe. A presumptive diagnosis is justified on the basis of remission of clinical signs with the avoidance of the suspected irritant as long as other differential diagnoses have been adequately ruled out.

Open or closed patch testing is seldom used for the purpose of identifying an irritant chemical or physical agent.

Treatment

Once a diagnosis of irritant contact dermatitis has been made, the best method of treatment is avoidance of exposure. Supportive therapy often is necessary until the lesions are in remission. If pruritus is a prominent clinical sign, oral (see Table 3-9) or topical (see Table 3-3) corticosteroids are indicated. Antibiotics should be used if there is concurrent bacterial infection.

Care must be exercised when applying topical agents to lesions caused by irritants. When heavy crusting is present, warm water soaks without the application of topical medicaments are often helpful. If keratolytic agents are not irritating to the lesions, they may be indicated to help control scaling and crusting.

Prevention of further self-trauma may be achieved with the use of an Elizabethan collar or similar device.

Prognosis

The prognosis for irritant contact dermatitis is usually favorable if the primary irritant agent is identified and avoided.

Solar Dermatitis (Actinic Dermatitis, Photodermatitis)

Solar dermatitis is defined as an actinic or photoaggravated reaction that occurs on white, depigmented, or sparsely haired skin.

Etiologic Factors

Solar radiation (ultraviolet light waves of 320 to 400 nm) and genetic predisposition are thought to play major roles in the cause of solar dermatitis. Several other factors, such as photodynamic agents and other diseases, can result in an indirect photosensitivity reaction that leads to the clinical signs of solar dermatitis.

Pathogenesis

The exact pathogenesis of solar dermatitis is unknown, although multiple factors are thought to be involved. Some evidence suggests that the ultraviolet rays alter deoxyribonucleic acid (DNA) synthesis and repair in the epidermis.

History

The usual history for a dog or cat with solar dermatitis is that the lesions are exacerbated with extended exposure to sunlight. The dorsal muzzle is the most common site of involvement in dogs while the tips and margin of the pinnae of white cats are the common sites for feline solar dermatitis. The lesions frequently improve as the exposure to direct sunlight is reduced.

Incidence of solar dermatitis varies with geographic areas. It is most common in areas with long periods of intense sunlight, although reflection from snow can also result in severe reactions. The lesions tend to worsen each succeeding year unless treated. There is a tendency for the involved area to be easily traumatized because of the epidermal changes.

Solar dermatitis has no age or sex predilection. Dalmatians and white bull terriers have a higher incidence of solar dermatitis of the trunk. In cats early lesions of solar dermatitis may be seen by 3 years of age, although the common transformation to squamous cell carcinoma usually is observed in cats over 7 years of age.

The drug history often includes either a complete or partial response to corticosteroids or sunscreens, especially if the lesions are less severe. Animals that show good response to these therapeutic agents should be evaluated for autoimmune disease, especially discoid lupus erythematosus, pemphigus foliaceus, and pemphigus erythematosus (see Chapter 5).

Clinical Signs

Initial lesions of canine nasal solar dermatitis are erythema and depigmentation at the junction of the haired and nonhaired areas of the dorsum of the nose or on the planum nasale (Plate IX-2). Erosions and ulcerations are frequently present. Variable degrees of alopecia, crusting, excoriation, and secondary infection are observed. If the lesions are in a healing stage, they are often covered with a thin, dry, alopecic epithelium. A significant feature of nasal solar dermatitis is the localization of lesions to the nares and dorsum of the muzzle. If there are lesions on the pinnae or commissures of the mouth, other differential diagnoses should be strongly considered, especially immune-mediated disease.

Truncal lesions occur on the white skin, usually of the flank and abdomen. The lesions are erythematous initially; with prolonged exposure to sunlight, these areas become thickened, eroded, or ulcerated. Squamous cell carcinoma may develop in the severe, chronic lesion.

In feline solar dermatitis there is an initial inflammatory reaction with erythema of the tips and margins of the pinnae. Alopecia, scaling, crusts, and pruritus follow as the lesions become more severe and chronic. The ear margins may begin to curl. The eyelid margins, lips, and nares may also be affected in chronic feline solar dermatitis. Squamous cell carcinoma usually develops after several years of sunlight exposure. The neoplastic lesions are characterized by persistent, ulcerative, locally invasive lesions of the pinnae.

Diagnosis

History and clinical findings are suggestive of solar dermatitis. Most of the diagnostic workup is for the purpose of ruling out other primary etiologic factors that often result in similar lesions. Diagnostic tests indicated for dogs include skin scrapings, fungal and bacterial cultures, and cutaneous biopsies. Immunofluorescent studies may be indicated for immune-mediated diseases. A biopsy of suspected lesions on the cat will differentiate between inflammatory and neoplastic lesions.

Treatment

Several different treatments have been suggested to control the lesions associated with solar dermatitis. These include confinement to an indoor or shady environment during direct sunlight hours, topical sunscreens, and topical (see Table 3-3) and systemic (see Table 3-9) corticosteroids. The most satisfactory treatment for canine solar dermatitis is tattooing with black ink. In cats surgical amputation of the tips of the ears in early cases or radical amputation of the pinnae in advanced cases is recommended.

Prognosis

Canine lesions require continuous treatment during periods of exposure to sunlight. The long-term prognosis for untreated feline solar dermatitis is guarded because most lesions develop into squamous cell carcinomas. Early excision of the lesions, however, results in a permanent remission in most cats because metastasis seldom occurs.

CONGENITAL AND HEREDITARY DISEASES

Cutaneous Asthenia (Ehlers-Danlos Syndrome)

Cutaneous asthenia is an uncommon hereditary connective tissue disease characterized by hyperextensibility of the skin.

Etiologic Factors

Cutaneous asthenia is usually an autosomal dominant trait in dogs and cats that results in dysplasia of the dermal connective tissue. A recessive cutaneous asthenia has been described in cats.

Pathogenesis

Activity of the enzyme procollagen peptidase is deficient, resulting in production of abnormal collagen molecules and weak connective tissue in the skin, thus causing the marked reduction of the tensile strength of the affected skin. Some secondary hyperplasia of the elastic tissue probably is involved because increased stretching of the collagen promotes elastofibrogenesis, but this has not been demonstrated histopathologically. The loss of rigidity and tensile strength predisposes the affected skin to excessive tearing.

History

The owner may first observe multiple lacerations on the animal with no knowledge of trauma. The onset of hyperextensibility is gradual and may not be recognized by the owner in a young animal. It is not unusual to see a dog or cat with multiple alopecic, scarred areas on the back and legs.

A breed predilection exists for the English springer spaniel and boxer. Cutaneous asthenia has also been seen in other breeds, including the beagle, dachshund, St. Bernard, German shepherd, and greyhound.

Clinical Signs

Marked hyperextensibility of the skin is the most striking clinical sign (Plates IX-3 and IX-4). Excess skin hangs loosely on the dependent portions of the body. Multiple lacerations with large open wounds often are seen. There is minimal hemorrhage on the surface. Subcutaneous hematomas may develop at sites of trauma. Old lesions usually heal with scarring.

Diagnosis

History and clinical signs are usually sufficient to make a diagnosis. Histopathologic findings are variable. The collagenous fibers in the affected skin are small and sparse compared with control sections.

Treatment

There is no specific treatment for cutaneous asthenia. Lacerations must be sutured using tension patterns. The animal should be protected from any minor or major trauma.

Prognosis

The prognosis is unfavorable because of the hereditary, chronic course of the disease and the predisposition to injury.

Dermatomyositis

Pathogenesis

Dermatomyositis is a debilitating genetic disorder of dogs transmitted as an autosomal dominant trait with variable expressivity. It is most prevalent in collies, Shetland sheepdogs, and their crosses. It is likely that earlier cases were reported as epidermolysis bullosa simplex.

Clinical Signs

Animals first begin to show signs at about 12 weeks of age. Lesions include vesicles, scaling, erosions, and scarring and are most evident on the face, ears, hocks, and elbows (Plate IX-5). Muscle wasting may also be evident, especially on the head and hindquarters.

Diagnosis

Diagnosis of dermatomyositis is made on the basis of breed predisposition, clinical expression, biopsies for histopathology, and electromyograms (EMGs). Well-chosen biopsies may reveal an interface dermatitis at the dermoepidermal junction while EMGs may display fibrillation potentials, positive sharp waves, and bizarre high-frequency discharges.

Treatment

Therapy is only symptomatic and can include vitamin E, corticosteroids, and topical emollients and/or astringents. The condition often follows its own course when the animal reaches maturity, with some animals getting progressively better and others getting progressively worse. Affected animals should not be used for breeding regardless of the severity of clinical signs.

Color-Mutant Alopecia

Synonyms for color-mutant alopecia include blue Doberman syndrome, fawn Irish setter syndrome, and blue dog disease. The disease is a hereditary abnormality characterized by color mutation, alopecia, and papules.

Etiologic Factors

The specific genetic basis of the disease is unknown. Defects in melanization and structure of hair cortex have been described.

History

By the time the animal is 6 months of age, the owner notices a sparse haircoat that is bluish-gray in color if the normal color is black, blond in color if the normal color is fawn, and liver-colored if the normal color is red. A gradual development of scales and papules, especially dorsally, is accompanied by thinning of the haircoat and partial alopecia. The lesions usually are fully manifested by 2 years of age, although the age of onset is occasionally 1 to 2 years. There is often a history of poor response to a therapeutic trial of thyroid hormone. Minimal pruritus is reported unless it is associated with dry skin or pyoderma.

Clinical Signs

Generalized thin, dry haircoat with patches of partial alopecia and multifocal papules on the dorsum are the most common signs of color-mutant alopecia. Dry scale may also be present. Secondary superficial folliculitis is common.

Diagnosis

A diagnosis of color-mutant alopecia is based on coat color, history, and clinical signs. Skin scrapings and fungal cultures are indicated. Thyroid function tests are recommended because a small number of color-mutant alopecic dogs have concurrent hypothyroidism and show some response to thyroid replacement. Cutaneous biopsies are helpful to confirm a clinical diagnosis. Cystic hair follicles, hyperkeratosis, and hypergranulosis are common microscopic findings.

Treatment

All treatments are palliative. Antiseborrheic shampoos (see Table 3-6) and oil rinses are usually helpful. Antibiotics (see Table 3-11) should be administered if bacterial folliculitis is observed. Systemic fatty acid supplements may be helpful.

Prognosis

The prognosis for a cure is unfavorable. Most dogs with color-mutant alopecia require symptomatic treatment for life.

Ichthyosis (Fish Scale Disease)

Ichthyosis is a congenital disorder characterized by extreme hyperkeratosis and exaggerated thickening of the digital, carpal, and tarsal pads. It is discussed under disorders of keratinization (see Chapter 10).

Lethal Acrodermatitis

Pathogenesis

Lethal acrodermatitis is a fatal disorder seen in bull terriers that is inherited as an autosomal recessive trait. Thymic hypoplasia may be involved as well as an underlying defect in trace mineral metabolism.

Clinical Signs

Affected animals normally are presented at about 1 to 3 months of age with splayed toes, lighter than normal pigmentation, pododermatitis, mucocutaneous crusting, and hyperkeratotic footpads.

Diagnosis

Unfortunately, the diagnosis is often only confirmed on postmortem examination when a markedly hypoplastic or absent thymus is evident. Skin biopsies are not diagnostic nor are blood tests.

Treatment

There is no successful treatment for lethal acrodermatitis and animals do not appear to benefit from zinc administration or any other symptomatic therapy.

Ectodermal Defect

Ectodermal defect is a hereditary congenital alopecia observed from birth. This defect has been reported in the miniature poodle, Lhasa apso, Belgian shepherd, beagle, whippet, and cocker spaniel breeds.

Pathogenesis

There is a total absence of hair follicles and associated adnexa in the alopecic skin. Abnormal dentition has been reported in several of these dogs.

History and Clinical Signs

The regions of alopecia include the dorsum of the head, most of the lateral and ventral trunk, and the extremities except for the feet. The alopecic skin often becomes scaly and darker as the animal ages.

Diagnosis

The clinical signs of alopecia from birth are suggestive of an ectodermal defect. Biopsies are necessary to confirm the diagnosis.

Black Hair Follicular Dysplasia

Black hair follicular dysplasia is a tardive (not apparent at birth) hereditary alopecia in black and white spotted dogs. It has been observed in mongrel, papillon, and dachshund breeds. The subject is covered in more detail in Chapter 10.

Pathogenesis

Dysplasia of the follicle in the alopecic areas of black skin occurs with resulting abnormal hair development and shedding. The white skin is not affected.

History and Clinical Signs

The puppies are normal at birth. As the dog matures, hair on several of the black patches of skin fails to grow. Sparse, fragile hair and scales are seen. The hair on the adjacent white skin grows normally.

Diagnosis

The clinical signs of alopecia limited to the black patches of skin on a spotted black and white dog are suggestive of follicular dysplasia.

DISEASES OF UNKNOWN OR MULTIPLE CAUSES

Acanthosis Nigricans

Etiologic Factors

The cause of acanthosis nigricans is not defined. Frictional, endocrine, allergic, idiopathic, and malignant factors have all been suggested as being possibly related to the clinical disease. There is a strong suggestion of a congenital and hereditary predisposition because of the predominant incidence of primary acanthosis nigricans at an early age in the dachshund.

Pathogenesis

The pathogenesis of acanthotic and hyperpigmented lesions is unknown. Various endocrine-related pathways are possible. Frictional acanthosis usually occurs when the conformation of the dog results in friction between the lower anterior chest and medial forearm. When the dog is obese, friction is exacerbated. Localized pruritus in the axilla and groin sometimes occurs in association with acanthosis nigricans–like lesions.

History

There is usually a history of a slowly progressing axillary hyperpigmentation that takes place over a period of months to years. A gradual thickening and increased scaling of skin in the axillae also occur. The primary complaint of the owner at initial examination may be axillary pruritus, irritation, and odor. The dachshund is the breed primarily affected, although the disease does occur in other breeds. Age of onset varies from 6 months to several years. Relapses are common.

Clinical Signs

The clinical signs are similar whether the problem is primary (idiopathic) or secondary acanthosis nigricans. The three clinical stages observed are juvenile, axillary, and advanced.

The juvenile stage is characterized by a bilaterally symmetric oval brown patch in both axillae. There may be a transitory inflammatory reaction. The axillary stage is a progression to larger, grayish-black, thickened, and lichenified plaques (Plate IX-6). Seborrheic dermatitis with a greasy surface and rancid odor may be present. Excoriation may follow pruritus. The lesions may be secondarily infected. In the advanced stage, the lesions are extended to the forelegs, ventral thorax, and inguinal and perineal regions. Ear pinnae, commissures of the mouth, and the ventral neck may be involved. Bacterial infections and seborrheic dermatitis are prevalent.

Diagnosis

The diagnosis of acanthosis nigricans is based on the history, clinical signs, and ruling out of other primary causes such as those of allergic, endocrine, bacterial, and traumatic origin. Biopsy results are nonspecific for acanthosis nigricans, but may rule out other specific primary causes.

Treatment

The most commonly used protocol for the axillary stage includes administration of alternate-day, low-dose corticosteroids (see Table 3-9) and frequent use of antiseborrheic shampoos (see Table 3-6). The juvenile stage and mildly active axillary stage often respond to topical corticosteroid creams. Antibiotics should be used when secondary infection is present (see Table 3-11). Melatonin, a pineal gland hormone, has been an effective treatment for acanthosis nigricans but is not commercially available. Other adjunctive therapies include vitamin E (200 IU twice daily) and weight reduction.

Prognosis

The prognosis for cure of acanthosis nigricans is unfavorable. Even with maintenance therapy, the disease tends to be slowly progressive, although there are usually periods of partial remission.

Canine Acral Lick Dermatitis

Acral lick dermatitis, lick granuloma, or acral pruritic nodule is a solitary lesion or multiple lesions on one or more extremities resulting from excessive and persistent licking.

Etiologic Factors

Many factors have been suggested to predispose to or cause lick dermatitis, including psychogenic causes, bacterial folliculitis, boredom, foreign bodies, neuropathy, local trauma, allergy, and joint or bone disease.

Pathogenesis

The specific pathogenesis is unknown. It is suggested that a primary folliculitis and release of mediators of pruritus are the major predisposing factors in acral lick dermatitis. Licking results in damage to the epidermis, leading to erosion and ulceration to a depth that elicits a chronic pruritic and/or pain sensation. Elimination of the epidermal protective barrier and continued trauma to the dermal tissue lead to deep folliculitis and dermal inflammation, involvement around apocrine sweat glands, and keratin plugging of the hair follicles. Epidermis on the periphery of the ulceration becomes hyperplastic, which leads to the development of a nodular plaque. Continued licking prevents normal reepithelization and perpetuates the dermal inflammatory response, and thus persistence of the itch-lick cycle.

History

The owner's primary complaint is the presence of lesions at sites of persistent licking. Large-breed dogs have a higher incidence of lick dermatitis. The most common site is the anterior carpal or metacarpal area. Onset of lesions can occur at any age, but it is more common in dogs over 5 years of age. Lesions tend to be recurrent, either at the same or different sites. There is often a history of poor or partial response to many therapeutic regimens.

Clinical Signs

Gross appearance of the lesions varies. Alopecia and some erosion or ulceration is usually present (Plate IX-7). In chronic conditions a nodular plaque is present, which may be mildly to markedly erythemic and moist or ulcerated. Most crusts are removed by licking.

Diagnosis

Diagnosis of acral lick dermatitis is based on the history, clinical signs, and elimination of other primary causes. Biopsy of the lesion is helpful in ruling out neoplasms and dermatomycoses. Fungal culture may also be indicated if a kerion is suspected. If joint or bone involvement is suspected, radiographs should be taken. If there is a history of generalized pruritus, either seasonal or nonseasonal, an allergy workup should be done.

Treatment

Many different therapies have been recommended for treatment of acral lick dermatitis. Almost all treatments have the primary goal of breaking the itch-lick cycle.

The psychogenic predisposition can be treated by such changes as more exercise, more human companionship, a new playmate, or a new environment. Phenobarbital has been used on either a short- or long-term basis. Other systemic therapies include narcotic antagonists, amitryptilline, and pimozide.

The most successful topical treatment is a combination of dimethyl sulfoxide (DMSO), fluocinolone acetonide (Synotic™—Syntex), and flunixin meglumine (Banamine™—Schering).

Intralesional injections with triamcinolone acetonide or methylprednisolone acetate have been used on small acral lesions. Surgical excision followed by protective bandages may be successful.

Antibiotics are often indicated, even if the surface of the lesion is not suggestive of a bacterial problem. Naltrexone, an endorphin blocker, has been used successfully in a limited number of dogs. Cobra venom and acupuncture may also be used.

All local or systemic treatment should be accompanied by use of an Elizabethan collar, bucket, or other device to prevent the dog from reaching to lick the lesions(s) until the itch-lick cycle is broken.

Panniculitis

Panniculitis is an uncommon inflammatory disease of the subcutaneous fat of dogs and cats caused by a variety of underlying disorders.

Etiologic Factors

The specific causes are many and varied but it is clear that some panniculitides are immune mediated while others may result from microbial, nutritional, metabolic, neoplastic, or undetermined causes. Potential underlying causes include pancreatitis, pancreatic neoplasia, lupus erythematosus, scleroderma, dermatomyositis, erythema nodosum, deep microbial infections, and steatitis.

History

The usual acute onset of subcutaneous nodules is often accompanied or preceded by intermittent fever and anorexia. Some nodules are painful, and some may ulcerate and drain. The drug history is that of poor response to therapeutic trials with antibiotics; corticosteroid therapeutic trials result in rapid improvement in immune-mediated cases. Dogs often respond to antiinflammatory dosages of glucocorticoids, while cats usually require immunosuppressive dosages. The age of onset of nodular panniculitis in dogs is usually under 6 months of age; however, mature dogs do contract the disease. Adult cats of 5 to 9 years of age are most commonly affected. The dachshund and collie breeds appear to be predisposed to nodular panniculitis. No breed predilection for cats or sex predilection for either species has been reported.

Clinical Signs

Multiple subcutaneous firm nodules, 0.5 to 5 cm in diameter, are found on the trunk and neck (Plate IX-8). Some nodules are fluctuant and some rupture, discharging an oily brown or blood-tinged exudate. There may be evidence of scarring in the area of the ruptured nodules, and a secondary staphylococcal infection may occur after rupture. The panniculitis observed in collies is most often a punctate lesion with the brownish discharge and an absence of the dermal nodules. Fever and bacterial cellulitis are commonly associated findings.

Diagnosis

History and clinical signs are suggestive of panniculitis. Cutaneous biopsy reveals inflammation of the subcutaneous fat that may be pyogranulomatous or mononuclear. A biochemical profile will help rule out systemic disease. If lupus erythematosus is suspected, an antinuclear antibody (ANA) test is indicated. A therapeutic trial with antiinflammatory dosages (dog) and immunosuppressive dosages (cat) of glucocorticoids is indicated. Bacterial cultures of unruptured nodules yield no growth, while *Staphylococcus* species may be cultured from draining nodules. Direct smear of the exudate reveals more fat droplets than expected with an abscess of primary bacterial origin.

Treatment

Administration of corticosteroids at 1 to 2 mg/kg daily for 7 to 14 days usually results in a rapid clinical response in dogs. In cats, 4 mg/kg daily of prednisone is recommended. The corticosteroids should be tapered on an alternate-day dosage schedule for an additional 7 to 14 days (see Table 3-9). Antibiotics should be given concurrently if the nodules are ruptured (see Table 3-11). Long-haired animals should be shaved if there are many draining nodules causing matting of the hair. The use of an antibacterial shampoo also is indicated.

Prognosis

Prognosis for the immature dog is good with minimal chance of relapse. Adult-onset nodular panniculitis in dogs and cats has a less favorable prognosis for cure because of a higher recurrence rate after discontinuance of therapy.

Calcinosis Circumscripta

Pathogenesis

Calcinosis circumscripta, or tumoral calcinosis, is a condition characterized by dystrophic mineralization of tissue not associated with systemic disorders or renal disease. The etiology is not known at this time.

Clinical Signs

The condition occurs predominantly in young, large-breed dogs, such as German shepherds, and presents as well-circumscribed nonpainful subcutaneous swellings with occasional ulceration and fistulation. Although lesions are usually found on the dorsum and extremities, they can occur anywhere, including the footpads and even in the oral cavity.

Diagnosis

Diagnosis is confirmed by histopathologic findings of dystrophic mineralization in the deep dermis and panniculus in the absence of systemic disease.

Treatment

Treatment at this time includes only surgical excision because the cause of the dystrophic mineralization currently is unknown.

Diseases of the Anal Sacs

Dermatoses involving the anal sac region of the dog are encountered with relatively high frequency.

Etiologic Factors

Predispositions to anal sac disease include thick secretions of large quantity, an abnormally small duct system, anal irritation, changes in muscle tone or fecal form, and as sequelae following diarrhea or estrus.

Several bacteria are associated with anal sac disease including *Streptococcus fecalis*, *Escherichia coli*, *Clostrid-*

TABLE 12-2

History and Clinical Signs Associated with Anal Sac Disease

Group 1: Signs directly related to the discomfort associated with anal sac impaction or infection

1. Tail-chasing or bottom-rubbing.
2. Ruptured abscess (acute severe infection)
3. Squatting and straining to defecate (subacute or chronic infection)
4. Scooting (chronic infection with an acute crisis)
5. Biting or incessant licking of flank or lumbosacral region (chronic infection with marked tenderness or pain)
6. Places weight on thigh, or begins to sit and then rises (chronic infection with marked tenderness or pain)
7. Yelping on sitting down (subacute infection with local erythema)
8. Rubbing back against chair or under a table (chronic infection with concomitant dermatitis)
9. Fixation licking without biting, applied to one or more areas of the body or limbs (low-grade chronic infection)
10. Lies supine and performs a snake-like movement to rub back or vertrum on floor or carpet (chronic infection and secondary generalized skin irritation)
11. Sudden and recent onset of aggressive attitude to handling of caudal half of the body, often attacking the approaching hand (chronic infection)
12. Chasing and biting tail, often holding tail in mouth

Group 2: Signs not primarily related to the anal sac disease, but which are often seen in association with it

13. Dermatitis, commonly on abdomen, in the axilla or in the groin (chronic infection)
14. Excoration over the lumbosacral area, usually 3 or 4 cm wide (chronic infection)
15. Dermatitis of hindlimb or perineum with erythema, pustules, crusts, and lichenification (chronic infection)
16. Dry, bland, gray or light brown band of skin surrounding the eyes, with partial or complete alopecia
17. Interdigital inflammation (chronic infection)

Group 3: Behavioral changes associated with the perianal irritation

18. At rest (lying down), suddenly jumps up; without warning, turns, and points muzzle toward its rump: then straightens and searches the air before returning to its resting position (infection and often impaction)
19. Walking or running, suddenly points to rump and rarely licks; short duration (impacted anal sacs)

Group 4: Results of tests aimed at confirming a diagnosis of anal sac disease

20. Sacs abnormally filled (consider enlarged if palpable through the skin of the perianal region)
21. Quantity of fluid obtained by expressing sacs exceeds normal volume
22. Nature of the fluid is abnormal in color, consistency, turbidity, or a combination of two or more
23. Frank exudate present
24. Sacs emptied only with difficulty with a plug observed in evacuated material
25. Local, marked inflammatory change in the perineal skin
26. Pathogenic bacteria cultured

Adapted from Halnan CRE: The diagnosis of anal sacculitis in the dog. *J Small Anim Pract* 17:527-535, 1976. Reprinted from Nesbitt GH: Diseases of the anal sacs: A review. *Vet Focus* 1:16–18, 1989, with permission.

ium welchii, *Proteus* spp., micrococci, *Staphylococcus* spp., and diptheroids.

Pathogenesis

The pathogenesis of anal sac disease and associated clinical signs are not fully understood. It is generally accepted that an initial anal sac impaction occurs followed by bacterial fermentation of the incarcerated material.

Conditioned hyperirritability (autosensitization dermatitis)—a phenomenon in which a dermatitis or an ulcerated lesion on one area of the body results in a more generalized hyperirritability of the skin, sometimes in areas distant from the primary site of inflammation—results in concomitant dermatoses.

History and Clinical Signs

The most common presenting history is that of scooting, biting, or licking (Table 12-2). In the majority of cases of anal sac disease there is a history of mild diarrhea 7 to 21 days before the onset of clinical signs.

Primary anal sac disease is commonly divided into four clinical entities: impaction, sacculitis, abscessation, and neoplasia. Distended anal sacs can often be palpated just lateral to and below the midpoint of the anus in "4 o'clock" and "8 o'clock" positions.

Normal anal sac fluid is described as pale yellow or straw colored, serous, clear to translucent, slightly viscous, and granular with a pungent odor, often with small brownish flecks. Abnormal fluid color varies from greenish yellow (pus) to red to brown to clay to black. Infected anal sacs are often associated with an opaque, thick, red- or greenish-colored fluid having a fetid odor. Impacted anal sacs are characterized by clay- or black-colored contents which are dry or pasty and have minimal odor. An abscessed anal sac (Plate IX-9) ruptures to the outside and is often associated with cellulitis surrounding the anal sac.

Several concomitant dermatoses are thought to be associated with the conditioned hyperirritability phenomenon, including anal pruritus and lichenification, acute moist dermatitis, chronic or recurrent pyoderma, otitis externa, pododermatitis, periorbital dermatitis, anal ulcers, and perianal fistula.

Apocrine and anal sac gland tumors are rare. They occur more commonly in aged females but have no breed predilection. Perianal swelling is the primary complaint. Ulceration of the perianal skin is observed in approximately 50% of the cases of anal sac tumors. Tenesmus is observed in a small number of dogs. Hypercalcemia and hypophosphatemia are variable. Metastasis to lumbar, iliac, and sacral lymph nodes occurs rather frequently.

Diagnosis

Manual expression and characterization of the anal sac contents must be completed. Evaluation of anal sac disease should include bacterial culture and sensitivity, direct microscopic evaluation, and occasionally biopsy.

Examination of normal anal sac secretions by direct smear reveals cellular debris and a few leukocytes, while secretions from diseased anal sacs yield a large number of leukocytes and numerous bacteria. Bacterial cultures and antibiotic sensitivity testing are indicated in chronic, nonresponsive, or recurrent anal sac infections. Biopsy of the anal sac is usually limited to those conditions in which neoplasia is suspected. Abdominal radiographs are also indicated in suspected anal sac neoplasia.

In dogs with concomitant dermatoses all other possible causes for the clinical signs should be ruled out, including allergy, skin fold dermatitis, idiopathic seborrheic dermatitis, psychogenic dermatitis, and tapeworm infections.

Treatment

Gentle expression of the sacs via rectal palpation is indicated in all cases of anal sac disease. If the contents are dry and cannot be expressed with gentle pressure, a softening or ceruminolytic agent, such as hexamethyltetracosane or mineral oil, can be instilled into the sacs using a blunt needle or lacrimal cannula. If purulent material is expressed, the sacs should be irrigated with a mild antiseptic solution, such as 0.5% chlorhexidine or 10% povidone-iodine solution. After emptying and/or flushing the sacs, they can be infused with an antibiotic solution, such as chloramphenicol cream, nitrofurazone lotion, or a corticosteroid-antibiotic ointment.

When an anal sac abscess is present with cellulitis but without rupture, a hot pack several times a day should be applied until the abscess is ready for drainage. The abscess then is lanced and the contents are expressed by rectal and external pressure. The anal sac duct must be opened, often requiring cannulation. When the abscess has ruptured or has been surgically opened, it should be flushed with 10% povidone-iodine and/or hydrogen peroxide daily until closed. Systemic antibiotics should be administered (see Table 3-11) and hot packs should be applied until inflammation resolves.

Anal sacculectomy is indicated in recurrent episodes of severe impaction or infection and abscesses of anal sacs, in chronic anal sac disease, neoplastic anal sac glands, adjunct surgical treatment for perianal fistulae, and when there are verified concomitant dermatoses that respond to anal sac treatment and then recur. Surgical excision of anal sac neoplasms is recommended.

Prognosis

The prognosis for anal sac impaction and anal sacculitis is generally good, although recurrences frequently occur. If anal sac abscesses are treated aggressively, there is a good prognosis. Malignant anal sac tumors have a guarded prognosis.

Otitis Externa

Pathogenesis

Otitis externa is a common disorder affecting the outer aspects of the ear canal and pinnae as a result of a variety of different causes. Primary microbial otitis externa is actually very uncommon while underlying problems, such as parasitism, conformational problems, immune-mediated conditions, hypersensitivities, keratinization disorders, metabolic disorders, environmental causes, and foreign body reactions, are more common.

Clinical Signs

Otitis externa usually manifests as head shaking, erythematous pinnae, and/or as an exudative process. Repeated trauma may even result in aural hematomas. The characteristics of the exudate produced are often helpful in determining the correct underlying cause.

Diagnosis

It is not difficult to diagnose otitis externa from the clinical signs but the true challenge is to determine the underlying cause. It is important to remember that bacteria and yeast often act as secondary invaders in inflamed ears and are rarely the primary culprits. Therefore, diagnostic efforts should be directed toward thorough otoscopic evaluation and cytology rather that microbial cultures. Undiagnosed tympanic membrane rupture is one of the major reasons for treatment failure. Most patients must be tranquilized or anesthetized for a comprehensive otoscopic examination.

Cytologic preparations from ear exudates are extremely valuable in the diagnostic process. Extracellular microbes are commonplace in an inflamed ear; numerous white blood cells with phagocytized microbes in their cytoplasm are proof of actual infection and likely tympanic membrane rupture and otitis media. Exudative material on microscope slides can be easily stained with hematologic preparations or Gram's stain before evaluation.

Microbial culture and sensitivity is overrated in cases of otitis externa and is only really of benefit when systemic administration of antibiotics is being considered for treatment of otitis media. Many organisms, including *E. coli*, *Staphylococcus intermedius*, and even *Pseudomonas aeruginosa*, can be recovered from inflamed ears and skin without necessarily being pathogenic.

More sensible diagnostic tests for chronic otitis externa, apart from thorough evaluation and cytology, might include intradermal allergy testing, hypoallergenic diet trials, thyroid profiles, complete blood counts, fecal evaluation for parasites, and biochemical profiles.

Treatment

Treatment should be directed at the underlying cause to be effective. If otitis media is present, a systemic antibacterial should be administered. Animals with inflamed ears of suspected allergic origin might benefit from the topical administration of corticosteroids on a short-term basis. It is cautioned that many topical corticosteroids are actually quite potent and may result in elevated blood levels of the active corticosteroid when used for as little as two weeks. Similarly, long-term use of potent antibiotics within the ear canal can lead to drug resistance and, potentially, adverse drug reactions.

Safe symptomatic therapies for inflamed ears while addressing the underlying problem might include acidic solutions (for example, 2.5% acetic acid), propylene glycol, docusate sodium or dioctyl sodium sulfosuccinate, antiseptics (for example, chlorhexidine, povidone-iodine), or even mild to moderate corticosteroid solutions. Parasites, such as mites and ticks, are usually easily controlled by a number of common antiparasitic products specially formulated for otic use. Yeasts, such as *Malassezia pachydermatis* (formerly *Pityrosporum canis*), are normal inhabitants of the ear canal and overgrow as long as there is exudate for them to feed on. They very rarely are involved directly in the pathogenesis of otitis externa. Yeasts can be effectively treated with acidic solutions such as acetic acid (vinegar and water) and rarely warrant specific antifungal therapies such as thiabendazole or clotrimazole. Nystatin is commonly included in combination products yet is much more effective against *Candida* in vivo than *Malassezia*.

As a final option, surgical intervention is sometimes warranted in chronically inflamed and hypertrophied ear canals or to establish drainage. Only about 50% of patients with lateral ear resections show improvement after surgery.

SELECTED READINGS

Ackerman LJ: Canine nodular panniculitis. *Compend Contin Educ Pract Vet* 6:818–824, 1984.

Anderson RK: Canine acanthosis nigricans. *Compend Contin Educ Pract Vet* 1:466–471, 1979.

Dodman NH, Shuster L, White SD, et al: Use of narcotic antagonists to modify stereotypic self-licking, self-chewing, and scratching behavior in dogs. *JAVMA* 193:815–819, 1988.

Jezyk RF, Haskins ME, MacKay-Smith WE, Patterson DF: Lethal acrodermatitis in bull terriers. *JAVMA* 188:833–839, 1986.

Mansfield PD, Boosinger TR, Attleberger MH: Infectivity of *Malassezia pachydermatis* in the external ear canal of dogs. *JAAHA* 26:125–128, 1990.

Nesbitt GH: Diseases of the anal sacs: A review. *Vet Focus* 1:16–18, 1989.

Scott DW, Walton DK: Clinical evaluation of a topical treatment for canine acral lick dermatitis. *JAAHA* 20:565–570, 1984.

Chapter 13

DERMATOSES UNIQUE TO THE CAT

Lowell Ackerman, DVM
Gene H. Nesbitt, DVM, MS

Feline dermatology has received much attention during the past decade. Many diseases affect both cats and dogs; however, several specific diseases or syndromes are unique to the cat. Diagnostic Key 13 (see end of Chapter 2), lists the pertinent history, clinical signs, and diagnostic tests for dermatoses unique to the cat.

FELINE EOSINOPHILIC GRANULOMA COMPLEX

Eosinophilic granuloma complex refers to a group of feline lesions of different gross and microscopic appearances that respond to similar therapeutic regimens. The "complex" includes indolent ulcer, eosinophilic plaque, and linear granuloma.

Pathogenesis

Evidence for an immunologically mediated disease is based on the histologic appearance of the lesions and the possible relationship between immune complexes and eosinophils. The response to immunosuppressive forms of therapy is also supportive.

History and Clinical Signs

Indolent ulcers usually are nonpruritic, ulcerative lesions in cats ranging in age from 9 months to 9 years. There is a higher incidence in females than in males. Approximately 80% of the ulcerative lesions are found on the lips (Plates X-1 and X-2), although they can occur on any part of the body and occasionally in the oral cavity. The lesions usually have a necrotic center and ulcerated margins. Indolent ulcers may gradually resolve without therapy but in most cases they are unrelenting. In some cats there is a history of increasing severity leading to squamous cell carcinoma or fibrosarcoma. Some cases may be associated with feline leukemia virus (FeLV) infection. An additional cause speculated is that the lesions might result from constant irritation, perhaps related to the rough tongue or sharp canine teeth.

Eosinophilic plaques are localized, raised, pruritic lesions occurring most often in cats ranging in age from 2 to 6 years. Approximately 80% of the lesions occur on the abdomen and medial thighs, although they can be found on any part of the body or in the oral cavity. The surface is often moist, ulcerated, and exudative (Plate X-3).

Linear granulomas (also known as collagenolytic granulomas) are seen most often in younger cats averaging about one year of age, and ranging in age from 6 months to 5 years. There is a higher incidence in females than in males. Most cats with linear granulomas are asymptomatic and spontaneous remission can occur. The lesions consist of well-circumscribed, raised, firm, dermal masses arranged in a linear pattern (occasionally) occurring on the posterior aspects of the hind legs. Lesions also can occur on the footpads and in the oral cavity. The surface is usually dry and yellow to pink in color (Plate X-4).

Diagnosis

Diagnosis of eosinophilic granuloma complex is usually made on the basis of history, clinical signs, and biopsies for histopathology. Blood eosinophilia is often associated with eosinophilic plaques, but is not usually observed in the other types of lesions. Tissue eosinophilia is prevalent with eosinophilic plaques but uncommon with indolent ulcer, and only associated with collagenolysis in linear granuloma. All affected cats should be assessed for concurrent FeLV infection although this is most commonly reported with indolent ulcer.

Most cases of eosinophilic plaque are associated with allergic reactions. Therefore, intradermal allergy testing and hypoallergenic food trials are indicated. Linear granuloma has been attributed to mosquito hypersensitivity.

Treatment

Lesions associated with the eosinophilic granuloma complex generally are responsive to glucocorticoids (see Table 3-7) and progestational compounds (see Table 3-14), but all patients should be treated on an individual basis.

Patients with eosinophilic plaques often have allergies as the underlying cause and may respond to hypoallergenic diets or immunotherapy depending on the exact cause.

If no specific cause can be determined daily immunosuppressive doses of oral prednisolone or prednisone frequently are required initially, followed by alternate-day treatment. Injectable methylprednisolone acetate given subcutaneously every 2 weeks usually is effective. Patients usually then can be maintained on injections given every other month or so. A minimum of 30 days of glucocorticoid therapy should be given initially, however, and then tapered as necessary.

Megestrol acetate is still sometimes prescribed for eosinophilic granuloma complex although it is not licensed for this use and side effects are commonly observed. Medroxyprogesterone acetate carries the same risks and warnings.

Radiation therapy has been effectively used to treat solitary lesions of indolent ulcer refractory to glucocorticoids and progestational compounds.

Nonspecific immunostimulants, such as levamisole, mixed bacterins, thiabendazole, and thymus gland extracts, have also been advocated for cases of eosinophilic granuloma complex. In many anecdotal reports, trimethoprim-sulfa has been credited with resolution of eosinophilic granuloma complex. The mechanics of such action have not yet been verified.

MILIARY DERMATITIS

Pathogenesis

Miliary dermatitis is a disease complex of multiple etiologic factors characterized clinically by small papules, crusts, and variable pruritus. External parasites, especially fleas, are the most common cause of miliary dermatitis, although *Cheyletiella* and *Notoedres* mites and lice occasionally are associated with typical lesions. Dermatophytosis is the second most common cause in many geographic areas. Other reported etiologic factors include inhalant allergies, bacterial dermatitis, intestinal parasitism, adverse food reactions, drug eruption, fatty acid deficiency, biotin deficiency, and idiopathic factors.

History and Clinical Signs

Pruritus is always a common denominator in cases of miliary dermatitis, manifested by scratching, biting, or licking. Hyperesthesia and personality changes have also been observed. No age, breed, or sex predilection is apparent.

Lesions consist of multifocal papules or small crusts

seen most frequently over the dorsum, although a generalized distribution is occasionally observed (Plate X-5). External parasites or flea excrement may be seen if these factors are involved in the condition.

Diagnosis

The diagnosis of miliary dermatitis is based on history, clinical signs, and a battery of screening tests for underlying disorders. Skin scrapings, fungal culture, Wood's lamp examination, fecal examination, hypoallergenic diet testing, and therapeutic trials with parasiticides are often indicated. Biopsies are often suggestive of, but rarely confirm, a diagnosis.

Treatment

Treatment for miliary dermatitis should be specific for the primary cause if identified. Most idiopathic miliary dermatitis lesions are not completely responsive to corticosteroids (see Table 3-7), although pruritus may decrease. Megestrol acetate (see Table 3-14) is also used but it is not approved for use in cats and has many potential side effects.

FELINE SYMMETRIC ALOPECIA

Pathogenesis

Feline symmetric (endocrine) alopecia should not be classified as an endocrine disorder at this time because no endocrine abnormality has ever been detected in affected cats. The name reflects the suggestive clinical and histopathologic appearance and the response to a variety of hormone supplements.

History and Clinical Signs

Feline endocrine alopecia is observed most often in male cats neutered at a premature age. About 10% of those cats affected are spayed females. There is no breed predilection. Feline endocrine alopecia is most common in the middle-aged cat; the reported age range is 2 to 12 years.

The owner usually observes a slowly progressive, symmetric thinning of the haircoat or total alopecia in the perineal and ventral abdominal areas (Plate X-6). Pruritus or excessive licking is usually not a feature of feline endocrine alopecia but it should be cautioned that many cats are "closet" groomers.

The condition presents as a bilaterally symmetric alopecia beginning in the perineal and ventral posterior trunk, the thorax, and forelimbs. Inflammation usually is not seen. Hair epilates easily in the involved areas.

Diagnosis

History and clinical signs are suggestive of feline endocrine alopecia. Results of biochemical testing are normal. Thyroid, adrenal, and sex hormone assays have not been diagnostic. Hairs plucked from affected areas are in resting phase (telogen) and not broken. Histopathologic findings, including thin skin with inactive hair follicles and minimal dermal cellular infiltration, are not specific for feline endocrine alopecia.

Treatment

Once diagnosis is assured, cats with endocrine alopecia require no specific treatment. Feline endocrine alopecia should be considered a cosmetic rather than a health concern and conscientious neglect is preferred to medical treatment options.

Feline endocrine alopecia is reported to respond to several different treatment protocols. Supplementation with triiodothyronine (T_3) is sometimes beneficial. Combined injections of a repository form of testosterone and stilbesterol are given intramuscularly and the injection is repeated in 6 weeks if there has not been good regrowth of hair. The possible transient side effects of such therapy include signs of estrus in females and aggressiveness and/or urine spraying in males. An overdose of either hormone can result in hepatobiliary disease, bone marrow suppression, and even death. An alternative form of therapy in castrated males is the injection of repository testosterone repeated two or three times at 2-week intervals (see Table 3-14).

Progestational compounds, such as megestrol acetate and medroxyprogesterone acetate (see Table 3-14), are also effective in treating affected cats but are not licensed for this use and have many side effects.

NEURODERMATITIS

Neurodermatitis (psychogenic alopecia) is a condition associated with excessive licking or scratching of a local area.

Pathogenesis

The traditional explanation for cats with neurodermatitis was that they suffered from anxiety neurosis or psychogenic insult. More recently, some cats with neurodermatitis have tested positive on intradermal allergy tests and been successfully managed with immunotherapy, offering another etiologic possibility. Once the cat starts licking or biting, the rough tongue surface causes superficial epidermal injury leading to inflammation, excoriation, and exposure of the sensory cutaneous nerve endings. Persistent irritation to the local area prevents healing of the surface.

History and Clinical Signs

A breed predilection for neurodermatitis is seen in Siamese, Burmese, Himalayan, and Abyssinian cats. A history of excessive licking, hair pulling, or scratching preceding or concurrent with the onset of the lesions usually is reported. The history may reveal some change in the cat's life-style immediately preceding the onset of clinical signs. Often there is a history of some displacement phenomenon, such as boarding, hospitalization, or a new pet or person in the household.

Feline neurodermatitis is manifested by two rather distinct clinical signs. Both signs need not be present in every patient. The first, or dermatitic form, is characterized by a solitary, discrete, excoriated, erosive, or ulcerated lesion, often with secondary infection. This lesion may be flat or raised, is usually moist, and varies in size. The dermatitic lesion is usually located on an extremity, the abdomen, or flank.

The second, or alopecic form, is characterized by solitary or multifocal areas of partial alopecia, broken hairs, and no inflammation of the skin (Plate X-7). The distribution may be a strip on the dorsal back, or alopecic areas in the perineal, genital, medial posterior thigh, and abdominal areas. The stubs of hair remaining do not epilate easily.

Diagnosis

The history and clinical signs are often suggestive of neurodermatitis. Further testing should include skin scrapings, fungal culture, fecal evaluation, and biopsies for histopathology. Intradermal allergy testing is worthwhile when no cause for neurosis can be discerned. Hairs can be plucked and examined under a microscope to check the status of the hair roots and shafts.

Treatment

Neurodermatitis is best treated by correcting the predisposing cause, if identified, and administering phenobarbital or progestational compounds (see Table 3-14) to break the itch-lick cycle.

If allergies are identified on allergy testing, then immunotherapy is warranted. Symptomatic therapy is often attempted with sedatives or progestational compounds. Phenobarbital (2 to 6 mg/kg twice daily) and diazepam (1.25 to 2.5 mg/kg twice daily) are commonly used but have unpredictable actions in cats. Chronic sedation also may not be a cat fancier's idea of a suitable alternative for psychogenic licking.

FELINE LEUKEMIA VIRUS INFECTION

Pathogenesis

Feline leukemia virus is a transmissible retrovirus that infects only cats and has a number of potential outcomes. The primary source of infectious virus in nature is the saliva of infected and virus-shedding cats. Environments that give cats the opportunity to "mingle" also increase the chance of exposure. Once contracted, the virus multiplies in the lymphoid tissue of the throat area, enters the blood en route to the bone marrow, and then spreads to other tissues.

Clinical Signs

Three different clinical syndromes are associated with FeLV infection: cancerous proliferation of virally transformed cells (for example, lymphosarcoma); degeneration of bone marrow progenitor cells, which causes anemia, leukopenia, and thrombocytopenia; and suppression of the immune system. More cats die from immunosuppression and its consequences than from cancer.

Cutaneous manifestations include chronic abscesses, susceptibility to other infections, and development of cutaneous horns on the footpads.

Lymphosarcoma, the most common feline neoplasm, accounts for about a third of all feline tumors. Younger affected cats are generally virus-positive and older cats are frequently virus-negative; however, it is believed that many cases of virus-negative feline lymphosarcoma are still caused by FeLV.

Diagnosis

Diagnosis is usually accomplished by tests for specific FeLV antigens or antibodies performed on whole blood, serum, plasma, or even tears.

Treatment

Treatment of FeLV infection depends on the clinical manifestation. About 50% of FeLV-positive cats die within 6 months and 80% within 3 years. Combination chemotherapy is often attempted with vincristine sulfate, cyclophosphamide (see Table 3-13), and prednisolone. Monitoring is critical because these drugs can have dangerous side effects. Cats with lymphosarcoma are much more responsive to chemotherapy than are cats with leukemia.

Immunotherapy represents one of the most recent advances in treatment, especially for immunosuppressed individuals. Several products have become available as immunostimulants, including bacterins, staphylococcal protein A, thymus gland extracts, levamisole, and thiabendazole.

Prevention of FeLV infection has always involved measures to discourage socialization, such as neutering and isolation. Transmission of FeLV requires fairly intimate contact. A subunit vaccine (Leukocell® 2—SmithKline Beecham Animal Health) has offered some solutions, but has also created much additional controversy.

FELINE IMMUNODEFICIENCY VIRUS INFECTION

Pathogenesis

The feline immunodeficiency virus (FIV) is a member of the subfamily Lentiviridae and resembles the human acquired immunodeficiency syndrome (AIDS) virus in morphologic features, protein structure, and the reverse transcriptase enzyme, although it is antigenically different. The virus was originally referred to as feline T-lymphotropic lentivirus but the name was changed to reflect internationally recognized nomenclature.

Transmission occurs by parenteral inoculation with blood, plasma or infective cell fluids, but contact transmission is only achieved slowly, and in utero and lactogenic transmission is unlikely.

Clinical Signs

The initial stage of FIV infection is characterized by fever and neutropenia beginning about 4 to 6 weeks after inoculation. Pronounced generalized lymphadenomegaly follows and persists for many months. Animals may then recover and appear normal for months or even years. Acquired immunodeficiency appears to develop months or years later, during the secondary stage of the disease.

The major clinical features of the immunodeficiency-like phase include oral cavity disease, including chronic gingivitis, periodontitis, stomatitis, tonsillitis, and glossitis; gastrointestinal tract disease; upper respiratory tract infections; and bacterial infections of the urinary tract, skin, and ears. Cutaneous lesions include chronic abscesses (Plate X-8), pyoderma, and generalized parasitic infestations, such as demodicosis and notoedric mange.

Diagnosis

Antibodies to FIV can be measured by enzyme-linked immunosorbent assay (ELISA) or immunofluorescence assay (IFA) tests. In addition, lymph nodes from FIV-infected cats display both hyperplastic and dysplastic changes on histopathology, while FeLV-infected cats show changes that are mainly hyperplastic.

Treatment

There are no cures available and therapy is only supportive. Therapy is directed primarily at the secondary or opportunistic infections.

POXVIRUS INFECTION

Pathogenesis

Cat pox is caused by a virus related to the cowpox virus. It is presumed that domestic cats might acquire infection from interaction with normal reservoir hosts, such as small rodents. It recently has been suggested that cat-to-human transmission might occur.

Clinical Signs

The clinical presentation begins with small crusty lesions that appear around the lips, eyes, paws, and head before progressing to cover most of the body. Lesions are usually erosive to ulcerative with raised indurated borders. After several weeks, there is usually complete recovery. The infection can result in a concurrent bronchopneumonia and occasionally an exudative pleuritis. Poxvirus infection can be progressive and fatal, however, especially if animals are young or have been administered corticosteroids.

Diagnosis

Tentative diagnosis is often based on the clinical presentation, but confirmation requires biopsies for histopathologic examination, virus isolation, or identification of specific serum antibodies to poxvirus.

Treatment

Treatment is symptomatic and supportive. Antibiotics can hasten healing of secondarily infected lesions and prevent pneumonia. Corticosteroids should not be used.

HYPEREOSINOPHILIC SYNDROME

Pathogenesis

Hypereosinophilic syndrome is a rare disorder characterized by persistent unexplained eosinophilia and diffuse infiltration of various organs by mature eosinophils.

Clinical Signs

Skin lesions may consist of pruritic maculopapular eruptions, crusts, and scales.

Diagnosis

Diagnostic testing should include skin biopsies, complete blood counts, and serial fecal examinations for internal parasites. The disease must be distinguished from eosinophilic leukemia, in which the eosinophils display malignant features.

Treatment

Treatment of hypereosinophilic syndrome has been universally unsuccessful.

PLASMA CELL PODODERMATITIS

Pathogenesis

Plasma cell pododermatitis is a rare disorder in cats and the cause is uncertain. No age, breed, or sex predilections are apparent.

Clinical Signs

Clinically, plasma cell pododermatitis presents as nonpainful swelling of multiple footpads without otherwise adversely affecting the health of cats (Plate X-9). Ulceration may result in some pain, secondary infection, and difficult ambulation. Some cats will have concurrent oral lesions.

Diagnosis

Diagnosis is based on clinical findings, cytology, negative cultures, and biopsies for histopathology. Neutrophilia, lymphocytosis, and hypergammaglobulinemia are not uncommon. Cytology usually reveals a mixed cell population with plasma cells predominating.

Treatment

Management is variable because some cases spontaneously remit while others remain refractory to treatment. Options include conscientious neglect, immunosuppressive doses of corticosteroids (see Table 3-7), or chrysotherapy (see Table 3-13).

XANTHOMATOSIS

Pathogenesis

Xanthomatosis is a rare disorder characterized by accumulation of lipids (fats) in large foam cells in the skin or other tissues. Primary xanthomatosis is associated with inherited disorders of lipid metabolism. The more common secondary xanthomatosis occurs secondary to factors that alter cholesterol or triglyceride metabolism, such as diabetes mellitus; hypothyroidism; diseases of the liver, kidney, or pancreas; or the administration of estrogens, progestagens, or corticosteroids.

Clinical Signs

The most consistent clinical presentation includes peripheral nerve paralysis and occasionally cutaneous nodules (xanthomas) and splenic enlargement.

Diagnosis

Xanthomatosis is diagnosed by biopsy and highlighted by a variety of special stains. Once a diagnosis has been made, further diagnostic tests should be undertaken to find the cause of altered lipid metabolism.

Treatment

Therapy should be directed at the primary cause of altered lipid metabolism.

SELECTED READINGS

Ackerman LJ: *Practical Feline Dermatology*, ed 2. Goleta, CA, American Veterinary Publications, 1989.

Beck ER, Harris CK, Macy DW: Feline leukemia virus: Infection and treatment. *Compend Contin Educ Pract Vet* 8:567–576, 1986.

Drolet R, Bernard J: Plasma cell pododermatitis in a cat. *Can Vet J* 25:448–449, 1984.

Gross TL, Kwochka KW, Kunkle GA: Correlation of histologic and immunologic findings in cats with miliary dermatitis. *JAVMA* 189:1322–1325, 1986.

Hardy WD: Feline T-lymphotrophic lentivirus: Retrovirus induced immunosuppression in cats. *JAAHA* 24:241–243, 1988.

Kiehl AR, Macy DW: Feline leukemia virus: Testing and prophylaxis. *Compend Contin Educ Pract Vet* 7:1038–1046, 1985.

Kwochka KW, Short BG: Cutaneous xanthomatosis and diabetes mellitus following long-term therapy with megestrol acetate in a cat. *Compend Contin Educ Pract Vet* 6:185–192, 1984.

MacEwen EG, Hess PW: Evaluation of the effect of immunomodulation on the feline eosinophilic granuloma complex. *JAAHA* 23:519–526, 1987.

McEwen SA, Valli VEO, Hulland TJ, et al: Hypereosinophilic syndrome in cats: A report of three cases. *Can J Comp Med* 49:248–253, 1985.

Miller WH Jr: Symmetrical truncal hair loss in cats. *Compend Contin Educ Pract Vet* 12:461–470, 1990.

Reedy LM: Feline miliary dermatitis with emphasis on dermatomycosis. *Compend Contin Educ Pract Vet* 2:833–838, 1980.

Scott DW: Feline dermatology 1983-1985: "The Secret Sits." *JAAHA* 23:255–274, 1987.

Scott DW: Feline dermatology 1986-1988: Looking to the 1990s through the eyes of many counsellors. *JAAHA* 26:515–537, 1990.

Sharpee RL, Berkenhauer WH, Baumgartener LE, et al: Feline leukemia vaccine: Evaluation of safety and efficacy against persistent viremia and tumor development. *Compend Contin Educ Pract Vet* 8:267–277, 1986.

Wilkinson GT, Bate MJ: A possible further clinical manifestation of the feline eosinophilic granuloma complex. *JAAHA* 20:325–331, 1984.

Yamamoto JK, Hansen H, Hu EW, et al: Epidemiologic and clinical aspects of feline immunodeficiency virus infection in cats from the continental United States and Canada and possible mode of transmission. *JAVMA* 194:213–220, 1989.

Chapter 14

AVIAN DERMATOLOGY

R. Dean Axelson, DVM

STRUCTURE AND FUNCTION OF AVIAN SKIN

The diseases of the avian dermis involve many different disease processes and encompass not only skin but feathers, cere, uropygial gland, spurs, wattles, combs, claws, and beak.

Avian skin, which consists of dermis and epidermis, is unlike that of mammals or reptiles in that it is very thin and tears easily. This has probably evolved to make birds lighter in weight to facilitate flight. The skin of the feet and legs is scaly and totally unlike the integument of the rest of the body. The only glands in the avian skin are the uropygial gland, which is a holocrine gland, at the base of the tail; holocrine glands in the external ear canal; mucus-producing glands around the vent; and the meibomian glands in the eyelid. Claws, beak, cere, wattles, combs, and scales on feet and legs are all modifications of the skin. Some of these modified skin structures are very colorful and can vary between the sexes.

Adipose tissue is located mainly in the subcutis. Feather follicles are attached by smooth muscles to deeper tissues and they control the movement of the follicles when birds fluff out their feathers. Dermocutaneous muscles raise the feathered crests on the head. The wing web is called the *propatagium*. During nesting, the mid-ventral skin of the chest modifies with increased vascularity and thickness to form a "brood patch" that provides extra warmth during egg incubation; this happens in the female or in both sexes, depending on the species. Bird skin is lightly attached to underlying muscles but is strongly attached to underlying bone structures on the head, extremities, and dorsal midline.

Feathers are part of the avian integumentary system just as hair is part of the mammalian system. The avian body is not totally covered in feathers; they grow in tracts or rows called *pterylae*. The bare skin areas between these tracts are called *apteria*. The avian body has two dorsal and two ventral pterylae that are placed roughly equidistant apart with the mid-ventral and mid-dorsal areas bare. These pterylae extend up the neck of most birds. Some species, such as pigeons, have denser groupings of feather follicles all around the neck with no apteria. The wings are feathered differently in rows. There are 10 primary wing feathers that are the most distal, long, flight feathers. Next to these are 10 secondary flight feathers. Flight feathers are also called *remiges*. Primary feathers are strongly attached to muscle, fascia, and bone of the wing by fibrous tissue and are not very moveable; secondary feathers have more mobility. The rest of the wing feathers are called *coverts* (Fig. 14-1). Right next to the body, but still involved with the wing, are the humeral feathers.

Feathers are necessary insulators in maintaining body heat, which in the bird ranges from 39° to 43°C (102° to 109°F). Feather follicles are the areas from which the feathers grow and are tubular invaginations of the skin. Feathers also provide flight, flotation, and waterproofing and are used in sexual display rituals during the breeding season.

The three main types of feathers are the ***contour feather*** (***penna***), the ***tufted bristle feather*** (***filoplume***), and the ***down feather*** (***plume*** or ***plumule***) (Fig. 14-2); three subtypes are the ***powder down feather***, the ***hypopenna***, and the ***semiplume***. Bristle feathers that act as eyelashes and vibrissae around nasal openings are called *setae*. Contour feathers cover the contour of the body, tail, and wings. Each area of the body has a fairly fixed number of contour feathers. Semiplume feathers have a longer *rachis* (the distal part of the shaft) than *barbs* (side branches of the shaft) and lie along the edge of feather tracts acting as insulators. Down feathers have a shorter rachis than barbs, are the first feathers that grow on chicks, may grow in the apteria, and provide insulation in adult birds.

The long axis of a feather is divided into the *calamus* (the thick hollow part closest to the body) and the *rachis* (which contains the branches of the vane), and together they make up the *scapus* (Fig. 14-3). The *vexilla* is formed by barbs growing at 45 degree angles from each

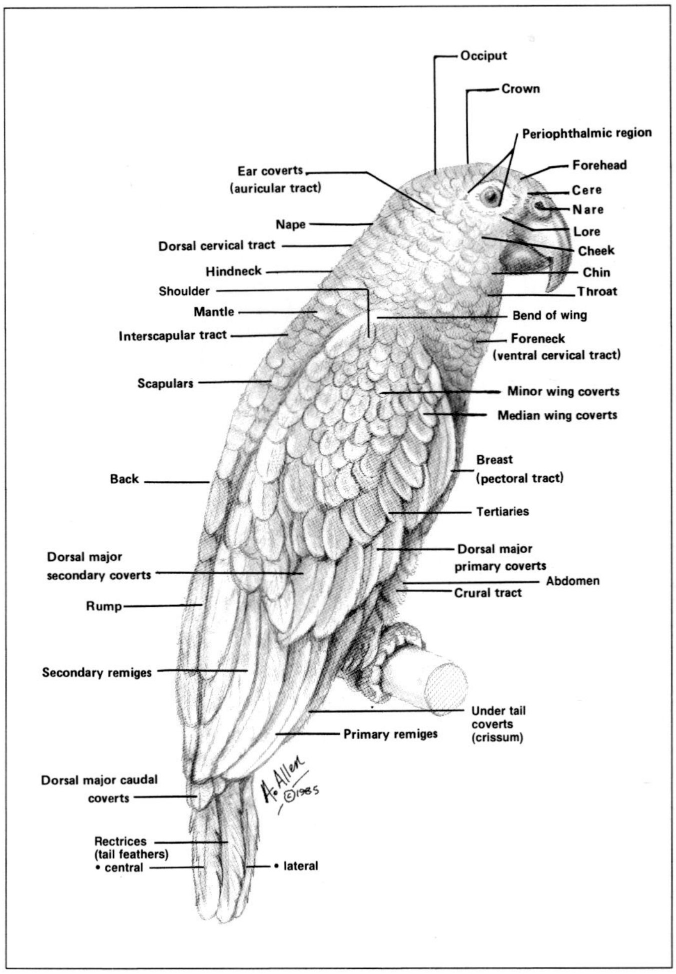

Figure 14-1. Topography of a bird showing normal plumage. (From Harrison GJ, Harrison LR (eds): *Clinical Avian Medicine and Surgery*. Philadelphia, WB Saunders Co, 1986. Used with permission of AR Allen)

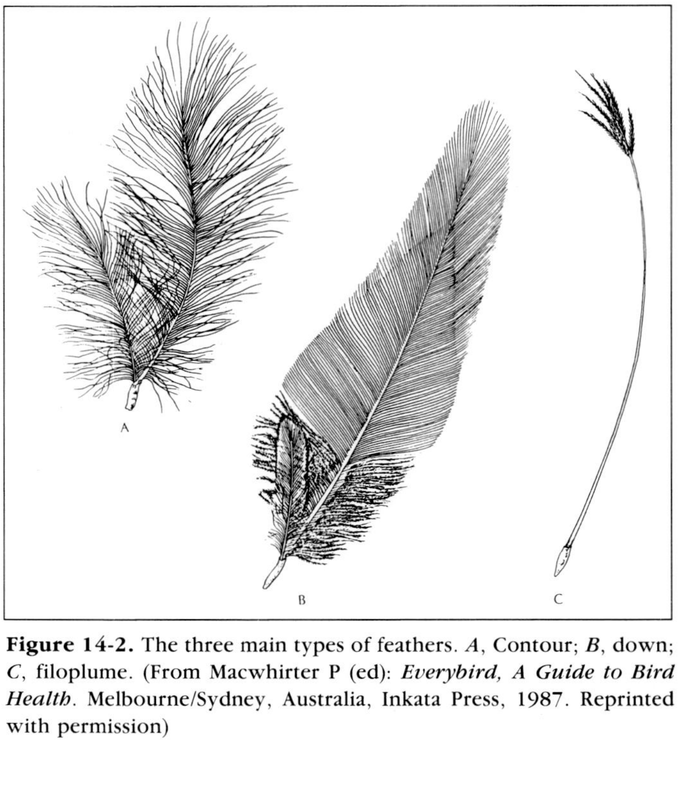

Figure 14-2. The three main types of feathers. *A*, Contour; *B*, down; *C*, filoplume. (From Macwhirter P (ed): *Everybird, A Guide to Bird Health*. Melbourne/Sydney, Australia, Inkata Press, 1987. Reprinted with permission)

side of the rachis. Arising from each side of the barbs are barbules which interlock with adjacent barbules from the neighboring barbs with a series of hooklets that latch onto a flange system from the next barb. One side of each barb has a row of barbules with hooklets, and the other side has a row of barbules with a flange system. The hooklets of one barbule attach to the flanges of the next barbule. This elaborate system keeps the feather parts together which allows the bird to move air and not collapse.

Down feathers (plumes) are characterized by a rachis that is shorter than the longest barb. Slender and noninterlocking barbules give them their fluffy appearance. These feathers grow from the follicles of contour feathers and lie next to the body under these larger feathers. Certain species have modified plume feathers called *powder down feathers*. Powder is a keratin material originating from cells on the surface of barb-forming tissue in the feather germ. These feathers break open, lose their powder, and then take on the appearance of regular plume feathers. Powder down feathers are the only feathers that grow continuously. The function of powder is not known.

Colors in feathers are controlled by pigments, such as melanins, carotenoids, porphyrins, and light diffraction on cells or layers of oil. These colors can be changed or modified by dirt, oils, hormones, bleaching agents, age, disease, diet, physical damage, and temporarily by water. White is produced by the refraction and reflection of all light wavelengths. Green is produced by the combination of yellow pigments and structural scattering in the feathers. Carotene pigments produce reds, yellows, and oranges; are in fat globules in the feathers; and originate from plant material. Porphyrins are synthesized by the bird and produce reds and some greens. Melanin produces brown, reddish brown, and black.

Molting is the process of losing old feathers and growing new ones. All birds molt annually, some twice a year and a few three times a year. Influential factors in molting are nutrition, reproduction, the time of year, temperature, natural and artificial light cycles, and the species or sex of the bird. Most birds molt after the end of the reproductive cycle. Some species, such as the Amazon parrot, molt continually during the year. Birds do not molt completely at one time, or they would be bald and incapable of flight. Certain areas lose feathers at different times than other areas so that there are always enough feathers in all areas to maintain body heat. Most birds also keep enough feathers on their wings to maintain flight, but a few species, such as some of the waterfowl, will lose all their flight feathers within a short time and become flightless until they regrow. Young birds generally molt their juvenile feathers just before they mature,

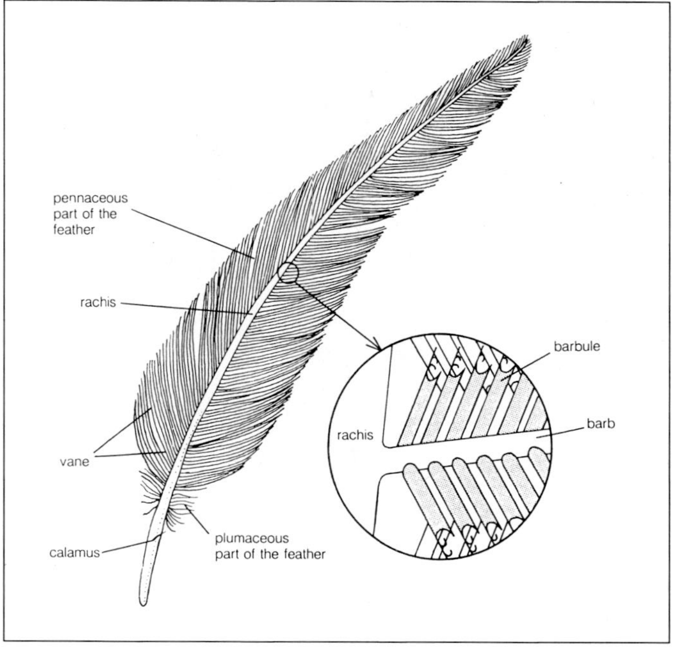

Figure 14-3. Anatomy of a feather showing the relationship of the interlocking barbules. (From Petrak ML (ed): *Diseases of Cage and Aviary Birds*, ed 2. Philadelphia, Lea & Febiger, 1982. Reprinted with permission)

and in some species this can extend over $1\frac{1}{2}$ to 2 years.

Molting usually starts with the inner primaries and follows a defined sequence in each bird. Cut feathers will not regrow until the feather shaft comes out during the next molt or is removed from the feather follicle. It takes about 6 weeks for feathers to regrow after they are lost or molted.

Molting is a stressful period for birds and it can lower their resistance, making them more susceptible to disease at this time. Feather growth puts an increased demand on body resources. Attention should be given to a better diet during molting.

PARASITIC DISEASES

Cere Mites

Pathogenesis. Cere mites, usually members of the genus *Knemidokoptes* or *Procenemidokoptes* (Fig. 14-4), are very small and are the most common mites parasitizing pet birds. Most budgerigars have this parasite on their bodies most of the time, having picked them up from their parents. Most of these birds are able to live asymptomatically with the mites as their immune system seems to be able to control the mite population. Under certain conditions of stress, malnutrition, or other disease, the immune system becomes impaired and the mites multiply and the infestation suddenly appears as a disease condition. Therefore, even with multiple birds in the same cage, not all will be affected.

Clinical Signs. Cere mites usually are first noticed around the bare areas of the face (Plate XI-1), spreading

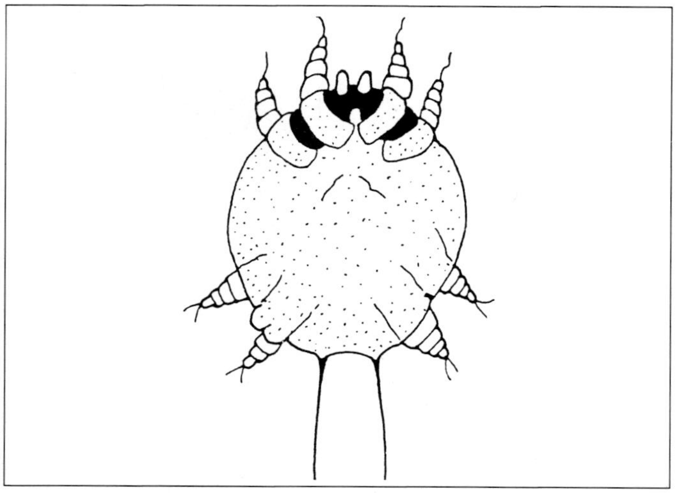

Figure 14-4. Knemidokoptic mite. (From Axelson RD: *Caring for Your Pet Bird*. Toronto, Canaviax Publications, 1981, with permission)

rapidly all over the face, around the eyes, cere, and beak. The bird spreads them to the feet and legs and around the vent in the process of preening and cleaning itself. A crusty proliferation of the outer layers of the epithelium builds up and on close inspection, the tiny burrows of the mites appear as a tiny honeycomb. If not treated, this crusty layer will get so thick that the bird will have trouble opening its eyes. The beak itself becomes honeycombed with mite burrows and will start to grow in a deformed manner. The normal curvature to the beak will lessen and the beak will begin to straighten out because of damage to the germinal cells at the base of the beak. Once this happens, the beak will remain deformed and will overgrow continuously; it will have to be ground or trimmed back to normal length on a regular basis. In severe cases, birds can end up with beaks that look like canary beaks; with regular assistance, these birds can survive. The feet, legs, and vent areas also can become very heavily crusted if the disease is allowed to progress for a long time without treatment. The uropygial gland area has been observed to be involved occasionally as well.

Diagnosis. Clinical signs usually are enough for a diagnosis but suspicions can be confirmed by taking a gentle scraping from one of the infected areas using a scalpel blade with a little mineral oil on it. Mites and eggs will be plainly visible on the slide under low-power magnification.

Treatment. A very effective method of eliminating a cere mite infestation is to lightly apply a mixture of 5% ivermectin in propylene glycol to the affected areas. The entire face, around the eyes, below and around the beak, the feet and legs, and the vent area should always be treated even if there is no evidence of crusting in all those places. If all of these areas are not treated, the problem may recur. My program includes one treatment per week for 3 weeks and one more a month later. This product is never dispensed to the client. There may be some maintenance problems after recovery, but rarely are these insurmountable.

In very severely infected cases, one drop of a 10% ivermectin and propylene glycol mixture is applied to the bare area of skin on both sides of the neck. It is absorbed through the skin and is also an effective treatment. A bovine preparation (Ivomec® —MSD AGVET) can be diluted 1:4 with propylene glycol and given at 0.05 ml/lb (0.1 ml/kg), with a budgerigar dose of 0.01 ml (per bird) given either orally or intramuscularly. Some clinicians put one drop of the pure bovine preparation on the neck of infected birds and have no problem with toxicity.

If an oil-based mixture is used to treat this disease, it must be applied *sparingly* so that the oil will not spread to the feathered areas. Too much oil (or glycerine) on feathers will cause them to stick together, impairing the bird's ability to maintain its body heat. The bird may then get chilled, and sicken and die. The main reason that I do not dispense this sort of product to clients is that they always apply too much, which can cause serious problems.

Red or Gray Mites

Pathogenesis. Red and gray mites (*Dermanyssus* spp.) are small but are visible to the naked eye. They generally do not live on the bird, but inhabit the cage environment, hide in cracks and crevices or nesting material, and come out at night to feed on the blood of the bird. A mite may be seen on the bird only occasionally.

Clinical Signs. Infested birds become irritated, itchy, have poor feather appearance, may preen excessively, or may become weak and anemic from excessive blood loss. A large number of mites can drain the blood of a nestling bird. Some skin irritation may be seen.

Diagnosis. These mites can be detected by covering the cage at night with a white cloth and later looking on the cloth's underside with a flashlight. Look for dark gray or red "spots" that move fairly quickly; cracks or crevices in the cage, nest box, or perches also should be checked.

Treatment. Strict cleanliness of the cage and environment are the best control methods. Clean out old nesting material. Dusting the bird and the cage with a mild insecticidal powder is effective in killing these mites. Products with a wide safety margin, such as pyrethrin and rotenone or pyrethrin combined with piperonyl butoxide, are effective and safe. Malathion and carbaryl in low concentrations also are fairly safe. In general, dusting powders that are safe for cats can be used on birds.

Depluming Mites

Clinical Signs. These mites (*Knemidokoptes laevis* and *Megninia* spp.) attack the feather shafts, causing broken, damaged feathers and feather loss. The damage starts in a small area and spreads to the head, neck, and legs (Plate XI-1). Psittacines are affected most often and infestation occurs in the summer. A scaly alopecia around the face often is a sign of *Megninia* mite infestation.

Diagnosis. The mites are found via scrapings or by acetate tape impressions of the affected area placed on a slide and observed with a microscope.

Treatment. Insecticidal powders should be applied; secondary bacterial skin infections can be controlled with antibiotic therapy.

Quill Mites

Pathogenesis. Several species of mites are involved, such as *Syrigophilus* spp., *Dermatoglyphus* spp., *Pterolichus* spp., and *Analges* spp.

Clinical Signs. These mites primarily attack new feathers and cause feather loss. The bottom part of the feather remains in the follicle and contains mites and debris.

Diagnosis. Mites can be demonstrated in the feather quill and can be squeezed out onto a slide with some mineral oil on it and examined microscopically.

Treatment. There is no totally effective treatment, but insecticidal dusts or sprays may help somewhat. Infested birds should be separated from healthy ones. An ivermectin spray may be helpful.

Fleas

Pathogenesis. Mammalian or avian fleas may infest birds on occasion if the population is high in a household or there is exposure to wild birds. Fleas are not commonly found on pet birds.

Clinical Signs. Affected birds may be irritable, scratch a lot, be unthrifty, and possibly be weak or anemic. Fleas might be seen running around on the body or embedded in the skin of the face, head, and neck.

Diagnosis. Finding fleas or flea feces is indicative of their presence. Nestlings are affected most often.

Treatment. The premises and environment should be cleaned using insecticidal powders and sprays. Other household pets should be treated as well. Residual sprays should be used in areas away from direct exposure to the birds. Direct access to wild birds should be prevented. Insecticidal powders should be applied to the flea-infested bird. Care should be taken in using sprays on birds. Repeat the treatment weekly as necessary.

Lice

Pathogenesis. There are several genera and species of biting, sucking, and chewing lice but they are not commonly found on house pets. Contact with wild birds is the usual source of these parasites. Lice usually are host-specific and do not survive very long off the bird.

Clinical Signs. Birds with lice may show feather damage, excessive preening, irritability, unthriftiness, and reduced productivity and vitality. Lice eggs or "nits" may be seen attached to the lower part of the feathers.

Diagnosis. Finding the lice or eggs confirms the diagnosis. They most commonly inhabit the neck, back, wings, and vent areas, and are elongated, fairly fast moving, light brown, flattened creatures.

Treatment. Spraying or dusting with safe insecticides will eliminate lice. Repeating in 2-week cycles for a few treatments will totally eliminate the lice.

Giardia

Pathogenesis. *Giardia lamblia* is the species found in birds; this is the same species that infects humans, thus there is some zoonotic potential. Giardiasis is seen most often in budgerigars and cockatiels and less often in toucans. It has been suggested that *Giardia* produces a malabsorption problem and allergic reaction that causes pruritus.

Clinical Signs. The birds may have soft green droppings, weight loss, and dry flaky skin, but the most significant dermatologic sign is that the pruritus leads to the bird scratching and chewing at itself until it actually chews lesions into the skin. These lesions can be very extensive and usually are found in the axillae, mid-dorsal back, or along the sides of the body under the resting wing. The lesions can become ulcers as the birds will not leave them alone.

Diagnosis. It is not always possible to demonstrate the presence of these parasites (Fig. 14-5). Attempt to find them with a wet mount sample of very fresh droppings. More than one sample may be required. The basophil count in a complete blood count (CBC) may be quite high in *Giardia* infections. Eosinophilia is common. Visualization of the parasite in the wet mount can be enhanced with the use of Gram's stain iodine or Lugol's iodine solution. False-negative results are common unless *very* fresh droppings are used (not more than 5 to 10 minutes old). The fecal trichrome stain may show a much higher sensitivity in finding positive samples; in this test, the sample must first be placed in polyvinyl alcohol, which is a preservative.

Treatment. At this time there is no sure cure for this parasite but there are drugs that will help reduce the population so that there will be some improvement in clinical signs. Dimetridazole (Emtryl® —Jensen-Salsbery) soluble powder (182 g/6.42 oz.) mixed in the drinking water at 1 teaspoon/U.S. gallon (3.8 L) should be given as the only source of water for 5 days only. This drug can

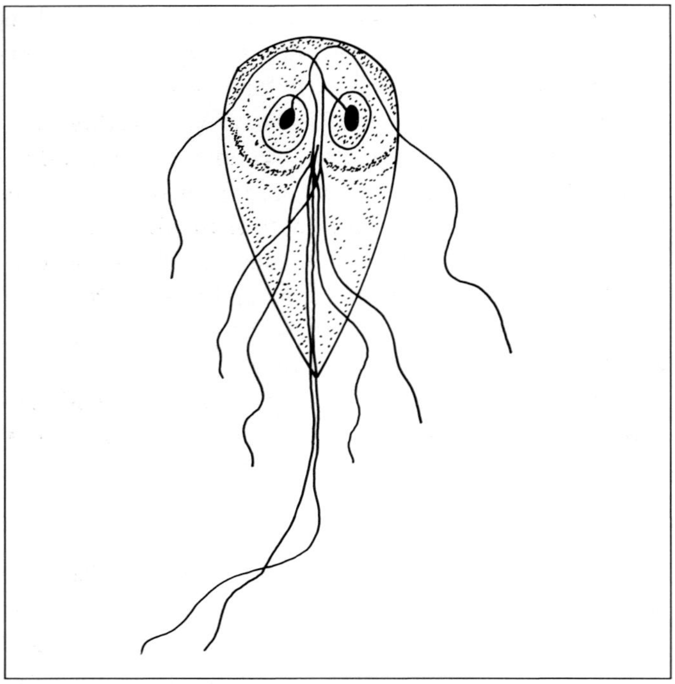

Figure 14-5. A *Giardia* organism.

be dangerous and this dosage and interval should not be exceeded or toxic levels may be reached. It is advised that breeding birds not be treated as toxic levels can be reached in the female if the male is feeding her. Ipronidazole (Ipropran®—Roche) soluble powder (61 g/2.65 oz.) mixed into drinking water at 500 mg/U.S. gallon and given for 7 to 21 days is another treatment. Metronidazole (Flagyl®—Rhone-Poulenc) in the human injectable form, given at 25 to 35 mg/kg three times daily intramuscularly for 2 to 5 days, can be effective also. Recurrence of clinical signs may occur after treatment.

The skin lesions also must be treated. It is necessary to break the self-trauma cycle long enough for healing to occur, which can take several weeks. An Elizabethan collar made of old x-ray film, custom fitted to the bird, will keep it from inflicting further injury to itself. The neck part of the collar should have a layer of adhesive tape along the edge to prevent the collar from cutting into the neck. If the skin damage is deep and extensive, the bird may require anesthesia so that an attempt can be made to debride and suture some of the worst areas. The skin edges should be freshened; some of the subcutaneous fascia will need to be dissected free to allow the skin to be moved to close the widest areas of damage. I use 4-0 Dexon® (Davis & Geck) with a CE-2 swedged-on needle; it is not necessary to remove these sutures as they will dissolve. Systemic and topical antibiotic treatment will keep secondary infection under control during healing. The topical use of aloe vera gel on all skin lesions in birds will decrease healing time, control local infection, and reduce scarring. It has antimicrobial, antiinflammatory, and tissue-regenerative properties and is in a nongreasy base.

It is advisable to leave the collar on for at least a few days after the area appears to be totally healed, which may take several weeks.

Strict hygiene is a must in controlling this organism. Be prepared for recurrences as giardiasis is a very difficult disease to eradicate. Chlorine as a disinfectant will effectively control *Giardia*. Water that has been put through a water heater will no longer contain live *Giardia*; temperatures of 60 °C (140 °F) will kill the organism.

Trichomonas

Pathogenesis. The flagellate *Trichomonas gallinae* causes disease in raptors, pigeons, canaries, finches, and budgerigars. Trichomoniasis in pigeons is commonly referred to as *canker*.

Clinical Signs. Caseous lesions are produced in the mouth as well as the esophagus and crop, and also can involve the commissures of the beak and the sides of the face. These signs may be confused with other diseases. Anorexia and weight loss also are evident.

Diagnosis. The characteristic lesions associated with the host species are fairly diagnostic. Removing some of the caseous material and making a wet mount from a scraping of the raw tissue lesion under it will confirm the diagnosis on microscopic examination. Motile, flagellated protozoa will be observed.

Treatment. Remove all the visible caseous material from the lesions. Local application of 5% Lugol's iodine daily, improved nutrition, and oral metronidazole at 10 mg/kg body weight daily for 5 days (up to 60 mg/kg) usually will be successful. Antibiotics for secondary infection may be necessary. Vitamin-mineral supplementation should be part of the improved nutrition.

VIRAL DISEASES

Avian Pox

Pathogenesis. The various pox diseases of birds are caused by varieties of the genus *Avipoxvirus*, a member of the poxviridae. These viruses produce intracytoplasmic inclusion bodies in the epithelial layer of the skin. *Avipoxvirus* is very hardy and is resistant to drying, humidity, and light. It can remain viable in soil for up to 1½ years. Mosquitoes play an important part in the transmission of the disease as they penetrate the intact epithelium and allow entry of the virus. Susceptibility and transmission depend on the virulence of the strain of virus but it generally spreads quickly, often with a high mortality in some species, such as canaries. Seventeen different types of poxvirus have been classified; most are host-specific but some are not.

Clinical Signs. This infection manifests itself in different forms, the most common being the "cutaneous form." Papular lesions appear mainly in the bare or unfeathered areas around the beak, nostrils, eyes, lower legs, and feet. It is unusual to find lesions in the feathered areas. The papules change color from yellow to dark brown and become crusty. If the bird survives, healing can occur after several weeks, often without scarring. Secondary bacterial or fungal infections can complicate the disease.

The wet or "diphtheroid" form of the disease starts out with papules similar to those of the cutaneous form, with the lesions appearing on the oral mucosa, larynx, and tongue. A fibrinous exudate is excreted which becomes caseous. Multiple small areas can enlarge to join and form large mucosal lesions that are difficult to remove without causing severe hemorrhage and tissue loss. These lesions make the bird very depressed and interfere with swallowing, and can cause dyspnea and even death by blocking the larynx with exudate (Plate XI-2).

Both the above forms of avian pox can appear in a given flock infection or even in one individual bird.

A "septicemic" form of the disease also exists, which starts with fluffed plumage, listlessness, cyanosis, and inappetence. Affected birds usually die within a few hours to 3 days.

In psittacines, a diphtheroid enteritis and/or necrosis of the myocardium may be seen along with or without the other forms of the disease. Amazon parrots may show a serous nasal discharge (coryza), which later becomes mucoid or fibrinous. This usually is attributable to secondary bacterial or fungal infection. Occasionally, in severe cases, an acute conjunctivitis occurs.

Tumors of the skin, lungs, or respiratory tract may develop in survivors as a result of the oncogenic properties of the poxvirus.

Diagnosis. Confirmation of the diagnosis of pox infection in birds usually is done histologically. Clinical signs are a good indicator that the disease is present, but finding the typical Bollinger intracytoplasmic inclusion bodies in skin lesions, pharyngeal mucosa, and growing pin feathers is pathognomonic. The septicemic and coryzal forms usually are only diagnosed by culture on embryonated chicken eggs, where lesions appear on the chorioallantoic membrane that contains Bollinger bodies. Several passages may be necessary with some strains of virus.

Treatment. No specific treatment exists for avian pox but risk can be minimized by controlling exposure to mosquitoes. Infected birds should be removed from the flock. Strict hygiene should be practiced and the premises kept clean and disinfected. Valuable birds can be given vitamin A at 2000 IU/kg body weight and vitamin C at 50 mg/kg body weight intramuscularly or per os. Antibiotics can be given for specific secondary bacterial infections. Be careful with empirical use of antibiotics as immunosuppression can be a side effect. Local use of chemical agents, such as mercurochrome or a mixture of tincture of iodine and glycerine, to the cutaneous or oral lesions may help. Be careful when using these products around the eye to keep them away from the eyeball. Antibiotic ointments can be used in the eye to help protect and lubricate it to keep the lids from adhering.

Vaccination with a pox vaccine in the face of an outbreak may have some beneficial effect in reducing the severity of the disease. A new killed virus, psittacine poxvirus vaccine has recently been released in the United States (Maine Biological Laboratories) and is distributed in Canada by P.V.U. Inc. A canary poxvirus vaccine is also available (Biomune). Preexposure use of these vaccines has great potential in controlling the disease.

Budgerigar Short Tail Disease

Pathogenesis. Thought to be of viral origin, this disease occurs in the lumbosacral and hip area, mainly in budgerigars. It is a gradually progressing disease and can involve other parts of the body. It appears initially in young immature birds and worsens as they mature.

Clinical Signs. The disease manifests itself as a folliculitis that causes the feathers to grow short, twisted, and deformed and several feathers to appear in one follicle that should only contain one feather. It usually is symmetric in pattern and varies from a few affected feathers to a large area of involvement. All birds in an infected aviary will not be affected but it does seem to be infectious.

Peachface lovebirds have a disease that causes multiple feathers to grow in one follicle and this is thought to be the same disease.

Diagnosis. Diagnosis can be suspected by the presence of typical signs and the failure to respond to all therapies.

Treatment. There is no known effective treatment. Control is by culling out all infected birds in a flock and practicing strict hygiene along with a disinfecting program.

Psittacine Beak and Feather Disease Syndrome

Pathogenesis. This disease is becoming a major economic factor in the pet bird industry in many parts of the world. One of the early names for this illness was *cockatoo beak and feather disease* as it was first seen in cockatoos, but it has now been recognized in many other species, such as budgerigars, cockatiels, lorikeets, rosellas, hooded parrots, lovebirds, king parrots, Mallee ringnecks, and Port Lincoln parrots. It has been called by several other names as well, including *adrenal gland insufficiency*.

Australian researchers report that the disease frequently occurs in wild Australian psittacines. It has not been recognized in species other than psittacines; it may manifest differently in different species. Young birds of both sexes are more often affected, but all ages can be affected.

Clinical changes in the beak, nails, and feathers are caused by a combination of hyperplasia and dystrophy in the epidermis during the growing phase. Hyperkeratosis of the sheath of the feathers and outer layers of the beak and nails follows. Powder down feathers grow almost continually and thus are often the first feathers to be affected. The reduction or loss of this powder makes the beak appear black and glossy. These changes are the result of apparent epidermal cell necrosis.

The virus has been isolated successfully and purified and transmission to other birds has been perpetuated by oral and intracloacal routes. This virus in now classed as a *Diminuvirus*, which is a new species of microvirus, the smallest virus known to date. It is very infectious, causing clinical signs within 7 days after injection into a susceptible host, and is shed by the fecal-oral route.

Clinical Signs. Beak involvement, feather changes only, or a combination of the two may be seen. Beak lesions can include progressive color changes from dull to glossy and growth pattern changes involving the appearance of fault lines, breakage, elongation, and other deformities. Large sections may break off. Secondary infections often invade the damaged beak and produce the so-called "beak rot" seen in some cases. Hemorrhage can occur in badly damaged beak areas. Necrosis of the palate and deformities of the toenails also can occur.

Feather changes are variable. The disease can occur as an overwhelming acute illness with symmetric loss of all growing feathers over a short period of time, followed by complete recovery, partial recovery, or death (Plate XI-3). It also can be a chronic progressive disease characterized by repeated loss and regrowth of feathers that are deformed and twisted, fail to mature, and are molted prematurely. Death can result from secondary infections. Green frothy diarrhea may be a symptom in some birds.

Initially, many of these cases are confused with feather picking (described under Miscellaneous Dermatoses). If the feathers of the head are involved in abnormal changes and/or the beak is affected, the psittacine beak and feather disease syndrome should be suspected.

Diagnosis. The proximal ends of affected feathers often show a characteristic "nipple-like" appearance when examined closely. A sampling of deformed growing feathers should be plucked, placed in formalin, and submitted to a laboratory for histopathologic examination. Skin biopsies are sometimes included. Some pathologists prefer to have at least one or more affected follicles along with the diseased feather. After preparing sections and staining with hematoxylin and eosin (H&E), intracytoplasmic inclusion bodies will be observed in macrophages and epidermal cells.

Treatment. No specific reliable treatment exists as yet for this disease. Immunostimulants, such as autogenous bacterins, appear to help some birds while in others no change is noted. Antibiotic therapy and supportive care, such as vitamins, minerals, fluid therapy, improved nutrition, anabolic steroids, parasite control, improved hygiene and environment, and segregation of affected birds, should be carried out in an attempt at treating these cases. Many will die, some fairly quickly and some as long as 2 to 4 years later.

Contaminated cages and aviaries should be thoroughly scrubbed and disinfected. Nest boxes should be replaced regularly. Control measures include not breeding very young, very old, or pairs of birds that have produced affected young. A rest of 1 or 2 years in the breeding program also may help. Researchers are in the process of developing a vaccine that will help prevent this devastating disease.

Papovavirus

Pathogenesis. Papovavirus has been described as being responsible for various skin lesions in birds. It has been isolated in papillomas on the legs of European finches, in proliferative skin lesions on the head and eyelids of African Grey parrots, and has been identified as the causative agent for budgerigar fledgling disease, which is considered a generalized papovavirus infection. The virus may have oncogenic potential and may be a factor in the high incidence of tumors in budgerigars. Gerlach states that budgerigar fledgling disease seems to occur in other species as well, such as macaws, amazon parrots, conures, pionus, African Grey parrots, sulfur crested cockatoos, and eclectus parrots. Most of these species contract the disease as hand-fed babies, but some parent-raised birds do get it as well. The virus is highly infectious.

Clinical Signs. Adult budgerigars are known to be carriers. Incubation of the disease in baby birds from time of hatching is 10 to 21 days. Diseased baby birds show a lack of or malformation of down feathers, retarded growth of tail and body feathers, and a distended abdomen. Dehydration occurs from polyuria. The skin may be a reddish color. It is an acute disease and secondary infections are common. Mortality can be quite high.

Diagnosis. On postmortem examination, hydropericardium, cardiomegaly, liver necrosis, and enlarged hyperemic kidneys are evident. Karyomegalic, clear or opaque inclusion bodies composed of virus particles are found in various tissues on histopathologic examination. Impression smears of liver, spleen, and other organs can be examined for these inclusion bodies.

Treatment. There is no known specific treatment. Several control measures can be implemented, such as depopulation of infected flocks and restocking with disease-free birds, cessation of breeding for several months, and isolating breeding flocks from cross-contamination. Strict hygiene, disinfection of the environment, and good nutrition are essential.

French Molt

Pathogenesis. French molt is not conclusively documented to be viral in origin and many other factors, such as parasites, nutrition, environment, and genetics, have been implicated. In Australia, French molt is thought to be caused by the psittacine beak and feather disease syndrome virus and in North America and Japan, the papovavirus seems to be involved. It appears that the two viruses produce a similar disease syndrome in the smaller species of psittacines.

Clinical Signs. In North America, French molt is a disease seen mainly in budgerigars, occasionally in lovebirds, and perhaps in some other small psittacines. It is a disease of baby birds and manifests itself primarily in the tail and long wing feathers (Plate XI-4). The feathers may break off at or beneath the skin surface, or are molted prematurely. In the more severe form of the disease, the birds never do grow normal feathers but continue to molt their bent and twisted ones. In the milder form, the bird begins to grow normal-looking feathers after one or two molts. Birds with damaged wing feathers cannot fly and are often referred to as "runners" or "creepers." The body feathers usually are not affected but can be in some birds.

Diagnosis. The condition can be suspected in young birds in which only the wing and tail feathers are affected.

Treatment. There is no effective treatment. Reproduction from infected birds is not recommended.

White Skin Wart Syndrome

Pathogenesis. The condition is also referred to as *herpesvirus warts* and is presumed to be caused by the herpes wart virus. This condition is seen primarily in cockatoos but also has been observed occasionally in Amazon parrots.

Clinical Signs. Usually one area of a single toe or sometimes two will have a patch of whitish skin, generally near the distal end of the toe. This white area usually involves the ventral surface of the toe and may encircle it, involving 10 to 25% of the toe. The ventral skin layers often become over-keratinized to the point where it is necessary to grind them down.

Diagnosis. The condition can be suspected on the basis of the distinctive clinical signs.

Treatment. I suggest soaking this area with 5% Lugol's iodine solution daily as required. The warts appear to be self-limiting and eventually disappear, with no apparent aftereffects.

Warts can appear on the feet of other species of birds as well and rarely require removal by surgery.

MICROBIAL DISEASES

Abscesses

Pathogenesis. Abscesses can occur in various places on the body but they are not a common problem in birds because of their high body temperature. Abscesses are accumulations of pus in pockets that are associated with infection or tissue irritation. Because birds lack lysozymes in their white blood cells that liquefy mammalian pus, most avian pus is caseous in consistency and is impossible to aspirate with a needle.

Clinical Signs. Subcutaneous abscesses often are associated with feather loss over the involved area if in a feathered area of the body. They can be the result of blocked sebaceous glands, damaged feather follicles, feather cysts, foreign bodies, infected wounds, pressure, friction, and spread of infection from other areas. A common site for abscesses in canaries, budgerigars, cockatiels, and mynah birds is the periocular region (Plate XI-5). Lesions can be isolated above or below the eyelids, involve both lids, or be extensions of an acute sinus infection and involve a large area of the face below the eye. A frequent site of infection in large psittacines is the hard palate along the margins of the choana and the base of the tongue. The mucous glands in these areas are involved as a result of hypovitaminosis A.

Cockatiels sometimes get an accumulation of a hard mass of pus under the nictitating membrane in conjunction with a conjunctivitis as a result of local infection.

The uropygial gland is another frequent site for abscess formation in small birds. Canaries and finches sometimes get abscesses on the top of the head. The condition can develop in feather follicles as well.

Parrots, especially the African Grey, and budgerigars are subject to abscess formation in the nares that often erodes the nasal opening and part of the cere to create a large pus-filled cavity (Plate XI-6). These abscesses may appear to be simply plugged, enlarged nares with some surrounding swelling. It is not until the huge mass of pus is removed that the full extent of the cavity is apparent. Response to treatment is good. A variety of organisms may be cultured from these lesions.

TABLE 14-1

Drug Dosages for the Avian Patient

Generic Name	Form	Route	Dosage	Comments
Amikacin	Injectable (250 and 500 mg/ml)	IM	15–20 mg/kg bid–tid (0.015 mg/g)	Must be diluted (1:4) for birds; for gram-negative infections; less nephrotoxic than gentamicin
Chloramphenicol succinate	Injectable (100 mg/ml)	IM IV	80 mg/kg bid or tid 50 mg/kg tid or bid	Rapidly excreted
Chloramphenicol palmitate	Oral suspension (25,30,50 mg/ml)	PO	50 mg/kg qid (0.1 ml/g bid–qid)	Erratic absorption; palatable
Erythromycin	Oral suspension (40 mg/ml)	PO	45–90 mg/kg bid × 5–10 days	Good for sinusitis
Gentamicin	Injectable (50 mg/ml)	IM	10 mg/kg bid–tid	Dilute 1:4 with sterile water; can be nephrotoxic; do not use for more than 7 days; transient polyuria possible
Piperacillin	Injectable (50 mg/ml)	IM	100 mg/kg	Good general purpose antibiotic
Tylosin	Injectable (50 mg/ml)	IM	10–40 mg/kg bid–tid	Nontoxic; good for respiratory disease

Chronic sinusitis with external abscessation may become very severe and involve both sides of the face with a joining passage inside the sinus cavity just above the cere in the frontal area. Serious curetting under general anesthesia may be required in such cases. Extensive chronic cases often require prolonged treatment to clear them up.

Diagnosis. The diagnosis of abscess is made clinically upon finding a pocket or accumulation of pus.

Treatment. Treatment of abscesses should include nutritional and environmental improvement, eliminating contributing factors, lancing and curettage of the lesion, local application of 5% Lugol's iodine if possible, local application of antibacterial creams (for example, chlorhexidine), and systemic antibiotics (Table 14-1). Most abscesses will respond rapidly to this sort of treatment. The use of bandages and possibly Elizabethan collars may be necessary.

Granulomatous Dermatitis

Pathogenesis. A nodular, granulomatous dermatitis that can be single or multiple is occasionally found on pet birds, mainly on the head. The etiology of these lesions may involve avian tubercle bacilli (*Mycobacterium* spp.), fungi, or other granuloma-inducing agents.

Clinical Signs. The skin thickens as a result of the accumulation of large macrophages in the dermis and subcutis. Bacterial granulomas from overwhelming disease processes may appear as small scabs in the mouth of sick budgerigars. Bacterial granulomas on the cere, beak, or other skin areas may closely resemble malignant tumors.

Diagnosis. Histopathologic evaluation often is necessary to confirm a diagnosis and to differentiate microbial granulomas from tumors. Acid-fast bacilli in large numbers can be found in macrophages in association with mycobacterial infections.

Treatment. Surgical excision of the lesions may be the best approach to therapy. The use of appropriate antibiotics may also be contemplated as an alternative to surgery (Table 14-1).

Fungal Dermatitis

Pathogenesis. Fungal dermatitis is rare in pet birds and birds in general, yet over 20 known species of dermatophyte fungi, including *Candida*, are capable of causing ringworm (also known as *favus*, *white comb*, *crete blanche*) by invading the keratinized layers of the skin and feathers. Birds with combs or wattles are more likely to be infected, especially in a wet, dirty environment.

Clinical Signs. Lesions are found mainly on the fleshy or thin-skinned areas of the head. Feather loss, scabs, and crusty areas appear. There may be extensive thickening of the epidermis producing crusty accumulations around the feather follicles. Neighboring feathered areas can become involved, resulting in extensive feather loss. The skin around the ears also may be involved. Fungal dermatitis may be secondary to other diseases in an immune-suppressed individual.

Diagnosis. A skin scraping using 10 to 20% potassium hydroxide solution may show the presence of septate hyphal fragments which will confirm the diagnosis. Fungal cultures can identify the species involved.

Treatment. Cleaning up and improving the environment are important steps in the treatment and control of this disease. It is infectious to other birds and possibly to humans. Infected birds should be removed and separated from the others. Local antifungal products, such as chlorhexidine, iodine, formalin, tinactin, mycostatin, and carbolic acid, may help. Oral griseofulvin at 125 mg/kg body weight can also be given at the same time.

NEOPLASTIC DISEASES

Tumors of the Uropygial Gland

The uropygial gland (preen gland, oil gland) is situated dorsally at the base of the tail. It is not present in all species of birds, and is not essential except in waterfowl, where it is needed to maintain feather condition and buoyancy. This gland is a common site for tumors, especially in the budgerigar and canary.

Enlargement of the gland and the appearance of a tissue mass in the area will draw attention to this problem. As the mass enlarges, the bird will often chew at it, causing hemorrhage and secondary infection.

Close visualization will determine if neoplasia is present. Differentiate from an abscess or blocked duct with simple enlargement. Histopathologic examination is necessary to identify the type of tumor tissue involved. The most common type of tumor found here is adenocarcinoma, followed by adenoma.

Surgical excision of the entire gland structure and tumor is essential to prevent recurrence. The use of an Elizabethan collar may be required as well during the healing period. Antibiotics and supportive care are usual accompaniments.

Papillomas

Papillomas, which are neoplasms originating from the nonglandular surface epithelium, occur most often on the skin of the feet, legs, neck, wing, eyelids, and uropygial area. The cause is not known, although they may have a viral etiology. Papillomas vary from finger-like projections to crusty, ulcerated masses and will bleed profusely when traumatized or excised. They can grow very large and usually are benign. Papillomas are subject to self-trauma and bleed easily.

The treatment of choice is complete surgical excision. Recurrence can be common. The use of an autogenous vaccine from some of the removed tissue has been suggested as an aid in preventing recurrence. The papovavirus group has been reported to cause papillomas in some parrot species.

Cloacal Papilloma

A cauliflower-like proliferation of tissue originating from the mucocutaneous junction of the vent, cloacal papillomas are most commonly observed in cockatoos, Amazon and hawk head parrots, and macaws, but have been reported in many species. Because it protrudes from the vent, the cloacal papilloma is often misdiagnosed as a cloacal prolapse. Cloacal papillomas vary in size from a small piece of exposed tissue to large masses completely circumscribing the vent (Plate XI-7). They are benign and thought to be of viral origin, and are very common in some geographic areas.

A high percentage of psittacines do not exhibit any clinical signs but these cases will progress rapidly when the birds are subjected to various causes of stress. Subclinical cases can be diagnosed by close inspection of the vent by gently everting the cloaca with a cotton applicator.

Clinical cases may show straining to defecate, smelly droppings, pasting of the vent, decreased fertility, bloody feces, anemia, or persistent bacterial infections. Applying 5% acetic acid on the cloacal lining will make the papilloma lesions show up white. Preparation H® (Whitehall) will help reduce the size of the cloacal lesion.

Improving the diet, reducing stress, and antibiotic therapy may help in some cases. Excision of involved tissue is the best therapy and can be done with cryosurgery or electrosurgery. Recurrence is common. Hemorrhage can be a problem unless care is taken. Some surgeons suture the defect closed. Care should be taken to prevent cloacal wall necrosis and strictures. Interrupted sutures are preferred rather than continuous sutures.

Controlling this disease by removing infected individuals in a breeding flock is important because of the infectivity of the disease and because breeding is impaired by it.

Inspection for cloacal papillomas should be a routine part of any complete physical examination of a potential breeding bird. The inside edge of the cloaca should be completely smooth all around, slightly moist, and pink in color.

Fibroma and Fibrosarcoma

Fibrosarcoma is a malignant tumor of fibrous connective tissue and fibroma is the benign form. Birds often get these tumors in the skin of the wings (Plate XI-8), legs, beak, and uropygial area. They usually are of firm consistency, oval or round in shape, and may have a necrotic center. They tend to be locally invasive but rarely metastasize. A beak tumor also may invade the mouth. Budgerigars, males particularly, may get fibromas on the sternum. Surgical excision is the best therapy but some tumors involve areas of the beak and face, making surgery impossible, and then euthanasia is recommended.

Lipoma and Liposarcoma

Lipomas and liposarcomas are neoplasms of adipose tissue; lipomas are benign tumors and liposarcomas are the malignant form. Budgerigars of both sexes seem to be more prone to these tumors than other species; there may be a genetic predisposition. Lipomas are more common than liposarcomas and both may be found anywhere there is subcutaneous fat tissue. The most common sites are the sternum, wings, abdomen, and rarely on the back, neck, and uropygial gland.

These tumors are more common on overweight birds, thus diet control and good nutrition are part of therapy. Lipomas typically are encapsulated and can be single or multiple, lobulated, subcutaneous masses. They should be differentiated from circumscribed lipogranulomas. Liposarcomas tend to be firm masses somewhat like fibrosarcomas and may be quite vascularized.

Surgical excision is the best therapeutic approach and most of these tumors can be successfully removed.

Hemangioma and Hemangiosarcoma

Derived from vascular endothelium, these tumors are not commonly seen, but are occasionally found as soft reddish to black subcutaneous swellings and often involve feather follicles. Hemangiosarcomas (the malignant form of the disease) can be locally invasive or metastatic. Treatment is by surgical excision.

Squamous Cell Carcinoma

Squamous cell carcinomas are found occasionally and occur mostly in the uropygial gland area and on the skin of the neck. Budgerigars appear to be the main host to these tumors.

Epidermal Cysts

An epidermal cyst occasionally may be found on a bird. These cysts are fluid-filled and collapse when punctured. I have seen epidermal cysts that contained a brownish fluid on the heads of canaries. An inclusion cyst in the area of the uropygial gland and a mucus cyst on the sternum, both in budgerigars, have been reported. Surgical removal is recommended.

Feather Cysts

Feather cysts are ingrown feathers that accumulate masses of necrotic feather material in the form of subcutaneous cysts that involve a feather follicle. They may occur as an isolated follicle that has been traumatized and healed over before the new feather grew out, or as generalized involvement of the feather tracts as seen on canaries (Plate XI-9). The long wing feathers are common sites for these cysts to occur, where the follicles are easily damaged.

Certain strains of canaries appear to be genetically susceptible to feather cyst formation. They may have an occasional cyst on the wings or the entire feather tracts of the body, dorsal and ventral, may be involved, producing extensive cyst formation.

Cysts show up as subcutaneous, whitish swellings over a feather follicle (often where a wing feather is missing) that become progressively larger. The birds may pick at and even damage these cysts. Multiple cysts can occur in one small area. When a cyst is opened, it contains whitish, often caseous, necrotic debris and curled-up feather structures sometimes are observed inside. One cyst can involve several feather follicles.

If possible, with a wing feather, it is best to incise the end of the cyst, gently tease out the necrotic tissue, and leave the base of the feather attached so it will continue to grow out of the incised end of the cyst to become a normal feather again. This may work in some cases; usually the whole mass, including the growing base, comes out in the mass of debris. If an opening is maintained in the end of the cyst, the new feather may grow out of the opening. Risk of infection is high and antibiotic ointment must be infused into the opening regularly. It may be necessary to remove the entire follicle surgically or destroy it with electrocautery in order to prevent frequent recurrence of the cyst.

In extensive feather tract involvement, it is pointless to try to surgically remove all the cysts. If the owners do not wish to keep a bird in this condition, euthanasia should be performed. If the owner is told that there is no cure and is willing to keep a heavily encysted bird, it will survive for a long time.

MISCELLANEOUS DERMATOSES

Disorders of the Feet and Legs

Leg Band Constriction

Leg band constriction is a common problem of small birds and occasionally is seen in large birds. Domestic-raised small birds usually have a closed band put on when they are a few days old. By the time these birds grow up the bands may become a little snug. All birds exfoliate the outer layers of the skin on the legs, more so in some species than others. The skin layers build up under the band, and gradually cause pressure between the band and the leg. This pressure triggers an inflammatory process that produces swelling. As the swollen tissue en-

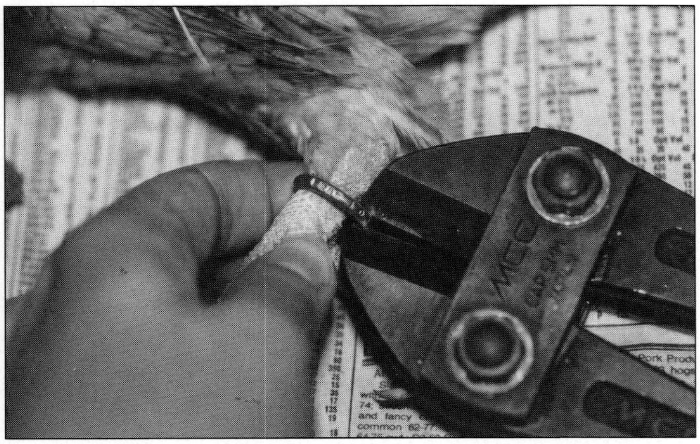

Figure 14-6. A safe way to remove heavy leg bands from large birds with a bolt cutter.

larges, more pressure develops under the band, circulation is impaired, infection develops, and all too frequently the leg dies from the band down. Dry gangrene results. The only treatment available at this point is amputation of the leg at the junction of healthy skin.

If found early in the progression of the problem, careful removal of the leg band with local and systemic treatment of the leg lesion will often restore the health of the leg. It is imperative that these leg bands be removed properly or the leg can be easily fractured at the site of the band. On small birds it is best to cut the band with a side cutter that cuts close to the edge of the tool by placing it on the band so that it cuts out a piece of the band in one cut without further injuring the leg. Do not try to get the tool under the band or the leg may get broken. Most small bird bands are made of aluminum or plastic and are easily cut. Large birds often have heavy stainless-steel bands that require the use of a heavy duty bolt cutter (Fig. 14-6); these usually are split bands so it is necessary to cut the band on the opposite side from the split.

Gout

Gout often is mistakenly diagnosed as abscesses of the foot. It is produced as a result of the body's failure to eliminate nitrogenous waste material from the blood via the kidneys. The result is the accumulation of urates, uric acid, and related substances in various parts of the body. This disease has been reported to be fairly common in southern Ontario, California, and Australia.

Birds suffer two different forms of the disease, visceral and articular gout. In visceral gout, the urates are deposited in and around the major internal organs, particularly the kidneys. Articular gout takes a more obvious form. The urates are deposited in the joints of the limbs, particularly the feet and legs (Plate XI-10). The birds become painfully crippled. Lesions (tophi) show up as whitish nodular swellings along the bare area of the legs, ankles, and toes, or more deeply involving the tissue around the joints. Affected birds exhibit acute lameness as the disease progresses. The joints become stiffened because of the mechanical encroachment of the deposits and tissue swelling. Polyuria may be evident.

If some of the whitish material is aseptically removed from a lesion and placed on a slide, the presence of uric acid crystals on microscopic examination will confirm the diagnosis. These crystals show up as thin, short, clusters of hair-like structures.

Attempts at surgically removing the deposits result in profuse hemorrhage and no benefit is gained from this approach. Correcting the diet by reducing the protein level and increasing the vitamins, particularly vitamin A, and giving fruits and vegetables may help prolong the life of the patient. Antibiotics should be given to control secondary opportunistic infections.

Few birds respond to treatment because of permanent kidney damage, but some have been known to recover when their dietary deficiencies are corrected and treatment begins early in the disease. The use of allopurinol may have varying effects in arresting the progression of the disease. Crush one 100-mg tablet in 10 ml of water (10 mg/ml). Give one drop per os four times daily, or 20 drops per ounce of drinking water. It will not cause resorption of the deposits but may assist in slowing the progression. The human drugs colchicine, an antigout drug, and probenicid, a drug used in venereal disease therapy, may provide additional options.

Self-Mutilation

Birds of many species have been known to start chewing on their feet and legs for no apparent reason. They may constantly work at them until they peel off large areas of epithelium, resulting in open sores that will not heal. The toes are a favorite site for this self-mutilation. These lesions may start from small wounds caused by trauma from something in the cage or may be the result of an overzealous neurotic feather picker. Stress of various sorts also can contribute to the problem.

Treatment involves correcting nutritional and environmental factors and breaking the chewing habit by applying an Elizabethan collar. The skin lesions can be treated with local chlorhexidine or antibiotic cream, protective bandages, and if necessary, systemic antibiotics. Once healing is complete, the collar can be removed. Medroxyprogesterone (Depo-Provera® —Upjohn) at 30 mg/kg given subcutaneously may help control these cases.

Nesting Fiber Constriction

A common finding, in finches particularly as well as canaries and some other small birds, is the presentation with one or often several swollen and sore toes. The end of the toe may even be gangrenous and dry. Under magnification, fine strands of plastic fiber can be seen in a circumscribed indentation in the skin of the toe, ankle, or foot. These strands originate from the synthetic fibers sold commercially as nesting material. Natural fibers used as nesting material are less likely to cause this problem than the synthetic fibers, although human hair is sometimes implicated. By carefully inserting a pointed scalpel blade under the fibers, they can be cut and removed. Once the fibers are removed, the damaged tissues heal quickly with topical treatment. The necrotic areas should be amputated and the foot bandaged for protection during healing. Systemic and local antibiotics usually are necessary.

Hyperkeratinization

This is a condition most commonly affecting canaries, finches, and mynah birds. It also has been observed in a few species of captive wild birds, such as starlings, crows, grackles, and evening grosbeaks. The condition results from excessive exfoliation of keratin on the skin surface and can result in scaling, swelling, irritation, cracking, and splitting (Plate XI-11). If a leg band is present, serious constriction of the band on the leg develops. In some species the abnormal keratinization is noted on the ventral aspects of the toes.

It is recommended that this material be removed manually on a regular basis before it develops to an advanced state. The layers of dead skin (keratin) can be carefully picked off using a narrow, blunt-pointed instrument, such as the pointed end of a small pair of suture removal scissors. The daily application of chlorhexidine cream or moisturizing cream will help soften this material and control infection. It should be rubbed into the feet and legs well until it disappears, not left on in excessive amounts. Vitamin A has long been known for its "normalizing" effect on keratinization and may be indicated in some cases.

Trauma

Trauma can take many different forms, such as bites, fractures, burns, scalds, and frostbite, and the feet and legs are commonly traumatized. These problems are treated according to the degree of injury, some requiring only cleansing and the application of antiseptics and others requiring more intensive treatment.

Burns from heat sources should have cold water put on them immediately. The treatment of burns should include initial shock therapy if needed, parenteral fluids (1 ml/100 g body weight) if lesions are severe, topical vitamin A and E creams, aloe vera gel, antibiotics, and bandaging of those areas that need protection and can be bandaged. Grease- or oil-based products should not be used. Treatment may be prolonged as severe burns take considerable time to heal. Some patients may require tube feeding or force feeding; an Elizabethan collar may be required as well.

Chemical burns are treated similarly except that acids must be neutralized with sodium bicarbonate solution and caustics with dilute white vinegar solution. Antihistamine and corticosteroid incorporated into a topical antibiotic cream initially may help reduce the shock and pain of the trauma. A moderately warm, humid environment is better than a hot dry environment.

Pododermatitis (Bumblefoot)

Pododermatitis is quite common in budgerigars, canaries, and cockatiels, and is occasionally seen in other species. The problem occurs on the ventral surface of the foot and may progress from there to involve other areas (Plate XI-12). It starts as a thinning of the epithelial layer; inflammation and swelling develop and then scabs and ulcers appear, along with a severe lameness. Progression of the lesion to involve the tendons and joints, as occurs in raptors at times, is rarely seen in psittacines or passerines. Contributing factors are hypovitaminosis (particularly vitamin A), dirty cages and perches, sandpaper perch covers, rough corrugated perches or sometimes perches that are too smooth, stress, hypothyroidism, and obesity. A variety of shapes and thickness of perches are better for birds than perches that are all the same size. A variety of perches that are round, oval, flat, and square in cross section are healthier for the feet than all round ones of the same size. The use of natural tree branches also can be of benefit.

It is necessary to debride these lesions and remove the necrotic tissue. Topical 5% Lugol's iodine and chlorhexidine cream followed by a protective bandage will assist in the healing of these areas. Bandages should be changed regularly during the healing period. The use of Vetrap® bandaging tape (3M Company) and systemic antibiotics administered parenterally initially, followed by oral dosing, will usually result in recovery (Table 14-1). Certain individuals appear to be highly susceptible to recurrences.

Padding of the perches with such materials as Moleskin tape (Dr. Scholl's Foot Products), which is available in any pharmacy foot products department, is quite helpful in protecting the bottom of the feet of affected birds.

Improvements in nutrition and environment are essential. Injections of B-complex and A, D_3, and E vitamins should be followed by continued use of oral supplementation of multivitamin–mineral–amino acid preparations.

Various organisms may be involved in these infections, such as *Staphylococcus* spp., *Streptococcus* spp., *Escherichia coli*, *Mycobacterium* spp., *Klebsiella* spp.,

Pseudomonas spp., *Proteus* spp., and *Candida albicans*. *Staphylococcus* spp. are the most common.

Nail Overgrowth

Nails that are allowed to overgrow (Fig. 14-7) may curl into a spiral shape and get caught in cages and toys and can result in broken nails, toes, or legs. Injured and misshapen toes often produce long nails that grow out straight or at abnormal angles.

The use of sandpaper perch covers or sandpaper on the bottom of bird cages is not recommended. It does not help to wear the nails down and it can cause abrasion and wear to the skin on the bottom of the feet, resulting in pressure sores and bumblefoot with secondary infection. A bird walking on sandpaper is comparable to a human walking on a gravel road in bare feet. It is better to put white, absorbent paper on the bottom of the cage, which will show the state of the droppings better and absorb moisture, which will keep the feet cleaner.

Placing gravel or grit on the bottom of the cage also does nothing to wear the nails down. The only purpose for gravel is for the bird to eat. It acts as teeth and helps to grind the food in the gizzard. A few grains a week are normally eaten, mainly by the smaller species. It is doubtful that larger psittacines require grit, but they could be offered it at least quarterly.

One way to help larger birds wear their nails and sometimes their beaks down normally is to place a brick or coarse rock on or in the cage. In the process of walking on the brick, the nails are worn down. They often rub their beaks on it as well which helps wear them down.

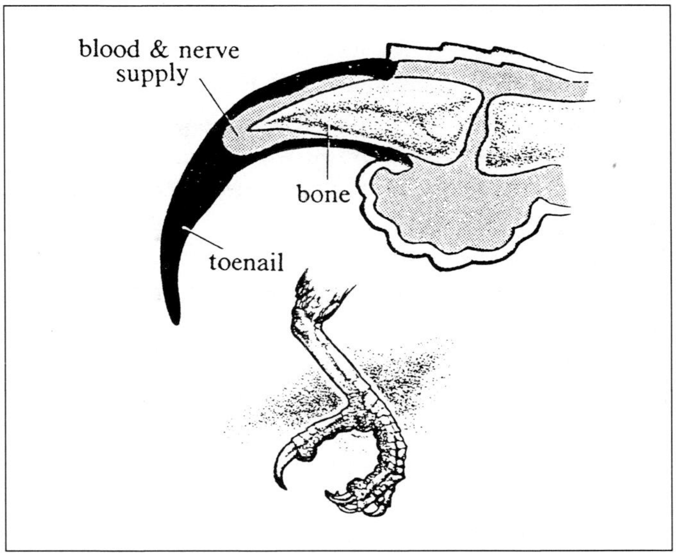

Figure 14-7. Cross section of a toenail. (From Axelson RD: *Caring for Your Pet Bird*. Toronto, Canaviax Publications, 1981, with permission)

Feather Disorders

Cockatiel Feather Syndrome

This disease can be very frustrating to the avian veterinarian, the owner, and particularly the bird. It is peculiar to cockatiels, and is commonly associated with giardiasis. A viral etiology also has been proposed. The bird is presented as a chronic feather picker, often starting in the carpal-metacarpal area, the flank, and legs. The birds often pick intensely and cry as if it hurts them. On examination, the birds may have atrophy of the pectoral muscles, dry flaky skin, feather loss in different areas of the body, chewed feathers, and watery droppings that may be diarrheic. As the condition progresses, the birds begin to actually chew the skin and produce large, nonhealing ulcers, especially in the axillae and on the back. Some birds work on the wing tips. These lesions often bleed and the sight of blood may alert the owner that there is a serious problem. Broken pin or blood feathers can be involved. Some of these birds may have secondary infections and may show anorexia and depression.

Diagnosis involves fecal assessment of fresh samples for *Giardia*, a complete blood count (CBC), fecal Gram stain, and perhaps a fecal culture. Eosinophilia may be a fairly consistent finding. Serum lactate dehydrogenase (LDH) and serum aspartate aminotransferase (ASAT/SGOT) levels often are elevated.

Treatment for *Giardia*, regardless of whether it was recovered, is usually the first therapeutic option. Nutrition should be evaluated closely. Supportive treatment (vitamins A, D_3, E, B-complex and selenium) should be started with injections and maintained orally. Antihistamines may provide temporary relief. The use of corticosteroids should be discouraged as many of these birds are already immunocompromised. Antibiotics should be given systemically or orally as some birds will respond to this therapy.

A shifting leg lameness may be present in some birds that seems to respond rapidly to injections of the above vitamins and selenium.

Skin lesions must be treated with topical nongreasy antibacterial agents, such as chlorhexidine cream. An Elizabethan collar usually will be required to keep the bird from continuing to chew at the open lesions. Recurrence is common.

Baldness

Balding disease is prevalent in canaries and is sometimes seen in finches. The feather loss starts on the back of the neck and spreads up onto the head, sometimes involving the entire head (Plate XI-13). The skin may become thickened or scaly and wrinkled. If this condition spreads to the eyelids, it may pose a physical problem for the bird. In general, the health of the bird is not affected by the baldness as it is a localized problem. Maintaining body temperature might be a factor but the feather loss usually is not severe enough for this. Owners tend to become alarmed when feather loss occurs.

The cause may be fungal or bacterial infections of the skin, thyroid deficiencies, or in male canaries, hormonal imbalances. It has not been proven that thyroid deficiencies are a contributing factor, but it is suspected and some birds do respond to treatment with thyroid replacement. It is thought that hereditary factors could be involved in some cases. In some birds, baldness is the result of an arrested molt. Birds that are "stuck-in-molt" lose the feathers on the head and neck, but do not grow replacements. The usual cause of this phenomenon is stress. Perhaps the hen has been forced into egg-laying through too rich a diet, or babies have been put through their stress of training before they finished their primary molt. Sudden weather changes may be enough stress to interrupt a bird's molt cycle. Poor nutrition and irregular photoperiods may predispose to this problem.

Some species, such as lutino cockatiels and cockatoos, have a genetic baldness on the top of the head under the crest. Another cause of baldness is over-aggressive birds that pick the feathers off the heads of their mates.

Birds that are "stuck-in-molt" often will regrow their lost feathers during the next normal molt cycle if their stress is reduced and nutrition improved. Treatment for the baldness in canaries and finches should include improved nutrition, vitamin-mineral supplements, hormone replacements (such as testosterone), thyroid replacement, and reduced stress.

Many cases will not respond to any treatment. These birds will remain bald permanently; their feather follicles appear not to be able to generate new feathers.

Feather Hemorrhage

Newly growing feathers have a thick, dark-colored base filled with blood and nerve supply. Those growing in on the tail and wings may be very large. These feathers are called *pin feathers* or *blood feathers*. At this stage in their development, they are very susceptible to injury. As these feathers grow out, they are covered by a protective sheath that is preened off by the bird before the feather fans out into its normal shape. Occasionally a bird will overzealously preen the sheath off too close to the distal growth area and cause some hemorrhage. These bleeders can be controlled with local clotting powders, such as Quick Stop or styptic powder (Rich Health).

Pin feathers often get traumatized down in the thick, vascular area and will bleed profusely. This hemorrhage is more difficult to control and it is better to pluck these feathers out by pulling the feather straight out in the line of growth. Do not bend or twist them. Moderate pressure and the use of clotting powder in the follicle area will soon stop the bleeding. It is better to grasp the feather near the skin when removing it to prevent it from breaking. Pliers may be needed for extra large feathers. Regrowth usually starts immediately after removal and takes about 6 weeks to complete.

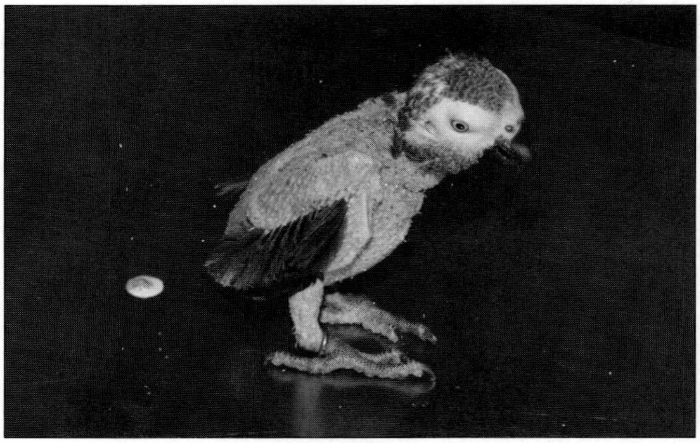

Figure 14-8. A badly feather-picked bird.

Stress Lines on Feathers

Stress marks can appear on feathers that are in the growth stage in a bird that undergoes severe stress, usually from some disease. They appear as lines or bands of incomplete feather development across the feather from side to side. These lines will appear in the same places on all the feathers that were growing in at the same time, and remain until those feathers are molted. Stress marks may weaken the feather somewhat and may be the site of feather breakage, but usually cause no problems. Variations in the nutritional supply to the feathers caused by the stress of the disease are a contributing factor.

Feather Picking

Feather chewing or plucking is a common problem in pet birds (Fig. 14-8), especially the psittacines, and can be very frustrating for both the owner and the attending avian veterinarian. It also has been observed in captive native North American wild birds.

Feather picking is most commonly seen in African Grey parrots, cockatoos, and cockatiels, but it has been seen in most psittacines and occasionally in other species as well (Plate XI-14). There are many contributing factors involved, many of which are environmental and behavioral irregularities. Some of the most common factors include nutritional inadequacies, boredom, emotional frustration, stress, insecurity, parasitism, infections (viral, bacterial, or fungal), and low humidity.

When wild birds are upset or frightened, they fly away

to escape. Caged birds cannot do this. Some are more nervous than others and like to have a place to hide. A privacy box, which is built like a nest box except it has a perch inside plus an open bottom, or an open paper bag in the cage will give the bird a place to hide and get away from some of its stresses. Covering the cage at night gives darkness if the owner has a light on while the bird is trying to sleep, and does provide some privacy.

Birds should be kept in a cage big enough to provide ample room for exercise. The bird that only eats and sleeps in its cage and is out all day can get along with a smaller cage than one that is kept caged all the time. Rectangular cages that are longer than they are high or wide are far superior to the tall, narrow, or round cages because most birds are not able to fly straight up and down like a helicopter.

Birds require 9 to 12 hours of sleep each night, preferably in darkness. Insufficient sleep can make a bird irritable, stresses it, and can cause it to start picking. Birds should be put in a dark room or have the cage covered at a reasonable hour at night. They awaken at dawn. Bird bed-time habits should be routine.

Abnormal increases or decreases in the various hormones can cause feather loss or trigger feather picking. This is most often seen as canary balding disease and hypothyroidism. Canary baldness can be caused by other factors as well.

Sexual frustration or a desire to breed and nest may induce a bird to feather pick. These birds should be sexed (surgically or otherwise) and paired with an appropriate mate in a breeding cage with nest box. Seasonal or intermittent picking can sometimes be controlled with injections of Depo-Provera or testosterone. Some birds that are paired already may only feather pick during their breeding cycle and may use their feathers to line their nest.

Self-mutilation can be a progression of feather picking or it can result from bacterial or fungal dermatitis, folliculitis, lacerations, ingrown feathers, *Giardia* infection, irregular photoperiods, allergic reactions, malnutrition, insect bites or stings, internal abscesses, tumors, arthritis, stress, puncturing foreign bodies, external parasites, thyroid problems, or foreign objects, such as fibers, wrapped around parts of the body.

Discomfort in an internal organ from infection, neoplasia, or other causes may induce a bird to chew the skin and or feathers over that area, but this is an uncommon situation.

Treatment must include a method to break the self-chewing cycle and an Elizabethan collar usually solves this problem. Local and systemic therapy must be combined with an attempt to find the original cause and correct it as well. Suturing may be required. The administration of Depo-Provera at 30 mg/kg subcutaneously may help control this problem in some birds; one of the side effects of this product, however, is obesity.

Preening Complications

Part of a bird's personal grooming procedure is to remove the feather sheaths that grow out around each feather. They also rearrange the feathers, lining up the hooklets and flanges on the barbules to assist the feathers in keeping their normal shape and appearance and to help keep them clean. This grooming procedure is called *preening* and usually is done with the beak.

Anatomical or physical disabilities, such as spinal injuries, fractures, malformation of the beak, long-term use of Elizabethan collars, or disinterest from illness, may interfere in a bird's ability to preen the feather sheaths off growing feathers or to accomplish other preening procedures. Birds often have difficulty in reaching their head and neck and prefer to rely on a cage-mate or owner to preen these areas. The bird may end up looking like a porcupine with quills sticking out of various parts of its body and tattered and unkempt feathers. The owner will need to remove these coverings by rubbing them between the fingers or allow another bird to do it. Young birds learn from their parents how to preen.

Canary Dysplastic Feather Syndrome

Canary dysplastic feather syndrome is also referred to as *straw feather disease* as the feathers somewhat resemble the appearance of straw. The disease affects all or most of the feathers of baby birds symmetrically in their first molt. The feathers often retain their sheaths and are very narrow as a result of improper development of the barbs and barbules. Dorsally the feathers appear glossy and ventrally they appear dull. These birds cannot fly and may not survive long as they have trouble maintaining body heat. Genetic factors are suspected as the cause and no treatment is known.

Hypothyroidism

History and Clinical Signs. One of the clinical signs of suspected thyroxine deficiency in some birds (mainly budgerigars and occasionally cockatiels) is an elongation of the down feathers. This phenomenon generally starts bilaterally on the lateral body under the wing (Plate XI-15); as it progresses, other parts of the body become involved. The down feathers grow longer than the regular feathers, and in an advanced case the bird will have fluffy down feathers sticking out all over its body (Fig. 14-9). Other clinical signs will develop later, such as nonpruritic feather loss, cardiac problems, and predisposition to bacterial and fungal diseases. Lethargy, depression, and sensitivity to cold may develop. Many of these birds become obese, which can occur before any feather changes. Hypothyroidism can occur in conjunction with thyroid hypertrophy (goiter) caused by iodine deficiency and insufficient thyroxine production.

Diagnosis. It is recommended that the confirmation of thyroxine deficiency be verified by using the thyroid-stimulating hormone (TSH) stimulation test rather than the measurement of a low thyroxine (T_4) level. The suggested protocol involves collection of baseline T_4 values followed by giving 1/4 to 1 IU of TSH intramuscularly (depending on the size of the bird), and collecting a second sample 6 hours later to measure the T_4 level again. Samples should be submitted to reliable avian laboratories. Serum cholesterol levels may be high.

Treatment. Empirical doses of thyroid replacement will often produce dramatic improvement. L-Thyroxine added to the water is quite effective. (I use a stock mixture of one 50-mg tablet in 1/2 ounce of water and give eight to ten drops per ounce of drinking water fresh daily.)

The long down feathers should be plucked out at the beginning of therapy as these can be a guide to monitoring the dose of L-thyroxine supplementation. If they start to grow in long again, this indicates that the dose needs to be increased. Thyroxine replacement should continue for the duration of the bird's life. Iodine in the form of one drop of 5% Lugol's iodine should be put in the drinking water daily or every other day as well.

If the bird is obese, the diet should be improved and the volume of food reduced. A vitamin–mineral–amino acid supplement is added to fresh water daily or sprinkled on moist fruit and greens. It is necessary to weigh the bird initially and at least monthly until the desired weight is reached. The volume of seed can then be adjusted so that this weight level is maintained. It usually is necessary to keep the bird on this controlled diet and thyroid replacement continuously with regular rechecks every 4 to 5 months.

As long as the overgrowth of the long down feathers and any other disease-related clinical signs are controlled, the dose of thyroid supplementation is maintained. Clinical signs of thyroid overdose will range from hyperactivity and nervousness to diarrhea and vomiting. Untreated birds will often progress to death over a fairly long period of time.

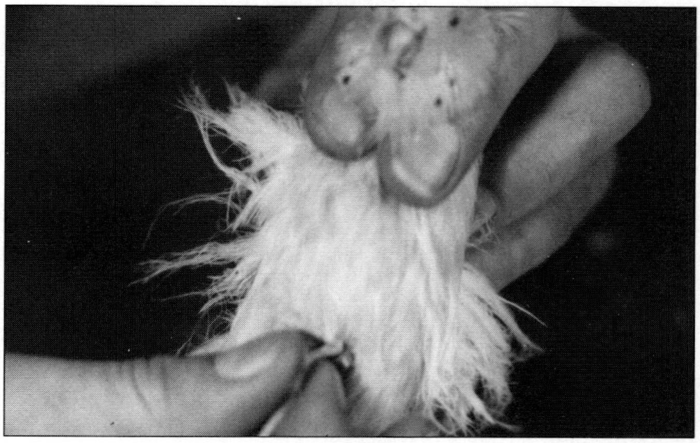

Figure 14-9. Budgerigar showing the long down feather syndrome that responds to thyroid supplementation.

Trauma

Breast or ventral chest sores are skin lesions found on the ventral chest over the sternal bone. They are actually decubital ulcers or pressure sores caused by a bird lying on its chest too much. After prolonged sternal recumbency the skin gets pressed between the sternum and the surface of whatever the bird is lying on. The constant pressure causes tissue necrosis and an ulcer develops. These sores are seen in birds that are chronically ill and weak and in birds recovering from fractures or leg problems that cannot stand properly. Breast sores also can occur from a bad fall or flying into a wall and the concussion splits the skin open in this area.

If not discovered early, the bird may self-traumatize the lesion with its beak and make it worse or prevent it from healing. Treatment involves a general anesthetic, debridement of the lesion, freshening the wound edges, disinfecting the area, and suturing the skin closed. It may be necessary to put an Elizabethan collar on until the skin heals. Antibiotic therapy will help control secondary infection.

Birds can fall prey to other household pets, such as dogs, cats, ferrets, and other birds, and receive skin lacerations varying in severity from minor scratches to extensive skin tears and punctures, even involving fractures.

Air movement fans that have no protective screen, especially ceiling fans, can do a great deal of damage to birds. They also can fly into walls, windows, and furniture and receive injuries. Birds that fly freely may swoop too high and scalp themselves on a rough textured ceiling. I have even seen birds that flew out a building door and were hit by a car as they crossed the street.

The area should be cleansed and the lesions sutured if needed. Local application of an antibacterial powder containing chlorhexidine or an antibiotic will help keep the area dry and control infection. Oral or systemic antibiotics along with multivitamin supplementation will help the injury to heal. General anesthesia may or may not be required.

Lipogranuloma

Budgerigars very commonly get lipogranulomas, which often are associated with obesity. In obese birds the fat is deposited primarily over the pectoral and abdominal areas. Fatty degeneration sometimes occurs in these fat pads, precipitating the formation of a small nodular granuloma which rapidly enlarges. Fat necrosis also can occur in the center of the mass. These granulomas are often confused with lipomas. It is best to surgically remove them and to strictly control the food volume consumption of the bird. Improved nutrition with proper control of volume consumed will bring the bird's weight down. Xanthomas (see below) may occasionally develop over a large distended obese chest or abdomen of a bird.

Xanthoma/Xanthomatosis

Pathogenesis. Xanthomas are relatively common in cockatiels and are seen less frequently in budgerigars, and may be seen occasionally in other species. The usual site of involvement in cockatiels is the tips of the wings. In humans and other animals, xanthomas represent alterations in lipid metabolism and although they are sometimes categorized as tumors, they should be considered metabolic disorders.

Clinical Signs. In the cockatiel, a thickening of the skin develops in the form of a lobular mass on the distal end of one or both wings. It gradually progresses down the wing toward the body (Plate XI-16). The lesion is yellowish-tan colored and gets thicker as it grows. It will surround the wing in its progression. As wing joints become involved and the mass gets heavier, the wing may droop and flight may be impaired. These masses can occur on other parts of the body as well. The bird may traumatize the mass as it enlarges and bleeding will occur. Xanthomas may occur as discrete tumor masses or as diffuse thickening of the skin as described above. Xanthomas often occur over protruding parts of the body, such as abdominal hernias, tumor masses, or obese fat pads.

Diagnosis. Xanthomas and xanthomatosis have a typical unmistakable appearance and can be confirmed by histopathologic examination.

Treatment. It is impossible to remove xanthomatosis and leave the wing intact. Usually by the time the owner notices it, the condition has progressed to the point that amputation of at least part of the wing is necessary. If the entire tumor is removed in the amputation, recovery is usually complete unless it starts in the opposite wing as well. Many birds have continued as useful pets with one or both wing tips removed.

If amputation is not done, the mass encroaches on the entire wing and severely inhibits the use of it. If the condition occurs as a discrete mass and as not the diffuse type, excision of the mass alone with some of the immediate surrounding tissue is possible.

Blocked Uropygial Gland

Occasionally the uropygial gland (commonly called the oil gland), which is located on the dorsal base of the tail, becomes blocked and distended from the build-up of the glandular secretion. This is most commonly seen in canaries, finches, and budgerigars. The gland may become quite large and cause discomfort to the bird, who may pick at the area, sometimes traumatizing the gland or the surrounding skin. The bird frequently plucks feathers out around the gland area and the base of the tail.

Very often the problem can be corrected by gentle pressure with the fingernails on the gland, forcing the contents out through the gland opening, which is a little protruding papilla. If the gland cannot be emptied in this manner, it may require lancing or even surgical removal. All species of birds do not have uropygial glands; they are absent in Amazon parrots and hyacinth macaws.

Local treatment of irritated skin should be done by applying soothing non–grease-based antiseptic creams.

Disorders of the Beak and Cere

Brown Hypertrophy of the Cere

The cere is the soft raised skin area surrounding some birds' nostrils. It is quite prominent in certain species, such as budgerigars, hawks, and falcons, and absent in other species, such as canaries and finches.

Brown hypertrophy or hyperplasia of the cere is seen mostly in budgerigars, most frequently in females, and is more common as they get older. The color of the cere may just turn a medium or dark brown, or it may build up excessive layers of keratin that can proliferate into a horn-like protruberance over the cere (Plate XI-17). Sometimes the nostrils are blocked in this build-up. Other than the blockage of the nares and the appearance of the build-up, there is little discomfort to the bird.

This build-up of dead skin layers can be gently removed by scraping or peeling it off the cere. Occasionally, overly aggressive removal may produce some hemorrhage that can be quickly controlled with clotting powder. Local application of chlorhexidine or moisturizing cream will soften the tissue and make removal easier if it adheres tightly. The build-up of cere tissue will recur. Regular removal of these layers is part of the maintenance program done on birds in my practice. The exact cause is unknown, but it may be associated with hormonal changes.

Demineralization of the Beak

Certain species, such as doves and pigeons, normally have a fairly soft beak. Demineralization of the beak to the point of being very soft, pliable, and rubbery can be the aftermath of pronounced malnutrition causing a severe nutritional secondary hyperparathyroidism, which produces this syndrome in the beak. Insufficient calcium, vitamin D_3, and methionine contribute to this process. Birds in this state also will often have a rubbery, twisted sternum and the ribs also may be deformed; this is seen most frequently in cockatiels, doves, and pigeons.

Correcting the diet and supplementing calcium, vitamins, and other minerals may save some of these birds. A badly twisted upper beak can be difficult to correct and may require some form of support splint to hold it straight while the beak firms up with remineralization. The ribs and sternum of some of these birds have so much deformity because of lack of rigidity that respiration is severely impaired and death may follow.

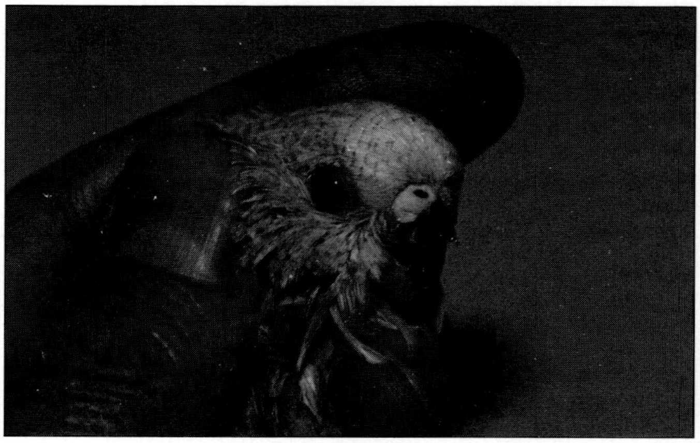

Figure 14-10. Budgerigar with upper beak chewed off to the cere by an Amazon parrot.

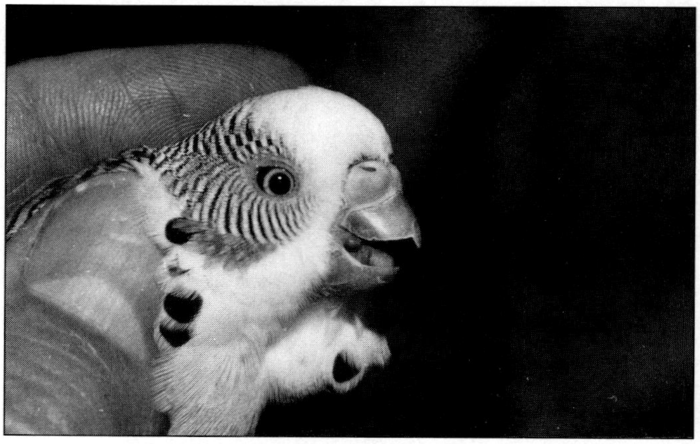

Figure 14-11. Same budgerigar as in Figure 14-10 with beak nearly completely grown back.

Beak Trauma

Beaks can be traumatized in a variety of ways. Birds can get their beak caught in metal clips, rings, and wires in a cage; be bitten by animals or other birds; or get caught in doors or other objects, as well as a multitude of other accidents that can happen.

Large birds can chew the beak of a smaller bird right off. Beakless birds cannot eat very well and usually have to be tube-fed until new beak tissue grows back, if in fact it does. I treated two budgerigars with this trauma and their beaks did regrow (Figs. 14-10 and 14-11). The beaks were chewed off, upper bill only, right back to the nostrils. The birds were tube-fed for many weeks. Gradually, the upper beak regenerated to be about three quarters of the original length, but the birds eventually were able to eat on their own.

Treatment of beak trauma can be relatively simple or quite complex. It may only require a little trimming or grinding plus some clotting powder, or a beak prosthesis may have to be made. Some beak defects can be repaired with 5-minute epoxy. Split beaks can be drilled and wired together with stainless-steel wire, which holds the pieces together as the beak grows out. Most glues and epoxies do not adhere to beak tissue very long as the outer layers continually exfoliate and detach the adhesive.

Beak prostheses can be made from dental acrylics, such as Cyano-Veneer (Cyano-Veneer kit—Ellman International Mfg.). A strengthening powder is mixed with the acrylic liquid and while it is pliable, it can be molded into the desired shape or molded to fit contours of the damaged beak. As the acrylic hardens, heat is produced and once it has hardened, it can be ground and polished. Coloring agents can be added in the early stage of preparation to match the tissue being repaired. The prosthesis can be attached to the beak stump with stainless-steel wire, Steinmann pins, K-wires, and epoxies or skin glue (Cyanodent or Tissue Glu—Ellman International Mfg.). As the damaged beak grows out, the prosthesis will often come off and have to be redone to fit again. The material can be molded around preset anchor pins or wires and then hardened quickly with a coating of quick-setting solution.

Medical acrylics that were originally developed for dentists can be very useful as adhesives and prosthesis material in birds (Fig. 14-12). Ethyl acrylic becomes very hard and is suitable for beak repair. Dental methacrylate can be used with exothermic catalytic polymerization. Super Glue is methyl acrylic and it contains ingredients that are toxic to tissue.

Damage to the growth area at the base of the beak usually will result in a permanently deformed beak. A fracture of the lower jaw that splits the lower beak will never heal again so that the beak is a solid unit. The split will always remain in the beak even though the bone of the jaw heals.

Even if the damaged beak cannot be repaired completely, many birds will learn to eat and adapt to a severe beak deformity.

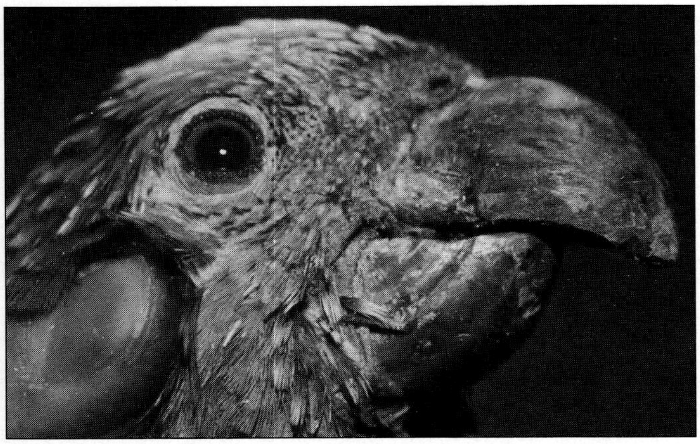

Figure 14-12. Acrylic prosthesis on an Amazon parrot with a severely damaged beak.

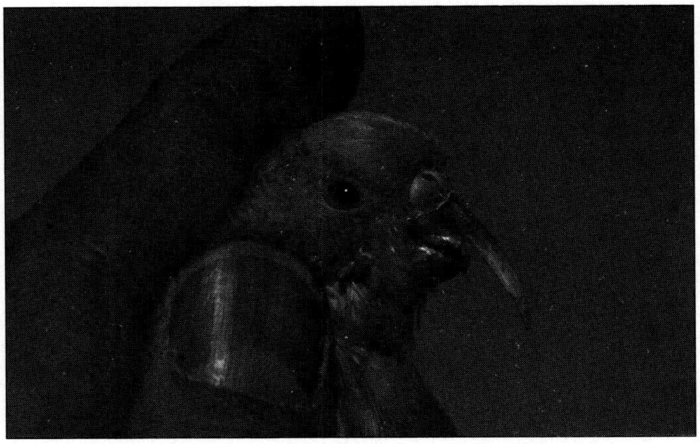

Figure 14-13. Budgerigar with beak deformed by *Knemidokoptes* mites.

Beak Overgrowth

Beaks often overgrow as a result of injury to the growth area or other trauma (Plate XI-18). Prolonged irritation from the *Knemidokoptes* mite will produce some bizarre beak shapes that need continual regular trimming or grinding (Fig. 14-13). Even normal undamaged beaks and nails will need regular maintenance care if they are not being worn down naturally. Overgrown upper beaks can grow long enough to impair eating and on occasion will grow into the neck in a long curve if neglected.

Beak tissues grow continuously and when they are trimmed, care must be taken to not cut them back too close or the inner "quick" area, which is the area containing the blood and nerve supply, will be exposed. When cut too short, these areas bleed profusely and are painful.

It is better to grind the beak and nails with a portable hand grinder using a small rotary grinding wheel about 1/2 inch in diameter. Flexible shaft grinders are available from jeweller's supply outlets and hand-held grinders from hobby shops or hardware stores. The beak can be shaped easily and quickly with these tools. If an area starts to bleed, it can be easily stopped by holding the grinder lightly on the bleeding spot for a few seconds, creating enough heat to quickly cauterize the bleeder.

Most psittacine birds produce flaking or crumbly build-up of beak tissue in the normal growth of the beak; in some birds this can leave unsightly platforms or steps of beak layers. This build-up should be ground off the beaks of larger birds and scraped off the beaks of smaller ones as a part of their regular maintenance program, which helps to maintain a healthier beak and better cosmetic appearance of the bird. Some birds require this more frequently than others but it should be done two to four times a year. A bird with a beak that is too soft and excessively flaky needs a mineral and vitamin supplement (especially calcium) plus dietary improvement (Fig. 14-14).

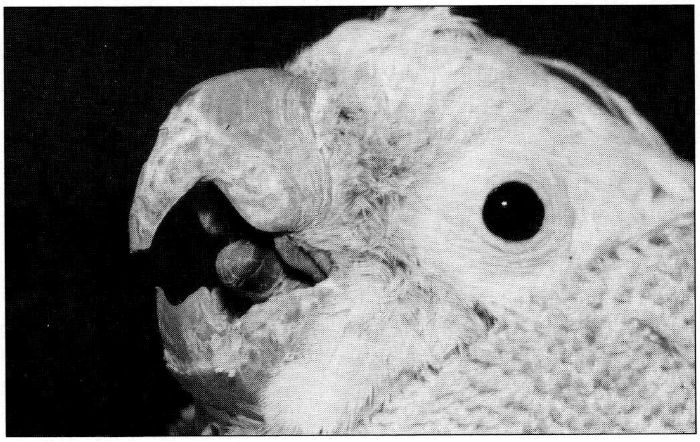

Figure 14-14. A Goffin cockatoo with excessive beak flakiness resulting from malnutrition.

A condition seen mostly in budgerigars and cockatiels causes the central part of the upper beak, including the point, to become longitudinally porous and crumbly. It may start as dark areas on the beak tissue, and usually results in a change in the angle of growth from the normal curve to a larger curve and sometimes a gradual straightening of the beak. Because the lower beak can no longer help to wear it down, the upper part will continue to grow and become very long unless a regular clipping or grinding program is maintained. Liver disease, vitamin deficiency, internal neoplasia, psittacine beak and feather disease syndrome, and even clotting abnormalities have been proposed, but the true cause is unknown. Once this problem starts, there is no way to reverse it and go back to normal tissue. Improve the general health of the bird with nutrition, test for liver disease, and continue to groom the beak regularly.

SELECTED READINGS

Altman RB: Conditions involving the integumentary system. In: Petrak ML (ed): *Diseases of Cage and Aviary Birds*, ed 2. Philadelphia, Lea & Febiger, 1982, pp 368–381.

Arnall L: Conditions of the beak and claw in the budgerigar. *J Small Anim Pract* 6:135–144, 1965.

Arnall L, Keymer IF: *Bird Diseases*. London, Bailliere Tindall, 1975.

Axelson RD: *Caring For Your Pet Bird*, rev ed. New York, Sterling, 1989, 160 pp.

Axelson RD: Possible chlorhexidine toxicity in finches. *Assoc Avian Vet Today* 1(5):208, 1987.

Campbell TW: Neoplasia. In: Harrison GJ, Harrison LR (eds): *Clinical Avian Medicine and Surgery*. Philadelphia, WB Saunders, 1987, pp 500–505.

Choudary C: Neoplasms, cysts, and obstructive diseases. In: Burr EW (ed): *Companion Bird Medicine*. Ames, IA, Iowa State University Press, 1987, pp 231–233.

Clubb SL: Therapeutics in avian medicine—Flock vs. individual bird treatment regimens. *Vet Clin North Am [Small Anim Pract]* 14:345–361, 1984.

Clubb SL: Therapeutics. In: Harrison GJ, Harrison LR (eds): *Clinical Avian Medicine and Surgery*. Philadelphia, WB Saunders, 1988, p 340.

Fudge A, McEntee L: A feather syndrome in cockatiels associated with giardiasis. Unpublished data, Sacramento, CA (private practice), 1986.

Fudge AM: Avian giardiasis: Syndromes, diagnosis, and therapy. In: *Proceedings of the Association of Avian Veterinarians' Conference, 1986*. E. Northport, NY, Association of Avian Veterinarians, 1986, pp 155–164.

Epple A, Stetson MH (eds): *Avian Endocrinology*. New York, Academic Press, 1980.

Gerlach H: Viral diseases. In: Harrison GJ, Harrison LR (eds): *Clinical Avian Medicine and Surgery*. Philadelphia, WB Saunders, 1986, pp 172–173.

Gough JF: Outbreaks of budgerigar fledgling disease in three aviaries in Ontario. *Can Vet J* 30:672–674, 1989.

Gould J: Liver disease in psittacines. In: *Proceedings of the Association of Avian Veterinarians' Conference, 1989*. E. Northport, NY, Association of Avian Veterinarians, 1989, pp 125–128.

Harrison GJ: Disorders of the integument. In: Harrison GJ, Harrison LR (eds): *Clinical Avian Medicine and Surgery*. Philadelphia, WB Saunders, 1987, pp 509–524.

Hillyer EV: Basic avian dermatology. In: *Proceedings of the Association of Avian Veterinarians' Conference, 1989*. E. Northport, NY, Association of Avian Veterinarians, 1989, pp 101–121.

Martin SL: Skin and feather diseases of pet birds. In Nesbitt GH (ed): *Contemporary Issues in Small Animal Practice. Dermatology*, vol 8. New York, Churchill Livingstone, 1987, pp 295–321.

McCluggage DM: Parasitology in caged birds. In: *Proceedings of the Association of Avian Veterinarians, 1989*. E. Northport, NY, Association of Avian Veterinarians, 1989, pp 97–100.

McDonald SE: Clinical experiences with cloacal papillomas. In: *Proceedings of the Association of Avian Veterinarians' Conference, 1988*. E. Northport, NY, Association of Avian Veterinarians, 1989, pp 27–30.

Paster MB, Isaacs M: Repair of damaged beaks in cherry-headed conures using cyanoveneer acrylic. *Bird World Magazine*, March 1983, pp 52–53, 55.

Perry R: Avian dermatology. In: Burr EW (ed): *Companion Bird Medicine*. Ames, IA, Iowa State University Press, 1987 pp 40–50.

Perry R: Skin, beak, claw and feather disorders. In: Macwhirter P (ed): *Everybird, A Guide to Bird Health*. Melbourne/Sydney, Australia, Inkata Press, 1987, pp 98–121.

Rosskopf WJ, et al: Normal thyroid values for common pet birds. *VM SAC* 77: 409–412, 1982.

Rosskopf WJ, et al.: Treatment of feather folliculitis in a lovebird. *Mod Vet Pract* 64:923–924, 1983.

Stunkard JA: *Diagnosis, Treatment and Husbandry of Pet Birds*, ed 2. Edgewater, MD, Stunkard Publishing Co, 1984.

Taylor TG: French molt. In: Petrak ML (ed): *Diseases of Cage and Aviary Birds*, ed 2. Philadelphia, Lea & Febiger, 1982, pp 361–367.

VanDerHeyden N: Psittacine papillomas. In: *Proceedings of the Association of Avian Veterinarians' Conference, 1988*. E. Northport, NY, Association of Avian Veterinarians, 1988, pp 23–25.

Chapter 15

DERMATOLOGY OF RABBITS, RODENTS, AND FERRETS

Petra Burgmann, BSc, DVM

It has been said that diseases in exotics are basically no different than those in any other species, and that the same principles of diagnosis apply equally well to these species as they do to any other. This is in fact true, but it is important not to extrapolate too far from one species to another. Just as there is no canine version of feline "endocrine" alopecia, one must recognize that certain species-specific peculiarities do exist.

The purpose of this chapter is to describe not only those skin diseases most frequently seen in the commonly kept exotics—rabbits, rodents, and ferrets—but to present them in such a way that the species-specific differences can be easily identified.

The Parasite Diagnostic Key (Table 15-1) lists the most commonly encountered skin parasites, while the Therapeutic Key (Table 15-2) lists the most common treatments. Certain parasitic skin diseases and some treatments are described more fully in the text because of their importance in that species.

Therapeutics in exotics is a controversial issue because practi-

TABLE 15-1

Parasite Diagnostic Key

Parasite	*Description*	*Distinguishing Features*	*Host*	*Usual Habitat*	*Life Cycle*	*Pathologic Effects*	*Other Health Significance*
Ornithonyssus bacoti	Blood-sucking mite, rare	750 μm long	Wild rodents, mice, rats, hamsters	Crevices, bedding, wild rodent burrows	13 days; female survives off host up to 70 days	Anemia, debilitation	Can harbour eastern equine encephalitis (EEE) virus, typhus, Q fever, plague, natural vector for tularemia, dermatitis in humans
Trombicula alfreddugesi	Chigger mite, rare	200–400 μm long; red to yellow, 6-legged larvae	Rodents, rabbits	Only larval stage is parasitic; other stages free-living in soil	On host only a few hours or days	Intense pruritus, swelling, lasting days to weeks	Painful bite, pruritus in humans
Fleas, various spp.	Common	1–3 mm long	Rabbits, ferrets, rodents	Pelage, bedding, environment	16–21 days; can survive off host for months	Pruritus, allergic dermatitis, anemia, debilitation	Vector for sylvatic plague, tularemia, intermediate host for tapeworms
Cuterebra spp.	Fly larvae, common	20–42 mm long	Rabbits, rodents, ferrets	Eggs at entrance to burrows	Enter via nose or mouth; migrate to subcutaneous location	Subcutaneous mass, weight loss, debilitation	None
Myobia musculi	Fur mite, common	300–500 μm long; single empodial claw on tarsi of second pair of legs	Mice	Pelage, especially head, ears, back	23 days; eggs hatch in 8 days	Inapparent to severe allergic dermatitis with pruritus, alopecia, ulceration	None known
Myocoptes musculinis	Fur mite, common	200–300 μm long; dark brown; 3rd and 4th leg pairs	Mice	Pelage, especially inguinal region, abdomen, and back	Probably 8–14 days; eggs hatch in 5 days	Inapparent to erythematous dermatitis, patchy alopecia	None known
Radfordia affinis	Fur mite, common	300–500 μm long; pair of subequal terminal claws on tarsi of second pair of legs	Mice	Pelage, especially head, back	Unknown, probably 21–23 days	Dermatitis, pruritus, alopecia	None known
Psorergates simplex	Follicle mite, rare	90–150 μm, rounded body	Mice	Fur follicles	Unknown	Dermal pouches on visceral skin surface, occasionally scabby dermatitis of ears	None

Polyplax serrata	Sucking louse, rare	0.6–1.5 mm long; eggs fastened near skin	Mice	Pelage, especially shoulders	13 days; eggs hatch in 5–6 days	Pruritus, dermatitis, restlessness, debilitation, anemia	Vector of murine haemobartonellosis, eperythrozoonosis, possible vector of tularemia
Notoedres spp.	Burrowing mite, rare	200–400 μm long; anus located dorsally	Hamsters	Ears, especially nose, feet, genitalia, tail	6–10 days	Papilloma-like yellow crusts, hyperkeratosis	None
Demodex criceti	Follicle mite, common	80–100 μm long; short stubby body	Hamsters	Skin follicles	Unknown; probably 10–15 days	Unknown	None
Demodex aurati	Follicle mite, common	150–200 μm long; cigar-shaped	Hamsters	Skin follicles	Unknown; probably 10–15 days	Moderate to severe dry, scaly alopecia usually nonpruritic	None
Demodex spp.	Follicle mite, uncommon	100–400 μm long	Gerbils	Skin follicles	Unknown; probably 10–15 days	Alopecia, dermatitis	None
Radfordia ensifera	Fur mite, common	300–500 μm long; pair of equal terminal claws on tarsi of second pair of legs	Rats	Pelage, especially head, back	Unknown	Dermatitis, pruritus, self-inflicted trauma	None known
Notoedres muris	Burrowing mite, rare	200–400 μm long; anus located dorsally	Rats	Especially ears, nose, tail; occasionally genitalia, limbs	19–21 days; eggs hatch in 4–5 days	Papilloma-like, yellow crusts on ears, nose; papular dermatitis; hyperkeratosis	None
Polyplax spinulosa	Sucking louse, rare	0.6–1.5 mm long; eggs fastened near skin	Rats	Pelage, especially back	26 days; eggs hatch in 5–6 days	Pruritus, dermatitis, restlessness, debilitation, anemia	Vector of murine haemobartonellosis, typhus between rodents
Chirodiscoides caviae	Fur mite, common	350–500 μm long; often joined in pairs	Guinea pigs	Deep in pelage, especially back	Unknown	Inapparent to pruritus, alopecia	None
Trixacarus caviae	Burrowing mite, common	200–400 μm long; anus located terminally	Guinea pigs	Especially neck, shoulders, lower abdomen	Probably 10–14 days	Intense pruritus, hyperkeratosis, alopecia, self-inflicted trauma, debilitation	Dermatitis in humans
Gliricola porcelli	Biting louse, common	1–1.5 mm long; narrow head and body; eggs fastened to fur	Guinea pigs	Pelage, especially around ears	Unknown	Pruritus, unthriftiness, alopecia	None known

TABLE 15-1 (continued)

Parasite Diagnostic Key

Parasite	*Description*	*Distinguishing Features*	*Host*	*Usual Habitat*	*Life Cycle*	*Pathologic Effects*	*Other Health Significance*
Gyropus ovalis	Biting louse, common	1–1.2 mm long; wide head, oval body; eggs fastened to fur	Guinea pigs	Pelage, especially around ears	Unknown	Pruritus, unthriftiness, alopecia	None known
Cheyletiella parasitovorax	Fur mite, common	350–500 μm long	Rabbits	Pelage, especially between shoulders, ears, back	14–21 days; female can survive off host 10–14 days	Mild alopecia, scaling to erythematous, oily dermatitis with pruritus	Transient dermatitis in humans
Listrophorus gibbus	Fur mite	300–500 μm long	Rabbits	Back, abdomen	Unknown	None	None known
Sarcoptes scabei cuniculi	Burrowing mite, rare	200–400 μm long; anus located terminally	Rabbits	Especially head, neck, ears, then generalized	17–23 days; eggs hatch in 3–8 days	Intense pruritus, alopecia	Dermatitis in humans
Notoedres cati var. *cuniculi*	Burrowing mite, rare	200–400 μm long	Rabbits	Skin of head, ears, neck, forelegs	21 days	Crusts, hyperkeratosis, pruritus, alopecia, self-inflicted trauma	Transient dermatitis in humans
Psoroptes cuniculi	Ear mite, common	400–800 μm long	Rabbits	Ear canals, occasionally face, neck, legs, inguinal region	21 days; eggs hatch in 4 days	Dry tan crusty exudate; when removed reveals moist, red painful otitis; pruritic dermatitis	None known
Haemodipsus ventricosis	Sucking louse, rare	1.2–2.5 mm long; eggs oval with operculum	Rabbits	Pelage, especially back and sides	30 days; eggs hatch in 7 days	Extreme pruritus, alopecia, anemia debilitation	Vector of *Francisella tularensis* in rabbits (cause of tularemia)
Sarcoptes scabei spp.	Burrowing mite, uncommon	200–400 μm long; anus located terminally	Ferrets	Feet, or generalized	17–23 days	Erythematous, swollen feet, or generalized alopecia, intense pruritus	Dermatitis in humans
Otodectes cynotis	Ear mite, common	450 μm long	Ferrets	Ear canals, skin	21–28 days	Otitis, occasionally pruritus	Zoonotic to cats, dogs

TABLE 15-2

Therapeutic Key

	Mice	*Hamsters*	*Gerbils*	*Rats*	*Guinea Pigs*	*Chinchillas*	*Rabbits*	*Ferrets*
Antibiotics								
Ampicillin	2–10 mg/kg IM/PO bid 5–7 days			2–10 mg/kg IM/PO bid 5–7 days				10 mg/kg bid IM/PO 5–7 days
Cephaloridine	10–25 mg/kg IM/SC sid 5–7 days	10–25 mg/kg IM/SC sid 5–7 days	10–25 mg/kg IM/SC sid 5–7 days	10–25 mg/kg IM/SC sid 5–7 days	10–25 mg/kg IM/SC sid 5–7 days	12.5 mg/kg IM/SC sid 5–7 days	10–25 mg/kg IM/SC sid 5–7 days	10–25 mg/kg IM/SC sid 5–7 days
Chloramphenicol succinate	30 mg/kg IM/SC sid 5–7 days	30 mg/kg IM/SC sid 5–7 days	30 mg/kg IM/SC sid 5–7 days	30 mg/kg IM/SC sid 5–7 days	30 mg/kg IM/SC sid 5–7 days	30 mg/kg IM/SC sid 5–7 days	30 mg/kg IM/SC sid 5–7 days	30 mg/kg IM/SC sid 5–7 days
Chloramphenicol palmitate	50 mg/kg PO bid 5–7 days	50 mg/kg PO bid 5–7 days	50 mg/kg PO bid 5–7 days	50 mg/kg PO bid 5–7 days	50 mg/kg PO bid 5–7 days	50 mg/kg PO bid 5–7 days	50 mg/kg PO bid 5–7 days	50 mg/kg PO bid 5–7 days
Enrofloxacin	2.5 mg/kg bid; should not be used in very young animals		2.5 mg/kg bid; should not be used in very young animals	2.5 mg/kg bid; should not be used in very young animals		2.5 mg/kg bid; should not be used in very young animals	2.5 mg/kg bid; should not be used in very young animals	2.5 mg/kg bid; should not be used in very young animals
Gentamicin	5 mg/kg IM/SC sid 5 days	5 mg/kg IM/SC sid 5 days	5 mg/kg IM/SC sid 5 days	5 mg/kg IM/SC sid 5 days	5 mg/kg IM/SC sid 5 days	5 mg/kg IM/SC sid 5 days	5 mg/kg IM/SC sid 5 days	5 mg/kg IM/SC sid 5 days
Sulfadiazine/trimethoprim combination	30 mg/kg SC sid	30 mg/kg SC sid	30 mg/kg SC sid	30 mg/kg SC sid	30 mg/kg SC sid	30 mg/kg SC sid	30 mg/kg SC sid	30 mg/kg SC sid
Sulfamethoxazole/trimethoprim combination	15 mg/kg PO bid	15 mg/kg PO bid	15 mg/kg PO bid	15 mg/kg PO bid	15 mg/kg PO bid	15 mg/kg PO bid	15 mg/kg PO bid	15 mg/kg PO bid
Tetracycline hydrochloride	10–20 mg/kg SC/PO bid 5–7 days	10–20 mg/kg SC/PO bid 5–7 days	10–20 mg/kg SC/PO bid 5–7 days	10–20 mg/kg SC/PO bid 5–7 days	10–20 mg/kg SC/PO bid 5–7 days	25 mg/kg SC/PO bid 5–7 days	25 mg/kg SC/PO bid 5–7 days	25 mg/kg SC/PO bid 5–7 days
Tylosin	10 mg/kg IM sid 5 days	10 mg/kg IM sid 5 days	10 mg/kg IM sid 5 days	10 mg/kg IM/PO sid 5–7 days				10 mg/kg PO sid 5–7 days
Antifungals								
Griseofulvin	25 mg/kg PO sid 14 days	25 mg/kg PO sid 14–28 days	25 mg/kg PO sid 14–28 days	25 mg/kg PO sid 14–28 days	25 mg/kg PO sid 14–28 days	25 mg/kg PO sid 4–6 weeks	25 mg/kg PO sid 4–6 weeks	25 mg/kg PO sid 4–6 weeks

	Indications	*Dosage (for all of the above species)*	*Route*
Antiparasitics			
Amitraz (Mitaban® —Upjohn)	*Demodex, Sarcoptes*	3–6 treatments 14 days apart	Topical
5% Carbaryl powder (Diryl® —Pitman-Moore)	Fur mites, fleas, lice	Dust lightly once weekly for 3–6 treatments	Topical
Dichlorvos-impregnated resin strip (Vapona® —Shell)	All external parasites	Hang in room once weekly for 6 weeks	Follow package directions for room size
Ivermectin (Ivomec® —MSD AGVET)	*Sarcoptes, Psoroptes, Otodectes*, fur mites, lice	200–400 μg/kg	Per os or subcutaneously
Lime sulfur	*Sarcoptes*, fur mites	Dilute 1:40 with water; apply once weekly for 6 weeks	Topical
Lindane (Rogar® —STB)	Fur mites	0.03% dip once weekly for 3 weeks	Topical
Malathion	Fur mites, lice	2% dip every 10 days for 3 treatments	Topical
Pyrethrin .05% shampoo (Vetatix® —Winthrop)	Mites, lice, fleas	Shampoo once weekly for 3–6 treatments	Topical
Tresaderm® (MSD AGVET)	*Otodectes, Psoroptes*	2–5 drops in each ear bid for 7 days; repeat in 2 weeks	Topical

cally none of the drugs commonly used are approved for use in these species. Because most treatments have evolved through a "hit and miss" type of system, there are great discrepancies in the literature concerning not only which drugs to use, but at what dose to administer them. The treatments listed are those that I have used myself, or that have had at least two references in the literature. A special caution must be given with reference to the use of antibiotics. Fatal reactions to antibiotics are common, as either a direct toxic effect or indirectly because of an alteration of the normal bacterial flora. If a certain drug is not listed for a particular species, try to choose one that has been listed.

MICE

Although they are one of the less frequently encountered exotic pets in private practice, mice are prone to a variety of unique dermatologic conditions.

Bacterial Conditions

Bacterial dermatitis and abscesses are most commonly caused by *Staphylococcus aureus* and *Streptococcus* spp. These infections are often secondary to a primary wound caused by fighting amongst males, or by self-trauma because of acariasis. Treatment consists of eliminating the inciting cause, lancing the wound if necessary, cleansing the wound with 3% hydrogen peroxide, and treating with an appropriate antibiotic. Topical preparations are often unrewarding in this species because of their fastidious grooming habits.

Corynebacterium kutscheri and *Pasteurella pneumotropica* have also been identified as infrequent, opportunistic pathogens of mice. *C. kutscheri* can produce septic emboli, causing infarction of dermal vessels that results in skin necrosis and ulceration. *P. pneumotropica* can cause superficial lesions and subcutaneous abscesses. Culture and sensitivity will aid in diagnosis and choice of an appropriate antibiotic.

Furunculosis in genetically nude mice has also been reported, but is obviously rarely encountered in private practice.

Viral Conditions

Mousepox (Ectromelia)

Although not uncommon in breeding stocks of mice in China, Japan, England, and Europe, mousepox is rare in North America and is unlikely to be encountered in private practice. It has been imported into laboratory facilities in the United States on several occasions via live mice, mouse tissues, or tumors, causing severe epizootics. Caused by an orthopoxvirus, the usual route of infection is via skin abrasions on the face, feet, or abdomen from virus-contaminated bedding or cage surfaces. Most susceptible mice die shortly after the primary eruption, but those that survive the acute infection often develop a dermatitis. The severity of the eruption is determined by the extent of secondary viremia. The lesion can be solitary or generalized. The eruption goes through a macular, vesicular, and pustular stage, and will recede within a few weeks. Necrosis of the dermal epithelium can produce a surface scab that heals as a hairless scar, but severe infection of the feet or tail can cause them to become gangrenous and drop off, hence the name *infectious ectromelia*.

Diagnosis is by microscopic examination of tissues revealing eosinophilic cytoplasmic inclusion bodies, or by electron microscopy revealing the orthopoxvirus. Treatment consists of eradication and disinfection, or vaccination with the vaccinia virus by scarification of the base of the tail.

Fungal Conditions

Several dermatomycoses have been reported to occur in mice, but these infections, commonly known as *ringworm*, are caused most often by *Trichophyton mentagrophytes*. Mice are often asymptomatic, but stressed or debilitated animals may exhibit clinical signs of a sparse haircoat or a well-demarcated crusty lesion with focal hair loss, erythema, and scaling. Lesions on the tail are common.

Diagnosis is by microscopic examination of skin scrapings macerated in 10% potassium hydroxide (KOH) for 30 to 60 minutes and identification of mycelia or arthrospores, or by growth of the fungus on dermatophyte test medium (for example, Fungassay® —Pitman-Moore). Because the organism grows slowly, cultures should be held for 3 weeks for a definitive diagnosis.

Treatment includes disinfecting the environment, clipping the hair around the lesions, and treating orally with griseofulvin. Griseofulvin should not be used in pregnant animals because of possible teratogenic effects. Topical creams are of little use in this species because of their fastidious grooming habits. It is always important to remember the zoonotic potential of dermatophytes, particularly because many of these "pocket pets" are carried around inside their owners' clothing, and *T. mentagrophytes* is highly infectious for humans. It is not unusual for lesions to be noticed first on an owner, while the rodent remains an asymptomatic carrier.

Parasitic Conditions

Mites are very common in mice and infestations are frequently encountered in private practice. *Myocoptes musculinis* is the most common ectoparasite, although it frequently is found in conjunction with *Myobia musculi*. When both mites are present on the same host,

Myocoptes tends to crowd out populations of *Myobia*. *Radfordia affinis* is also frequently encountered.

Lesions consist of varying degrees of alopecia and ulceration, usually involving the neck, lateral thorax, and flank regions (Plate XII-1). The scabby to ulcerative dermatitis of *Myobia* is actually caused by self-trauma, induced as a pruritic response to the mite allergen. It has been found that certain genetic strains of mice are more susceptible to an allergic response to the mites than other strains. In these mice even a very low parasite burden can cause extensive skin lesions. The mite is spread by direct contact, usually from parents to offspring, but lesions usually do not develop until the mouse reaches maturity, indicating that a period of sensitization is required even in susceptible strains. Once the hypersensitivity has developed, however, exposure to even a few mites will result in an anamnestic response, with lesions developing within 1 to 2 days of exposure. The lesions of *Myocoptes* are also pruritic, but tend not to be as ulcerative as those of *Myobia*. It has been said that the mites are difficult to eliminate, but I suspect that in those cases treatment likely was not intensive enough.

Diagnosis is by skin scrapings and mite identification (Plate XII-2). The main differences between the three mites are described in the Parasite Diagnostic Key (Table 15-1).

Treatment consists of a weekly light dusting with a 5% carbaryl powder, thorough cage disinfection, and the use of a dichlorvos-impregnated resin strip hung in the pet's room for 24 hours once a week for 6 weeks. Certainly this approach is not applicable in a laboratory setting, but it can be quite efficacious for treatment of an individual pet. Because of the 23-day life cycle of the mite *Myobia* and the resistance of the egg to insecticides, treatment in a laboratory setting must consist of at least two treatments, with the second treatment occurring between 8 and 10 days after the first. A 1 x 2-inch piece of a dichlorvos-impregnated resin strip placed on the cage for 24 hours for two treatments is the most widely advocated treatment for the laboratory setting. An alternative treatment consists of two subcutaneous injections of ivermectin given at 200 μg/kg 8 days apart. Concurrent treatment of the environment is still advisable.

Polyplax serrata, the mouse louse, is rare, but when encountered is significant because of its zoonotic importance as a possible vector of tularemia. It is spread by direct contact. Treatment is the same as that described for mites.

Nutritional Conditions

Recognition of nutritional deficiencies in rodent species encountered in private practice is rare. Most of the deficiencies described in the literature have been experimentally induced; the most important of these experimental findings have been included for the sake of completeness. Mice have an absolute requirement for linoleic and arachidonic acids. Chronic essential fatty acid deficiency can lead to hair loss and dermatitis with scaling and crusting of the skin. Zinc deficiency can cause hair loss on shoulders and neck.

Several varieties of rodent chow are commercially available and are nutritionally complete; however, owners must be reminded that freshness and quality should be considered when purchasing these foods.

Neoplastic Conditions

Spontaneous skin tumors are rare in mice, although many have been experimentally induced. Of those encountered naturally, squamous cell carcinoma appears to be the most prevalent. Spontaneous tumors of the Harderian gland occur frequently. These tumors appear late in life and grow slowly, but may cause proptosis of the eye.

Miscellaneous Conditions

Facial Hair Loss

Facial hair loss resulting from friction on cage bars or feeders, or barbering of the vibrissae or head by a dominant mouse or cage-mates during crowding or stress, is common in mice (Plate XII-3). A thorough history and examination of the cage will often provide a simple solution, such as separating cage-mates or removing offending objects from the environment. In most cases hair regrowth will be complete in 30 days, although some small patches of alopecia can remain for up to 90 days depending on the phase of the hair cycle.

Dry Gangrene

Dry gangrene of the ear tips in mice was reported in one instance, and appeared to be associated with cold environmental temperatures as well as self-trauma caused by parasite infestation. An area of hyperemia was first noted in the distal third of the ear, followed by a distinct line of demarcation and a gray ear tip that would slough within a few days. The lesions were self-limiting once the inciting causes had been eliminated.

RATS

Chromodacryorrhea

Of all the rodents, rats are the species most frequently presented because of chromodacryorrhea. Chromodacryorrhea refers to the ability of various rodents to secrete a porphyrin-containing pigment from the eyes. The red pigments are produced in the Harderian gland and are secreted in response to parasympathetic stimulation under stress or as a result of certain diseases. Discharge from the eyes can be profuse and can also stain the forepaws, and is often mistaken for blood by the owner. Treatment consists of identifying and removing the underlying cause of stress, or identifying and treating the disease state. Sialodacryoadenitis virus can also cause marked Harderian gland secretion and is described below.

Bacterial Conditions

An ulcerative dermatitis caused by *Staphylococcus aureus* is common in rats, particularly in young males. Lesions begin on the neck and shoulders and appear as irregularities in the haircoat with small focal areas of alopecia or ulceration, and can progress to involve the entire anterior trunk with extensive ulcerations. Some lesions scab and regress spontaneously, while others are pruritic and stimulate scratching and self-mutilation. Treatment includes cleaning the wounds with hydrogen peroxide, choosing an appropriate oral antibiotic, and clipping the toenails to reduce self-mutilation. Underlying acariasis may be a contributing factor and should be considered in the etiology of the lesions.

Pasteurella pneumotropica has also been implicated as a cause of skin abscessation, although it often occurs as a secondary opportunist. Treatment is the same as that described above.

Ulcerative pododermatitis is also encountered from time to time in private practice. The cause is unknown, but wire-bottomed cages or rough cage surfaces may be contributing factors. One report implicated exercise wheels used in their experiments as a contributing factor. The lesions are often difficult to treat; bandaging to allow healing may be of use in severe cases as well as eliminating the inciting cause and treating with an appropriate antibiotic.

Viral Conditions

Sialodacryoadenitis, a very common disease in research facilities, is caused by a coronavirus. Transmission occurs by direct exposure to virus-laden nasal secretions or fomites. Clinical signs include profuse chromodacryorrhea, cervical lymphadenitis, sneezing, keratoconjunctivitis, and corneal lesions. Clinical signs develop within 8 to 10 days of exposure to virus-infected rats. Complete recovery usually occurs within 30 days, and no latent carrier state is known. Diagnosis is by the characteristic clinical signs, virus isolation, or acute and convalescent antibody titers. Immunity is conferred for one year after exposure. No vaccine exists, and prevention is best accomplished by preventing exposure.

Pox infection in rats has been reported but is extremely rare. Lesions are similar to those described for mousepox.

Fungal Conditions

Dermatophyte (ringworm) infections are rare in rats. If present, *Trichophyton mentagrophytes* is the most commonly encountered fungus. Rats usually are asymptomatic, but a patchy alopecia with scale, papules, and pustules is sometimes seen, primarily over the back. Diagnosis and treatment are the same as that described for mice.

Parasitic Conditions

Radfordia ensifera is a commonly encountered fur mite of rats. Small scabby lesions around the head and shoulders are caused by self-inflicted trauma as a result of the pruritus caused by the mite allergen. Diagnosis and treatment are the same as that described for mice.

Polyplax spinulosa, the blood-sucking louse of rats, is rarely encountered in private practice, as is the mite *Notoedres*. Both are described in the Parasite Diagnostic Key (Table 15-1). Treatment for lice is the same as that described for fur mites in mice. Treatment of *Notoedres* consists of bathing the affected area with a 0.05% pyrethrin shampoo and applying lime sulfur topically to the affected areas with a cotton swab. Two oral doses of ivermectin given at 200 μg/kg a week apart will also be beneficial in treating this condition.

Nutritional Conditions

Of all the species maintained under laboratory conditions, the most is known about the dietary requirements of rats. Again, dietary deficiencies are seldom reported in private practice, but are included here for completeness. Deficiencies in linoleic, linolenic, or arachidonic acids have been reported to result in reduced hair growth, alopecia, scaly skin, and cutaneous ulceration in rats. As is reported for hamsters, vitamin A deficiency may result in a thin, coarse haircoat and keratinizing squamous metaplasia. Deficiency in vitamin B_2 (riboflavin) can cause dermatitis and alopecia, whereas deficiency in vitamin B_6 (pyridoxine) can cause hair loss and achromotrichia (loss of hair pigmentation). Achromotrichia is also reported in copper deficiency in rats. Biotin deficiency can cause dermatitis, alopecia, and achromotrichia.

Neoplastic Conditions

Spontaneous tumors of the skin and subcutis are uncommon in rats; when they do occur, they usually are found around the head, tail, or paws. Papillomas, basal cell carcinomas, and squamous cell carcinomas are the most frequent types. Basal cell tumors may be locally invasive, but tend not to metastasize. Squamous cell carcinomas are locally invasive and may metastasize to other areas. Squamous cell carcinomas of the face and head are highly invasive but seldom metastatic and often start as a sebaceosquamous tumor from the glands of Zymbal in the ear.

Subcutaneous mesenchymal tumors, such as fibromas, fibrosarcomas, lipomas, and undifferentiated sarcomas, are more common than epithelial tumors. Benign mammary fibroadenomas are the most frequently encountered tumors in rats in private practice, and can occur in both males and females.

Treatment of all tumor types is surgical excision where applicable. A subcuticular line of closure will prevent the rat from chewing out the stitches.

Miscellaneous Conditions

Ringtail describes a condition in which there are one or more annular constrictions of the tail (Plate XII-4). Distal to the constrictions the tail can become edematous, then necrotic, and, if sloughed, usually heals without complications. The condition occurs most often in unweaned rats 7 to 15 days of age and is caused by housing the animals in less than 20% humidity. Seen most frequently in winter as a result of the use of heating systems, treatment consists of raising the humidity level to 50%, reducing air turnover in laboratory facilities, and providing solid-bottomed cages with nesting material for nursing dams. Ringtail is rarely encountered in private practice.

HAMSTERS

Hamsters have two well-developed dark-pigmented "hip glands" located on either side of the midline in the flank region (Plate XII-5). Poorly developed and scarcely visible in the female, the glands are more prominent in the male. Thought to be used for olfactory identification of territory, when the male becomes sexually excited the fur around the gland becomes wet and he scratches and rubs at the gland. This activity often is incorrectly interpreted as pruritus of a skin lesion by the owner, who is often unaware that these glands exist.

Bacterial Conditions

Skin and cheek pouch abscesses caused by *Staphylococcus aureus* and *Streptococcus* spp. are fairly common in hamsters (Plate XII-6). Treatment is the same as that described for mice.

Viral Conditions

A papovavirus has been identified as a cause of cutaneous epitheliomas in hamsters. The lesions usually are wart-like, and occur most often around the eyes, mouth, or perianal area. The condition is rare but the virus is highly contagious, has a long incubation period, and is very resistant. It has also been implicated in several other disease processes in infected colonies. No individual treatment for this condition has been described, but its presence in a laboratory setting could have serious consequences; therefore, depopulation and strict sanitation is advised.

Fungal Conditions

Dermatophytosis (ringworm) is rarely reported in hamsters but it can occur. As in other rodents, *T. mentagrophytes* is the most likely cause. Treatment is the same as that described for mice.

Parasitic Conditions

Demodex is particularly common in hamsters older than 1.5 years of age and is frequently secondary to immunosuppression, malnutrition, or concurrent systemic disease. Two types of demodectic mange mites are recognized in hamsters. *Demodex criceti* is a short stubby-bodied mite that generally is considered to be nonpathogenic. *D. aurati* is a cigar-shaped mite that burrows in the pilosebaceous component of the skin, causing a moderate to severe, dry, scaly alopecia which starts over the back and can extend to involve the entire body (Plate XII-7). Transmission occurs from mother to young during the time of suckling. Diagnosis is by recovering mites from skin scrapings, although examination of clinically normal hamsters has revealed mild to moderate infestations with *D. aurati* and in other cases the mites have been difficult to demonstrate on skin scrapings.

A variety of different miticidal preparations have been used with varying success, but in my experience it is important to recognize that the mange is more likely indicative of an underlying problem that has predisposed the hamster to the condition than a serious disease entity in its own right. Weekly bathing of the hamster with a benzoyl peroxide shampoo will stimulate follicular flushing and reduce the mite load, followed by topical application of a miticidal preparation, such as amitraz, by cotton swab to the most severely affected areas. Lime sulfur is an additional option.

Nutritional Conditions

As with most of the commonly kept small rodents, dietary deficiencies are seldom seen if the animal is maintained on a fresh, good quality, commercially available rodent chow. Several nutritional deficiencies have been produced experimentally, however, and are included here for the sake of completeness. Essential fatty acid deficiency causes hair loss, tight skin, and increased ear wax production in hamsters. Vitamin A deficiency results in a thin, coarse haircoat and keratinizing squamous metaplasia. Deficiency in vitamin B_2 (riboflavin) results in dermatitis and alopecia, whereas deficiency in vitamin B_6 (pyridoxine) results in hair loss and achromotrichia. Achromotrichia is also recorded in copper deficiency. Niacin deficiency has also been reported as a cause of alopecia and rough haircoat.

Neoplastic Conditions

Adenomas and carcinomas of the adrenal cortex and thyroid gland are common in hamsters, and it is reasonable to assume that they may present with some of the same cutaneous manifestations as do other species. Melanomas are also common, with a much higher incidence in males than females. Several other neoplasms have been described, although their incidence is sporadic. Diagnosis of these tumors can be made by skin biopsy. Treatment consists of surgical removal of the tumor where applicable.

One interesting report of cutaneous lymphoma resembling mycosis fungoides in humans was described in three pet hamsters. Clinical signs included erythema, alopecia, pruritus, and flaking skin, progressing to plaques or tumors (Plate XII-8). Anorexia, lethargy, and weight loss were also noted. No treatment was described.

Miscellaneous Conditions

Allergic dermatitis attributable to cedar or pine shavings has been seen by the author. Lesions consist of swelling of the face and feet with associated pruritus. In one instance several cases occurred in the course of one month. All the owners had recently purchased a fresh bag of shavings produced by a leading pet company. When the animals were housed on plain newspaper the lesions regressed spontaneously. Since then I have seen several more cases in which people have purchased bulk shavings from landscaping or nursery outlets. Presumably the shavings have been chemically treated in some way that causes a contact allergy.

One report described another lesion caused by wood shavings. In this case the footpads became thickened and developed granulomata. Histologic examination revealed a foreign body, giant cell reaction with wood shavings and sawdust seen within the lesions. When shredded paper was substituted for the shavings, no more lesions developed. A similar case recently presented to the author resolved with removal of the shavings.

GERBILS

Gerbils have an ovoid hairless ventral midline sebaceous gland which is especially pronounced in the male and is used for scent marking (Plate XII-9). The area is normally a tan color and has a clearly defined smooth border. This area is frequently involved in bacterial infections and tumors. Other than the conditions described below, skin conditions are less frequent in gerbils than in other species.

Bacterial Conditions

Nasal dermatitis in gerbils is a common problem affecting 5% of the gerbil population. The lesions, which begin as erythemic, small crusts, or alopecia, surround the external nares, but often go on to involve the entire face, forepaws, and sometimes the abdomen with extensive moist dermatitis and alopecia (Plate XII-10). If not resolved, gerbils may become unthrifty and anorectic and die. Various theories have been presented to explain this phenomenon, including abrasion on rough cage surfaces, or staphylococcal or streptococcal infections. A recent theory postulates that hypersecretion of the Harderian gland or failure to spread the material by grooming leads to the dermatitis. The worst damage appears to be self-inflicted, as scratching with the forepaws leads to bleeding, scabbing, and alopecia. Treatment involves (1) cleaning the lesions of moist dermatitis with 3% hydrogen peroxide; (2) oral antibiotics to treat the secondary bacterial infection if present; and (3) permitting sandbathing to decrease the amount of Harderian gland lipids on the pelage.

The midventral sebaceous glands can become infected and abscessed, most often with staphylococci or streptococci. Because of the fastidious grooming habits of gerbils, topical ointments are not advised. Cleaning the lesions with 3% hydrogen peroxide and administering an appropriate oral antibiotic are more efficacious.

Fungal Conditions

Dermatophytosis (ringworm) is extremely rare in gerbils, although it can occur. Diagnosis and treatment is the same as that described for mice.

Parasitic Conditions

Apart from one reported case of demodicosis, external parasites are extremely rare in gerbils. In the one case of demodicosis reported, alopecia and focal ulcerative dermatitis was seen, but, as with hamsters, debility of aging appeared to be the predisposing factor in this case.

Nutritional Conditions

Information on the nutritional needs of gerbils is sparse; presumably they would exhibit clinical signs of deficiency similar to those of other rodents.

Neoplastic Conditions

Tumors have been reported in various sites in gerbils; the most frequent site of tumor development is the scent gland area. Sebaceous gland adenomas are most common, but basal cell and squamous cell carcinomas also occur. Treatment is by wide surgical excision of the tumor.

Miscellaneous Conditions

Gerbils are known for their sleek, smooth haircoat; however, when relative humidity is greater than 50%, the hair will often appear greasy and stand out instead of lying smoothly. Pine shavings can also cause this appearance.

Biting near the base of the tail causing denuded spots is common in overcrowded conditions. Tail chewing can occur because of boredom.

GUINEA PIGS

Skin diseases in guinea pigs are frequently encountered in private practice, particularly in recently purchased pets or in older males. A complete physical examination will often reveal at least one of the conditions listed below.

Bacterial Conditions

Ulcerative Pododermatitis

Ulcerative pododermatitis is caused by the organism *Staphylococcus aureus*. It is most frequently seen in obese animals housed on rough or soiled wire mesh floors, and presents as firm, ulcerated masses on the plantar surfaces, most commonly on the forefeet. If not treated, it can progress to osteoarthritis as the infection penetrates the tendon sheaths and joints. Amyloidosis of many organs has also been reported as a common sequel to severe infection.

Treatment consists of moving the animal to a smooth, clean cage surface, or in severe cases, housing the animal on 2 to 3 inches of clean, soft bedding. The nails should be trimmed and the feet treated topically. In cases of osteoarthritis, systemic antibiotics and bandaging may be of benefit.

Cervical Lymphadenitis

Cervical lymphadenitis is caused most frequently by the organism *Streptococcus zooepidemicus*. Soft, fluctuant subcutaneous masses appear in the ventral cervical region. These abscessed cervical lymph nodes can rupture spontaneously, exuding a thick, cream-colored pus. Diagnosis can be easily made by examination of a Gram stain of the material, which will reveal chains of gram-positive cocci. The organism is believed to be transmitted by a variety of routes, through small abrasions in the oral cavity caused by coarse plant feeds, such as hay or oats; through cutaneous bite wounds; or via the respiratory tract or conjunctiva. Septicemia is not an uncommon sequel, and in young animals may cause a fatal, generalized disease. The mortality rate is lower in older animals, although generalized lymphadenitis, pleuritis, pericarditis, arthritis, and nephritis have been described. Treatment consists of surgical drainage and debridement of the wound where required. Culture and sensitivity of the organism is warranted; chloramphenicol palmitate given at 50 mg/kg orally for 5 to 7 days is often the first drug of choice because it is one of the few antibiotics that is relatively safe in guinea pigs. Affected animals should be isolated to prevent the spread of infection.

Slobbers

Slobbers describes a condition in which excessive drooling, dysphagia, and weight loss are the predominant signs. The excessive drooling leads to matting of fur under the chin which may lead to a secondary bacterial dermatitis. Several causes have been suggested, the most likely of which is malocclusion because of the lower molars bridging over the tongue, or some other dental condition. Treatment consists of a thorough examination of the oral cavity under general anesthesia to determine the underlying cause, and cleaning the skin lesions with hydrogen peroxide and topical ointments.

Fungal Conditions

Spontaneous dermatophytosis has been reported to occur frequently in young guinea pigs, but any age group can be affected. Most often caused by *Trichophyton mentagrophytes*, the lesions usually involve the nose, face, and ears with a scaly alopecia. More generalized infection with moist, raised, hairless lesions called *kerions* can occur. Tufts of hair lifted from these lesions provide excellent specimens for examination. Fungal by-products diffused into the vascular tissue can be deposited as antigens in other parts of the skin. These lesions, usually found on the dorsal trunk or underside of the limbs, contain a sterile, clear liquid and represent an immune-mediated hypersensitivity reaction. Diagnosis and treatment is the same as that described for mice. An alternative treatment consists of using a 1.5% solution of griseofulvin in dimethyl sulfoxide (DMSO) applied daily to the lesions for 5 to 7 days. Topical antifungal preparations, such as miconazole nitrate (Conofite® —Pitman-Moore), are useful in guinea pigs.

Parasitic Conditions

The lice *Gyropus ovalis* and *Gliricola porcelli* are both very common in guinea pigs. Distinguishing features are listed in the Parasite Diagnostic Key (Table 15-1). Mild infestations can be asymptomatic, although the nit eggs are readily visible attached to the shafts of the hairs around the ear and eye region (Plate XII-11). Severe infestations may cause alopecia and pruritus.

The fur mite *Chirodiscoides caviae* is also considered common, but infestations usually are asymptomatic. The small, nonburrowing mites can be found deep in the fur, usually over the dorsum. Pruritus and alopecia have been observed in heavy infestations.

Both of these parasite types can be treated with weekly insecticide baths, followed by a light dusting with a 5% carbaryl powder for six treatments. Disinfecting the environment and once weekly 24-hour exposure to a dichlorvos-impregnated resin strip hung in the pet's room for 6 weeks is also advisable.

The sarcoptic mange mite *Trixacarus caviae* causes a severe dermatitis with alopecia, epidermal scaling, hyperkeratosis, and intense pruritus (Plate XII-12). Lesions are first seen on the neck, shoulders, lower abdomen, and inner thighs, but can progress to a generalized, debilitating dermatitis. Diagnosis is best accomplished by deep skin scrapings cleared with 10% potassium hydroxide to reveal the sarcoptic mite. Weekly bathing with an antiparasitic shampoo, followed by 1:40 lime sulfur dips for 6 weeks or three weekly applications of 1% lindane, is usually effective. Ivermectin given at 200 μg/kg orally is also effective. This disease is also important because of its zoonotic potential.

Nutritional Conditions

As is well known, scurvy is an important condition in guinea pigs, and may first present as a roughened haircoat, anorexia, and a mild white crusty discharge from the eyes. A complete description of this condition is available in other reference texts.

Metastatic soft tissue calcification has often been reported over the years, but to date no clear cause has been identified. An imbalance in the relationship between calcium, phosphorus, and magnesium is suspected as the cause. Clinical signs include mineral deposits in soft tissue near the elbows and ribs, in the spinal column, gastrointestinal tract, and skeletal muscle. Stiff and sore carpi and small white foci of calcium phosphate crystals in the footpads also occur. No treatment is known.

Fatty acid deficiency has been known to cause dermatitis, fur loss, and skin ulceration. Rough haircoat and skin atrophy have been seen with riboflavin deficiency.

Endocrine Conditions

Diffuse hair loss over the flanks and back in sows in late pregnancy is quite common, as is thinning of the haircoat in weanlings during the time of transition from baby fur to adult fur.

Marked shedding during stress is also very common. When a guinea pig is frightened or very ill, it is easy to epilate an entire spot of hair when tenting the skin for an injection.

Neoplastic Conditions

Neoplasms of the skin and subcutis occur infrequently in guinea pigs. Of these, benign trichofolliculomas occurring over the lumbar area appear to be the most common. They are described as unencapsulated multiloculated cysts lined by stratified squamous epithelium with abortive hair follicles. They are confined to the hypodermis and often contain hair, keratin, and sebum. Fibrosarcomas, sebaceous adenomas, and fibrolipomas have also been reported.

Miscellaneous Conditions

Overcrowding or stress often leads to barbering, either self-inflicted or by a cage-mate. Inadequate roughage can also cause this condition. Separating incompatible animals and adding alfalfa hay to the diet may help.

Mature males can produce a sebaceous secretion around the circumanal region that can almost occlude the anus. The plug can be softened with soap and water and removed. Washing the area periodically will prevent recurrence.

Mature males can also develop preputial infections when foreign materials, such as bedding, become entrapped in the preputial folds after mating. Bedding is drawn into the preputial fornix by adhering to the moistened prepuce. Once there it can cause a severe foreign body reaction. Removing the foreign body and treating the area locally with an antiinflammatory cream is usually sufficient to resolve the lesions. Preputial dermatitis can also be caused by physical irritation from rough cage flooring and subsequent fecal contamination or urine scalding. Cleaning the wounds and treating locally with zinc oxide ointment is usually sufficient.

Guinea pigs also have a tendency to develop small horny growths on the lateral aspects of the front footpads. Keeping the toenails trimmed and occasionally trimming back the nonvascular portions of the growths will keep these lesions under control.

CHINCHILLAS

Chinchillas are known for their soft, thick haircoats and are mentioned here briefly because of several common skin conditions.

Fungal Conditions

Dermatophytosis (ringworm) is relatively common. Most often caused by *Trichophyton mentagrophytes*, lesions tend to start around the face, axilla, groin, and base of the tail. Erythema, white flaky dermatitis, and easy fur epilation are the predominant clinical signs. Diagnosis is the same as that described for mice. Treatment consists of removing all the affected fur at the periphery of the lesions, bathing the chinchilla with an iodine-based shampoo, such as Welladol® (Pitman-Moore), and using oral griseofulvin and topical antifungal preparations. As with other species, environmental sanitation by thorough vacuuming and disinfection will prevent recurrence and minimize the zoonotic potential.

Miscellaneous Conditions

Fur Chewing

Fur chewing is a common vice in chinchillas. The cause is unknown, but environmental stress, overcrowding, heredity, dietary deficiencies, a low-roughage diet, boredom, and nesting activity have all been implicated as possible causes. Treatments described have been varied, but providing fresh alfalfa hay, proper chinchilla pellets, and reducing stress should help.

Fur-Slip

Fur-slip is the term used to describe the chinchillas' ability to shed large tufts of fur suddenly when frightened or attacked. The loss of fur causes no pain to the animal, although large patches of bare skin may be exposed. It can take 3 to 5 months for the fur to regrow, however, so it is a situation best avoided. Quiet surroundings and calm, gentle handling will minimize the chances of occurrence.

Fur Ring

Fur ring describes a condition in which a ring of fur becomes entrapped within the prepuce, causing paraphimosis. Treatment consists of lubricating the penis to free up the ring of fur and trimming the fur away.

Chinchillas tend to have fewer coat problems if sandbathing with chinchilla dust, which is available commercially, or Fuller's earth. The dust should be poured 2 inches deep in a tray large enough to accommodate the chinchilla and allow rolling. Bathing should be allowed for half an hour two to three times a week. To prevent the possibility of fungal spores contaminating the dust bath, regularly placing the dust bath in an oven for 20 minutes at 300 °F (148.8 °C) has been suggested.

RABBITS

Rabbits are prone to a number of dermatologic conditions. One of the most significant effects of these conditions, however, is the tendency of rabbits to develop gastric trichobezoars. Because of the rabbit's inability to vomit and its narrow pyloric antrum, these trichobezoars do not always respond well medically, and surgical intervention is almost invariably fatal. For this reason, any dermatologic condition in which ingestion of hair is a component must be treated and resolved swiftly to prevent this secondary condition.

Bacterial Conditions

Ulcerative pododermatitis, also known as "*hock sores*," actually involves the ventral metatarsal region. It is often encountered in heavy rabbits kept on wire mesh or rough or dirty flooring, or in any rabbit in which the plantar fur pad is too thin. For this reason, it is often encountered in Angora rabbits after they have been groomed or trimmed because the desire to trim the matted, soiled fur from this region is natural. The lesions appear as well-circumscribed, ulcerated areas covered by a dry scab. Abscess formation under the scab occurs frequently, and infection can spread to nearby joints causing a septic arthritis. Treatment consists of providing a clean, smooth environment, and treating topically with an appropriate antibiotic and bandaging the wounds. If an abscess or arthritis is present, culture and sensitivity and systemic antibiotics are required.

Sore dewlap refers to a localized submandibular dermatitis, caused by drooling from malocclusion or by drinking from an open pan or crock. Treatment consists of removing the inciting cause by trimming the affected teeth, or by replacing the crock with a sipper tube waterer, and treating the dermatitis topically with hydrogen peroxide and an appropriate cream.

Staphylococcus aureus, Pasteurella, Salmonella, and *Streptococcus* have all been implicated as causes of dermatitis or abscessation (Plate XII-13). Self-trauma can be an important cause of progression of these lesions. Treatment consists of cleaning or debriding the wounds and treating with an appropriate antibiotic.

Venereal spirochetosis is caused by the spirochete *Treponema cuniculi*. It is transmitted by direct contact, especially during mating or by infection of the offspring at birth or during nursing. The rabbit is the only known natural host for the organism. The most common clinical signs are hyperemia and edema of the vulva or prepuce, followed by macules, papules, erosions, ulcers, and crusts on the external genitalia, perineal areas, eyelids, nose, and lips. Affected rabbits remain alert, and the disease regresses after several weeks. Lesions may heal with minimal scarring or persist as proliferative areas suggestive of papillomas. Diagnosis is by finding fine spiral-shaped bacterium 10 to 30 μm long on dark field examination of skin scrapings; or by the use of serologic tests, although a positive titer might not occur until 5 to 6 weeks after lesions have already appeared. Treatment success has been reported using three subcutaneous injections at 7-day intervals of 42,000 IU/kg penicillin G benzathine–penicillin G procaine.

Necrobacillosis, or Schmorl's disease, is caused by the organism *Fusobacterium necrophorum*. Clinical signs include ulceration and abscessation of the skin and subcutaneous swellings about the face, neck, and oral cavity. The lesions have a foul odor and may be present for weeks or months. Affected animals are usually pyrexic and anorectic as a result of the lesions in and around the mouth. The organism is a gram-negative, non–spore-forming, pleomorphic anaerobe present in the digestive tract of rabbits and other animals. Infection occurs under filthy conditions in which continuous fecal contamination of feet or wounds is possible. Diagnosis is by anaerobic culture of the organism. Treatment consists of cleaning and debriding the wounds and treating with an appropriate antibiotic. Prevention is easily accomplished by practicing proper husbandry; thus, this condition is rarely encountered in commercial facilities or in private practice.

Pseudomonas aeruginosa has also been identified as a cause of a dermatitis that has been referred to as "blue fur" because of the blue-green pigment produced by the organism. *Pseudomonas* is a ubiquitous gram-negative bacillus readily found in water and soil. Most infections are opportunistic, and are associated with immunosuppression or prolonged broad-spectrum antibiotic administration. Chronic wetting of the fur, usually caused by pan waterers or dripping water bottles, appears to be the major contributing factor. Skin lesions are often edematous, hemorrhagic, and necrotic. *Pseudomonas* is resistant to a number of different antibiotics; therefore, culture and sensitivity is imperative in establishing a proper therapeutic approach. Clipping the hair, debriding the wounds, and treating locally with 3% hydrogen peroxide may slow the spread until proper antibiotic therapy is instigated.

Viral Conditions

Myxomatosis is primarily an arthropod-transmitted poxvirus endemic in wild rabbits but is of great importance to domestic rabbit owners in Europe, Australia, and the western United States. Because the disease is transmitted by arthropod vectors, the incidence varies greatly from year to year based on the number of arthropods parasitizing the species. Birds, plants, and fomites can also act as mechanical vectors in the transmission.

Natural attenuation of the virus has led to the development of various strains, ranging from a mild avirulent fibroma-causing strain to an almost uniformly lethal strain. Clinical signs associated with the California strain most often include erythema, palpebral edema, purulent conjunctivitis, and gelatinous subcutaneous swellings of undifferentiated mesenchymal cells, especially of the face, ears, and external genitalia. Death usually occurs 8 to 12 days after exposure, but in those that survive, the lesions usually regress in 1 to 3 months. Diagnosis is based on the clinical signs and characteristic histopathologic lesions. Virus isolation and identification by fluorescent antibody technique is required in those cases in which lesions do not provide a definitive diagnosis. No treatment is known, and prevention is best accomplished by keeping pets in insect-proof enclosures and eliminating exposure to wild rabbits. Vaccinating with an attenuated vaccine prepared in the face of an outbreak may be helpful in rabbitry situations.

The Shope fibroma virus is a poxvirus antigenically related to the myxomatosis virus. Usually regarded as a cause of benign, localized fibromas in cottontail rabbits throughout North America, the virus has caused severe epizootics in commercial rabbitries in the United States. The disease is transmitted primarily by arthropod vectors, although mechanical transmission can occur. Tumors usually occur on the legs and feet, but may be seen on the muzzle or eyes of infected rabbits. The tumors are subcutaneous, localized, benign fibromas, and may persist for months without causing any other clinical signs. Diagnosis is by the characteristic clinical signs and histopathology of the lesions, or by virus isolation and identification. No treatment is known, but because arthropod vectors are important in the transmission, eliminating exposure to wild rabbits and insect-proof enclosures will aid in prevention.

The Shope papillomavirus causes wart-like lesions most frequently found on the neck, shoulders, or abdomen of cottontail rabbits. The virus causes a benign disease of cottontail rabbits in the midwestern United States, but has also been seen in domestic rabbits in that area. The warts begin as red, raised areas at the site of infection, then grow to become papillomas with rough, rounded surfaces, or large keratinized horny growths. These lesions usually regress spontaneously within 6 months, but occasionally go on to form malignant squamous cell carcinomas. Diagnosis is by the characteristic clinical signs, or by histopathology of the affected tissue. Because the infection appears to be transmitted by arthropod vectors, eliminating exposure is the best prevention.

Rabbit pox is caused by a poxvirus only distantly related to the other poxviruses of rabbits. Only six outbreaks have been recorded since the 1930s, so it is unlikely that disease would be encountered in private practice. Skin lesions begin as erythematous or macular eruptions which progress to form papules all over the body. Extensive edema of the face and oral cavity and purulent conjunctivitis are also seen frequently. Death usually occurs 7 to 10 days after infection. Diagnosis is by clinical signs, histopathology, and virus isolation and identification. Depopulation and strict sanitation is advised.

Fungal Conditions

Dermatophytosis occurs more frequently in pet rabbits than in the laboratory setting. *Microsporum canis*, *M. gypseum*, *M. audouinii*, and *Trichophyton shoenleini* infections do occur, but *T. mentagrophytes* is the most common cause of ringworm in domestic rabbits. Often appearing first on the head, face, or forelimbs, lesions on the back are also common (Plate XII-14). The lesions appear as an irregularly coin-shaped alopecic area, with a ridge of acute inflammation and mild to moderate crusting around the periphery. An area of central healing and hair regrowth is characteristic. The lesions are often pruritic. Secondary bacterial infection of hair follicles is common. Diagnosis and treatment is the same as that described for chinchillas.

Parasitic Conditions

Psoroptes cuniculi is an obligate, nonburrowing ear mite that is extremely common in domestic rabbits (Plate XII-15). The lesions first appear inside the ears at the bottom of the ear canal, then gradually extend higher up as a dry, tan, crusty exudate which, when removed, exposes a moist, red, very painful skin surface (Plate XII-16). Head shaking, intense pruritus, self-mutilation, and secondary bacterial infections are common. The ear mite's life cycle is 3 weeks under favorable conditions, and owners may insist that the lesions were not there a week ago despite the fact that the ear canal is full of debris. Although usually confined to the ears, lesions can also be found on the external genitalia or on the face, neck, and limbs in conjunction with the ear lesions. Many authors maintain that simply instilling a few milliliters of mineral oil/miticide in the canal, repeating the process in 7 to 10 days, and allowing the rabbit to shake out the crusts itself is sufficient. Because the condition is extremely painful, I feel that anesthetizing the rabbit, flushing the ear canal with a dilute chlorhexidine solution, and then using an antibiotic-antiparasitic-corticosteroid otic preparation, such as Tresaderm® (MSD AGVET), is the preferred method of treatment in private practice. Ivermectin given orally at 400 μg/kg is also effective, but secondary bacterial infection of the canal should still be treated if present. The mite can exist off the host for a short period and is very contagious between rabbits; therefore, it is also advisable to treat the environment with an insecticide for 4 weeks to reduce the chance of spread.

Cheyletiella parasitovorax is a nonburrowing fur mite found very commonly in private practice in certain geographic regions. Clinical signs include thinning of the fur and scaling between the shoulder blades, progressing to reddened, oily, hairless patches over the back and head if not treated. Lesions are mildly to moderately pruritic in rabbits and can cause a transient dermatitis in humans. Treatment is the same as that described for fur mites in guinea pigs. Because the female *Cheyletiella* can exist for 2 weeks off the host, treating the environment with an insecticide for several weeks is also advised.

Listrophorus gibbus is an obligate, nonpathogenic fur mite of the rabbit found throughout the world. It is considered to be nonpathogenic and thus is often not mentioned in the literature. It is included here for the sake of completeness. Treatment would be the same as that described for *Cheyletiella*.

Haemodipsus ventricosis, *Notoedres cati*, and *Sarcoptes scabiei* can occur in rabbits but are rare and are described in the Parasite Diagnostic Key (Table 15-1). Treatment is the same as that described for lice and mange in guinea pigs.

Cuterebra larvae are common, particularly in rabbits housed outdoors. In northern climates there is a marked seasonality to myiasis. Flies usually emerge in June or July, and mating and egg laying follow within 7 to 8 days. Eggs are laid at the openings of rabbit burrows or around the rabbit hutch. The ova hatch in response to rapid increases in environmental temperature and moisture, likely caused by the immediate presence of the host. Larvae enter the host through nasal or oral openings, and larval development and migration occur in about one month. When the larvae are mature they exit the host, fall to the ground, and burrow in the soil to pupate and overwinter. Development resumes in the spring. The peak incidence of myiasis thus occurs in the late summer and early fall. No such periodicity is seen in southern climates, where myiasis can occur year round. The lesions consist of painful, 2- to 3-cm masses with fistulae in the center surrounded by moist matted fur. Treatment consists of anesthetizing the rabbit and lancing the lesion or enlarging the fistula to facilitate removal of the larvae. It is very important not to rupture the cystic cavity containing the larvae during this process because an anaphylactic reaction could ensue. After removal, the wound should be thoroughly cleansed and treated with an appropriate topical antibiotic.

Fleas are common in rabbits housed outdoors. Of the 1500 or so known species of fleas, approximately 25 have been identified as attacking wild or domestic rabbits. Of these, however, only *Cediopsylla simplex* (the common eastern rabbit flea) and *Odontopsyllus multispinosis* (the giant eastern rabbit flea) have been reported frequently in domestic rabbits. *C. simplex* is found most commonly around the head and neck region, while *O. multispinosis* is most common on the hind end. Infestation leads to pruritus and self-inflicted trauma, and severe infestations can be debilitating. Treatment consists of bathing with an insecticidal shampoo, and treating the rabbit and environment with insecticidal preparations suitable for cats. It is important to remember that fleas found on rabbits can serve as vectors of tularemia, myxomatosis, plague, and Rocky Mountain spotted fever as well as other diseases of zoonotic potential.

A number of ticks have been known to affect rabbits, but of these, only *Haemaphysalis leporis-palustris* (the continental rabbit tick) has been reported with any frequency in North America. Ticks are voracious blood suckers and are most important as vectors of disease, including Q fever, tularemia, and Rocky Mountain spotted fever. Treat with any commercially available tick spray suitable for cats.

Nutritional Conditions

A lack of roughage in the diet is an important cause of fur chewing in domestic rabbits. Rabbit pellets supplemented with fresh alfalfa hay must form the basis of the diet, with fresh fruits and greens, oats, and other treats added only in small amounts as supplements. Most diets contain 16 to 20% fiber, but diets with 25% fiber are required in some cases.

Several dietary deficiencies have been produced experimentally in rabbits. Pyridoxine deficiency resulted in scaling and thickening of the skin around the ears, and encrustations of the nose and paws. Biotin deficiency resulted in dermatitis; hair loss on the back, lips, eyelids, and tail; and scaliness and flaking of skin. Magnesium deficiency has been reported to cause alopecia and changes in fur texture and luster. Zinc deficiency resulted in achromotrichia and patchy alopecia 6 to 9 weeks after being on a zinc-deficient diet. Copper deficiency can cause achromotrichia, alopecia, and dermatosis.

Endocrine Conditions

Fur plucking for nest building by preparturient does is very common and usually begins several days before kindling. Hair is most often plucked from the dewlap, underbelly, or sides. Diagnosis is made by eliminating any other cause of the lesions. No treatment is required.

Neoplastic Conditions

Other than those tumors already described under Viral Conditions, spontaneous tumors of skin in rabbits are relatively rare, although both squamous cell carcinoma and basal cell adenoma do occur. Treatment of these two tumor types is by surgical excision where applicable.

Miscellaneous Conditions

Both male and female rabbits possess two sebaceous scent glands on either side of the vulvar/testicular region that secrete a brown waxy debris. This secretory substance can build up from time to time, and can be easily removed by gentle traction or soap and water. Hutchburn is caused by urine scalding of the perineal region because of an unclean environment or inability of the rabbit to void without soiling itself, such as after a fractured limb or a spinal injury (Plate XII-17). Washing the wounds with an antiseptic and applying zinc oxide cream has been remarkably successful in mild cases. In severe cases in which a limb or spinal injury is involved, baby diapers to absorb the urine, zinc oxide, and an Elizabethan collar to prevent the rabbit from pulling off the diaper are very effective until the inciting cause has healed, but owner compliance is essential.

FERRETS

Of all the species described in this chapter, the pet ferret is the most similar to dogs and cats. Because ferrets have become popular only in recent years, information on dermatologic conditions seen in this species is relatively sparse. Nonetheless, several conditions are seen regularly in private practice and are described below.

Bacterial Conditions

Bite wounds to the neck by cage-mates during play or during mating are common. Mild lesions often appear as a thinning of hair or a scabby, erythematous area around the neck and shoulders that can be mistaken for self-trauma resulting from pruritus if the history of contact with another ferret is unknown. Separating the ferrets will usually result in complete resolution of the lesions without medical intervention. Severe bite wounds may result in subcutaneous abscesses, most often caused by *Streptococcus* spp. or *Staphylococcus aureus*. Diagnosis is by cytology or culture and sensitivity of the organism. Treatment consists of lancing and flushing the wound and treating with an appropriate antibiotic.

Viral Conditions

Canine distemper is a highly infectious disease in domestic ferrets that has several very distinctive skin lesions. Caused by a paramyxovirus, it is spread via aerosolization of viral particles from nasal secretions or saliva from infected dogs or other ferrets. The incubation period ranges from 4 to 10 days, with clinical signs appearing 7 to 9 days after exposure. A mucopurulent conjunctivitis is usually one of the first signs, progressing to erythematous eruptions on the chin, footpads, and inguinal region over the next few days. Vesicle formation and secondary pyoderma are common, as is pruritus. Hyperkeratosis of the footpads is highly suggestive of canine distemper, but should not be confused with sarcoptic mange (described under Parasitic Conditions). Anorexia, fever, and respiratory and gastrointestinal signs are common, and animals surviving the acute phase may develop central nervous system signs before death. Death occurs anywhere from 2 days to a month after exposure. Infection with distemper offers a poor prognosis, as mortality approaches 100%. Prevention is best accomplished by annual vaccination with a modified live chick embryo origin vaccine. Canine cell origin vaccines should not be used, as they have been implicated as causing the disease in ferrets.

Fungal Conditions

Dermatophytosis (ringworm) in ferrets is most frequently caused by *Microsporum canis* or *Trichophyton mentagrophytes*. Clinical signs include circumscribed areas of alopecia and a scaly dermatitis most frequently seen around the eyes, nose, or limbs. *Microsporum canis* will sometimes display positive green fluorescence under a Wood's lamp, but diagnosis is best accomplished by microscopic examination of skin scrapings macerated in 10% potassium hydroxide (KOH) for 30 to 60 minutes and identification of mycelia or arthrospores, or by growth of the fungus on dermatophyte test medium. Because the organism grows slowly, cultures should be held for 3 weeks for a definitive diagnosis. Treatment includes disinfecting the environment, clipping the hair around the lesions, bathing with an iodine-based shampoo, and using topical creams and oral griseofulvin. Griseofulvin should not be used in pregnant animals because of possible teratogenic effects.

Parasitic Conditions

The mite *Otodectes cynotis* is very common in pet ferrets. It is transmitted by direct contact with infected ferrets, dogs, or cats. Clinical signs of head shaking and scratching may or may not be present, but waxy brown sebum and demonstration of the mites or eggs on an otic smear is diagnostic. The mites can exist on other areas of the body or off the host for short periods of time; therefore, whole body treatment with an insecticide is recommended as well as an otic preparation suitable for use in cats. Ivermectin given at 200 μg/kg twice at 14-day intervals is also effective.

Fleas are found on ferrets, and are often associated with homes that are infested with fleas as a result of the other pets in the household. Pruritus is the most common clinical sign, and lesions are consistent with self-trauma. Heavy flea burdens can cause severe anemia and debilitation. Treatment with a 0.05% pyrethrin or 0.5% carbaryl shampoo followed by a weekly light dusting with 5% carbaryl powder is effective, as long as the environment is also treated. The environment may be treated with any of the commercially available premise insecticides, but ferrets should only be treated with products considered safe for use in kittens.

Sarcoptes scabiei is an uncommon parasite of domestic ferrets. Infection is more common in areas where ferrets are used for hunting rabbits and may be exposed to the parasite in rabbit burrows. Transmission is by direct contact with an infected animal or by exposure to a contaminated environment. Two forms of infestation have been described. The most frequently encountered form involves the feet and toes, which are swollen, erythematous, and may become ulcerated as a result of self-trauma. If left untreated the ferret can lose its claws. In the more generalized form, skin lesions predominate, with focal to generalized alopecia, hyperkeratosis, and intense pruritus. Diagnosis is best accomplished by deep skin scrapings cleared with 10% potassium hydroxide to reveal the sarcoptic mite. Treatment consists of weekly insecticide shampoos followed by lime sulfur dips for at least six treatments. Soaking the feet before removing the affected portion of the claw and debriding the foot lesions is helpful. Ivermectin given at a dose of 200 μg/kg is also useful in treating this condition. Because of the zoonotic potential, thorough disinfection of the environment and use of dichlorvos-impregnated resin strips is also advised.

Cuterebra spp. infestation can occur in ferrets housed outdoors or used for hunting, but is rare in house pets. Treatment is the same as that described for rabbits.

Nutritional Conditions

The most common cause for alopecia and dull, dry haircoat in ferrets is poor dietary practices. Many misconceptions exist in the general population concerning what constitutes an adequate diet for ferrets. Ferrets are no different than dogs and cats in their need for good quality protein and essential fatty acids for maintenance of a healthy haircoat. They are different in that their very short digestive tract provides them with only a limited ability to digest fiber. Food passage averages 3 to 4 hours in ferrets; therefore, diets high in protein and fat but low in fiber are important. I believe that most of the commercially available cat foods are not adequate for ferrets, and that top quality nutrition, such as commercial ferret food, Hill's Science Diet Feline Maintenance®, or IAMS Cat Food, is required as well as a fatty acid supplement containing both linoleic and α-linolenic acids. No data are available concerning specific vitamin and mineral deficiencies in ferrets, but it is reasonable to assume that they may exhibit clinical signs similar to those seen in dogs and cats. Biotin deficiency has been seen in practice resulting from the feeding of raw eggs in the diet. Clinical signs include alopecia, hyperkeratosis, and achromotrichia.

Endocrine Conditions

Bilaterally symmetric alopecia of the ventral abdomen and tail area, enlarged vulva, and possible superficial perivulvar dermatitis are all part of the estrogen-induced aplastic anemia syndrome of unspayed female ferrets. Diagnosis is easily made by the obvious clinical signs. Treatment consists of spaying the ferret and improving the level of nutrition to aid in the recovery. Another treatment consists of the use of 50 to 100 IU of human chorionic gonadotropin (HCG) given subcutaneously to take the female out of heat as a temporary measure until she can be spayed, or bred on a subsequent heat.

A heavy shed can be seen in female ferrets after the first heat of the season, and in males during October and November. Hair regrowth occurs spontaneously provided that the diet is adequate.

Hyperadrenocorticism caused by a functional adrenal adenoma, carcinoma, or a pituitary tumor causing bilateral adrenocortical hyperplasia occurs infrequently in domestic ferrets. Clinical signs include progressive hair loss, muscle atrophy, and a thin skin with prominent blood vessels (Plate XII-18). Muscle weakness, polydipsia, and polyuria are infrequent findings. Skin biopsy reveals sparse hair follicles with irregularly arranged collagen. Dexamethasone suppression tests or resting cortisol levels are not always rewarding in trying to make a diagnosis, although they can be attempted. The disease seems to progress slowly, and currently there is no well-recognized method of treatment. Surgical removal of the tumor may be attempted. Little data be difficult because of the large fat pad surrounding the kidney and adrenal gland in the ferret. Chemotherapy with the antineoplastic drug o,p′-DDD may be attempted. Little data are available concerning dosages used or success rates. A dose of 50 mg/kg given once daily for 7 days and then twice weekly until signs resolve has been suggested.

Neoplastic Conditions

Skin tumors are the third most common tumor type reported in ferrets. Of these, squamous cell carcinoma is the most common, followed by poorly differentiated sebaceous gland adenocarcinoma. Mast cell tumors, myxosarcoma of the subcutis, basal cell carcinoma, neurofibroma/sarcoma, histiocytoma, sebaceous gland adenoma, and hemangioma have all been reported. Diagnosis is by cytology, or biopsy and histopathology. Treatment consists of surgical excision where applicable.

Miscellaneous Conditions

An unusual condition that I have seen in practice but not reported in the literature is a condition I refer to as "blue ferret syndrome." Male or female ferrets, neutered or unneutered, present with a history of "bruising" on the abdomen. Though the skin has a bluish discoloration, no obvious hematomas are evident. The lesion is bilaterally symmetric, and usually progresses over several weeks to involve most of the abdomen. There is no pain or pruritus associated with the lesion, the ferret's behavior does not change in any way, and the lesions regress spontaneously over the course of a few weeks. To date no hematologic or histologic abnormality has been identified. The cause of the condition is unknown, though rupture of subcutaneous blood vessels has been suggested. No treatment is necessary.

SELECTED READINGS

Ackerman LJ: *Trixacarus caviae* infestation in a guinea pig. *Can Vet J* 28:313, 1987.

Anderson LC: Guinea pig husbandry and medicine. *Vet Clin North Am [Small Anim Pract]* 17(5):1045–1060, 1987.

Barthold SW, Bhatt PN, Johnson EA: Further evidence for papovavirus as the probable etiology of transmissable lymphoma of Syrian hamsters. *Lab Anim Sci* 37(3):283–288, 1987.

Battles A.: The biology, care, and diseases of the Syrian hamster. *Compend Contin Educ Pract Vet* 7(10):815–825, 1985.

Besch-Williford CL: Biology and medicine of the ferret. *Vet Clin North Am [Small Anim Pract]* 17(5):1155–1183, 1987.

Besch-Williford CL, Wagner JE: Bacterial and mycotic diseases of the integumentary system. In: Foster HL, Small JD, Fox JG (eds): *The Mouse in Biomedical Research. Volume II: Diseases*. New York, Academic Press, 1982, pp 55–74.

Burke TJ: Rats, mice, hamsters, and gerbils. *Vet Clin North Am [Small Anim Pract]* 9(3):473–486, 1979.

Collins BR: Dermatologic disorders of common nondomestic animals. In: Nesbitt GH (ed): *Dermatology. Contemporary Issues in Small Animal Practice*, vol 8. New York, Churchill Livingstone, 1987, pp 235–294.

Cunliffe-Beamer TL, Fox RR: Venereal spirochetosis of rabbits: Description and diagnosis. *Lab Anim Sci* 31(4):366–371, 1981.

Davidson M: Canine distemper virus infection in the domestic ferret. *Compend Contin Educ Pract Vet* 8(7):448–453, 1986.

Estes PC, Richter CB, Franklin JA: Demodectic mange in the Golden hamster. *Lab Anim Sci* 21(6):825–828, 1971.

Flynn RJ: *Parasites of Laboratory Animals*. Ames, IA, Iowa State University Press, 1973.

Fox JG: *Biology and Diseases of the Ferret*. Philadelphia, Lea & Febiger, 1988.

Fox JG, Goad MEP, Garibaldi BA, Wiest LM: Hyperadrenocorticism in a ferret. *JAVMA* 191(3):343–344, 1987.

Fox JG, Cohen BJ, Loew FM (eds): *Laboratory Animal Medicine*. Orlando, Academic Press, 1984.

Frisk CS: Bacterial and mycotic diseases. In: Van Hoosier GL, McPherson CW (eds): *Laboratory Hamsters*. Orlando, Academic Press, 1987, pp 112–133.

Harkness JE, Wagner JE: *The Biology and Medicine of Rabbits and Rodents*, ed 3. Philadelphia, Lea & Febiger, 1989.

Harkness JE: Rabbit husbandry and medicine. *Vet Clin North Am [Small Anim Pract]* 17(5):1019–1044, 1987.

Harris IE: Rabbits: Medicine and other veterinary aspects. *Austr Vet Pract* 18(1):6–11, 1988.

Jacobson E, Kollias GV, Peters LJ: Dosages for antibiotics and parasiticides used in exotic animals. *Compend Contin Educ Pract Vet* 5(4):315–325, 1983.

Olsen GH, Turk MAM, Foil CS: Disseminated cutaneous squamous-cell carcinoma in a ferret. *JAVMA* 186(7):702–703, 1985.

Ryland LM, Bernard SL, Gorham JR: A clinical guide to the pet ferret. *Compend Contin Educ Pract Vet* 5(1):25–32, 1983.

Saunders GK, Scott DW: Cutaneous lymphoma resembling mycosis fungoides in the Syrian hamster. *Lab Anim Sci* 38(5):616–617, 1988.

Small JD: Drugs used in hamsters. In: Van Hoosier GL, McPherson CW (eds): *Laboratory Hamsters*. Orlando, Academic Press, 1987, pp 179–199.

Wagner JE, Farrar PL: Husbandry and medicine of small rodents. *Vet Clin North Am [Small Anim Pract]* 17(5):1061–1087, 1987.

Chapter 16

DISEASES OF THE INTEGUMENTARY SYSTEM OF REPTILES

Elliott R. Jacobson, DVM, PhD

A great variety of infectious and noninfectious integumentary diseases have been reported for reptiles. Many of these diseases primarily affect the integumentary system while others are generalized infections with both systemic and cutaneous involvement.

To appreciate abnormalities of the reptilian integument, an understanding of the normal structure is imperative. The first part of this chapter includes a brief review of the anatomy and histology of the reptilian integument. Infectious and noninfectious diseases of the integument are reviewed next, followed by a discussion of diagnostic techniques.

ANATOMY AND HISTOLOGY

Reptiles are the first truly terrestrial group of vertebrates. To avoid excessive water loss in a dehydrating environment, one of the major modifications that evolved over the ancestral amphibian plan included the integumentary system. For the most part, amphibians have a thinly keratinized skin containing an elaborate array of mucus and poison glands. In some amphibian species, the skin acts as a respiratory structure. The thin moist skin of amphibians restricts these animals to living in macro- or microenvironments that are moist or humid. With the evolution of reptiles, the integument went through some significant modifications to prevent dehydration and allowed the ancestral reptiles to radiate out into many untouched habitats. Invasion of aquatic systems resulted in further modifications. While crocodilians, lizards, and snakes all have a structurally similar integument, chelonians (turtles and tortoises) have developed a biologically unique integumentary structure, the shell. The chelonian shell evolved early in the evolutionary history and had a great selective value because it has changed minimally over millions of years.

From the standpoint of diagnostic work, the chelonian shell is extremely difficult to biopsy and evaluate histologically compared with the soft integument of other reptiles. The chelonian shell consists of outer epidermal scutes overlying a series of dermal plates. In most species, the epidermis is quite hard and is covered by a keratin-like material. In tortoises, new areas of growth are seen at the suture lines equidistant between the embryonic shields.[1] These growth lines may be more obvious in the plastron than the carapace (Plate XIII-1). The dermal bone is metabolically active[2] and in calculating dosages of medicaments to be administered, the weight of the shell must be considered in the calculation. The dermal bone of the chelonian shell integrates with the ribs and the vertebral column. In green turtles, Rathke's glands exit through small openings in the axillary and inguinal portions of the inframarginal scutes.[3] While terrestrial chelonians shed the outer portions of their shell as small, often imperceptible, flakes, many aquatic turtles shed the outer portions of entire scutes (Plate XIII-2).

The soft tissue of the integument shows similarities between the various orders of reptiles. The skin is composed of several layers of epidermal cells overlying a dermis composed of loose and dense connective tissue (Fig. 16-1). Many species of crocodilians have bony plates within the dermis called *osteoderms*; the best developed osteoderms are in the cervical region. Overlying the epidermal cells is a thin layer of keratin. In turtles the skin is covered by a keratin-like substance and is unique among vertebrates in composition.[4] A multitude of chromatophores are located within the dermis immediately below the basement membrane and consist of melanophores, erythrophores, xanthophores, and iridophores (Plate XIII-3). The reptile integument has relatively few glandular structures and typically is dry. The scent glands that do exist in reptiles probably function to ward off predators or function in sex discrimination and species recognition during the breeding season.

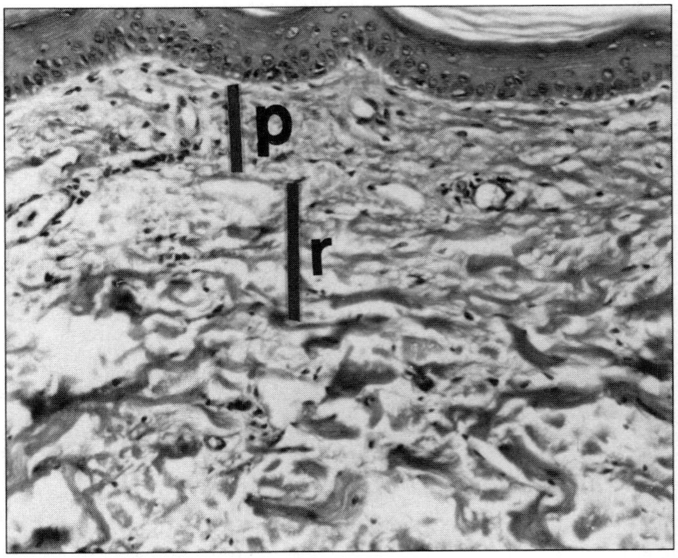

Figure 16-1. Histologic section of skin of a green turtle. The epidermis is approximately four to seven cells thick and is covered by a thin keratin-like substance corresponding to the stratum corneum. Immediately below the papillary layer (*p*) is the reticular layer (*r*), which is composed of large collagenous bundles. (H&E stain, x160) (From Jacobson ER, Mansell JL, Sundberg JP, et al: Cutaneous fibropapillomas of green turtles (*Chelonia mydas*). *J Comp Pathol* 101:34–52, 1989, with permission)

Lizards and snakes have a unique method of periodic epidermal ecdysis (skin shedding). In snakes and some lizards (night lizards, some geckos) the cornea is covered by a spectacle, which is also involved in the shedding process. In this process only the superficial portion of the skin is lost. In snakes ecdysis is characterized by six stages of epidermal development.[5] Clinically, as a snake enters a cycle of ecdysis the skin and spectacle take on a bluish tinge. During this time a new epidermal generation is laid down and matures. Approximately 4 to 7 days after the height of development of this dullness to the skin, the snake's color rapidly brightens and the spectacle of the eye clears completely and shedding occurs. After shedding, the epidermis enters a resting phase composed of the following three subdivisions: (1) postshedding resting phase, (2) perfect resting phase, and (3) late resting phase.[6] Subsequently, a renewal phase (lasting approximately 14 days) begins and the cycle repeats itself. If the snake goes one day beyond the normal time of shedding, the skin becomes roughened and somewhat dehydrated in appearance.

INFECTIOUS DISEASES

Viral Skin Diseases

Gray Patch Disease of Green Sea Turtles

A virus with the morphologic appearance of herpesvirus has been shown to be the causative agent of epizootics of skin lesions termed *gray patch disease* in young green turtles (*Chelonia mydas*) between 56 and 90 days after hatching in aquaculture.[7] Skin lesions commenced as small circular papular lesions which coalesced into spreading patches (Plate XIII-4) containing epidermal cells with basophilic intranuclear inclusions. Electron microscopy revealed inclusions to consist of viral particles having an electron-dense core. Particles were found enveloping from nuclear membranes and mature enveloped particles found in the cytoplasm measured 160 to 180 nm. The most severe epizootics occurred in the summer under stressful environmental conditions of high water temperature (>39 °C [102 °F]), crowding, and organic pollution. In controlled experiments turtles that were subjected to a gradual temperature increase from 25 to 30 °C (77 to 86 °F) with subsequent maintenance at 30 °C and those that were abruptly shifted from water temperatures of 25 to 30 °C showed a significantly shorter period before the onset of clinical signs and an increase in the severity of the lesions compared with control turtles.[8]

Poxvirus Skin Disease of Caimans and Nile Crocodiles

The first report of a virus-associated disease in a crocodilian is that of a poxvirus skin disease of captive caimans (*Caiman sclerops*).[9] Infected caimans were found to have gray-white circular skin lesions scattered over the body surface (Plate XIII-5). Oral proliferative lesions also were seen on the tongue and hard palate. While in some caimans severe lesions resulted in digital sloughing, other individuals only had focal lesions often involving only the palpebrae. By light microscopy large eosinophilic intracytoplasmic inclusions were seen within hypertrophied epithelial cells. Numerous inclusions were present in an extremely thickened keratin layer. By electron microscopy inclusions were found to consist of myriads of viral particles that were morphologically typical of poxvirus. The size of 200 x 100 nm was smaller than previously reported poxviruses of vertebrates and insects. A similar poxvirus disease was identified in juvenile farm-reared Nile crocodiles (*Crocodylus niloticus*) in Zimbabwe[10] and South Africa.[11]

Desert Tortoise Poxvirus

An amelanotic California desert tortoise (*Xerobates agassizi*) with multiple raised papular-to-vesicular lesions on the skin of the head, neck, and legs was found by light microscopy to have ballooning of the epidermal cells in the stratum granulosum.[12] Large intracytoplasmic inclusions were seen in many of these cells with hematoxylin and eosin (H&E) staining. Although the author of that report considered these inclusions to be consistent with those of poxvirus infection, there was no confirmation of this interpretation because no supportive electron photomicrographs were provided. Accumulations of protein and/or keratin within the cytoplasm of a dysplastic epidermal cell can be confused with intracytoplasmic viral inclusions.

Papillomavirus of Bolivian Side-Neck Turtles

Papilloma-like viral crystalline arrays were observed in skin lesions of recently imported Bolivian side-neck turtles (*Platemys platycephala*).[13] The turtles were submitted for examination with circular papular skin lesions that in some animals coalesced into patches (Plate XIII-6). The gross appearance of this disease was similar to that seen with herpesvirus infection of green turtles and poxvirus of caimans. Light microscopic evaluation of skin lesions, however, revealed hyperkeratosis and hyperplasia with acanthosis; no inclusions were noted. Electron microscopic examination of skin biopsies revealed intranuclear crystalline arrays of hexagonal particles measuring approximately 42 nm. These aggregates were morphologically consistent with those of papillomavirus. The lesions were more benign in appearance than papillomavirus-induced wart lesions of mammals.

Lacertid Lizard Papillomas

Cutaneous papillomas are commonly seen in lacertid lizards (Plate XIII-7). Raynaud and Adrian presented a detailed report on the distribution of papillomas in European green lizards (*Lacerta viridis*) maintained as a breeding colony.[14] The papillomas ranged in diameter from 2 to 20 mm and numbered 2 to 25 per individual. In females the papillomas were most commonly found in the caudal lumbar area of the body, in the vicinity of the tail base; papillomas were rarely found around the head. In males the papillomas had a dorsocranial distribution around the base of the head. Neither sex had papillomas associated with ventral scales. The authors associated the distribution to the reproductive behavior whereby males inflict bite wounds on females at the base of the tail and combative behavior between males during which males inflict bites at the base of the neck of other males. Histopathologic examination of papillomas showed hyperkeratosis and hyperplasia of epidermal cells. The nucleus of epidermal cells was often hypertrophied with margination of chromatin material and intranuclear inclusions. Papillomas submitted for electron microscopy revealed three morphologically distinct virus particles resembling papovavirus, herpesvirus, and reovirus.

Treatment/Management of Viral Skin Diseases

There are no vaccines available for any of the viral diseases of reptiles. In most cases the lesions are colonized by bacteria and fungi that often contribute to the severity of the lesions. Biopsies and microbial culture of these lesions allow selection of the most appropriate chemotherapeutic agent for treatment of these secondary invaders. Ill reptiles should be removed from healthy cage-mates and maintained under ideal environmental conditions. For aquatic species water quality control is imperative; water should be changed at least daily.

Bacterial Skin Diseases

Bacterial Shell Diseases of Chelonians

Septicemic cutaneous ulcerative disease of turtles was first described by Jackson and Fulton[15] and is commonly seen in freshwater turtles of the genera *Pseudemys* and *Chrysemys* that have been recently purchased from biologic supply companies. Often these turtles are kept under suboptimal environmental conditions and have not been fed adequately. Clinically the disease is seen as necrotizing ulcerative cutaneous lesions with both shell and skin involvement. Typically there is a septicemia with lesions in the liver, heart, kidney, and spleen. Although the organism *Citrobacter freundii* has been incriminated as the etiologic agent, *Serratia* may be necessary to initiate the infection.[15] Unfiltered aquatic systems with excess accumulations of fecal material will exacerbate the disease. Good water quality and a good feeding schedule are necessary for controlling this problem. Chloramphenicol was recommended as the antibiotic of choice. Wallach subsequently described an ulcerative shell disease of several species of aquatic turtles, with softshell turtles (*Trionyx* spp.) being most severely affected.[16] The gram-negative bacillus *Beneckea chitinovora* was cultured from these lesions on blood agar at 24 °C (75.2 °F) but not at 37 °C (98.6 °F). The disease was experimentally produced in softshell turtles and painted turtles (*Chrysemys picta*), and it was demonstrated that a prior injury to the shell was necessary for the bacteria to cause the disease. *B. chitinovora* is commonly isolated from shrimp and crayfish fed to turtles and the author recommended that these food items be avoided.

Middle Ear Infections of Chelonians

This disease is seen as a bulging of the skin (tympanic scale) overlying the middle ear.[17] It has been seen in free-ranging eastern box turtles (*Terrapene carolina*), either unilaterally or bilaterally (Plate XIII-8). I have also seen this disease in freshwater turtles and the green sea turtle. The lesion consists of caseous laminated material surrounded by mixed inflammatory cells. In advanced cases osteomyelitis may occur. *Citrobacter*, *Enterobacter*, *Morganella morgani*, *Providencia rettgeri*, *Pseudomonas*, and *Pasteurella* have all been cultured from these lesions. Treatment consists of removing the caseated material and flushing the area with a dilute organic iodine solution. In severe cases use of an injectable broad spectrum antibiotic is recommended.

Subcutaneous Abscesses

Subcutaneous abscesses of bacterial origin are commonly encountered in lizards and snakes (Plate XIII-9). In snakes, subcutaneous abscesses are most often secondary to trauma from prey items biting the snake, bite wounds from cage-mates, or penetration of foreign bodies. An adult mangrove snake (*Boiga dendrophila*) with a large subcutaneous abscess was found to have a tooth from another snake within the center of the abscess. A mixture of gram-negative organisms, including *Pseudomonas*, *Providencia*, *Escherichia coli*, and *Proteus*, have been cultured from these lesions. In the Cuban anole (*Anolis equestris*), *Serratia anolium* has been isolated from subcutaneous abscesses.[18] Subcutaneous abscesses associated with *Serratia marcescens* have been seen in a green iguana (*Iguana iguana*) and spiny-tailed iguana (*Ctenosaura acanthura*).[19] In the same report, *Salmonella marina* and *Micrococcus* were also cultured from subcutaneous abscesses in a green iguana and spiny-tailed iguana. Recently a *Neisseria* species was isolated from tail abscesses in green iguanas and from the oral cavity of healthy iguanas.[20] Bite wounds inflicted by oral carriers were believed to be the source of the infection. The abscesses could not be effectively managed with either systemic antimicrobial therapy or localized treatment; thus, the *Neisseria* was considered a highly pathogenic organism. I have also isolated *Corynebacterium pyogenes* from an iguana with a subcutaneous abscess (Plate XIII-10) and a variety of anaerobes have also been isolated from abscesses of reptiles.[21]

Whatever their origin, subcutaneous abscesses should be surgically removed. In some situations the abscess may be a single large focal lesion surrounded by a fibrous capsule, while in other cases abscesses may be miliary and diffusely found in surrounding tissues. After removal, it is not uncommon for abscesses to recur at the same site, especially if they are in the miliary form. Antibiotic therapy includes use of a broad spectrum antibiotic and if an anaerobe is present, an appropriate drug such as metronidazole.[21]

Necrotizing Bacterial Dermatitis

Necrotizing skin lesions colonized by *Pseudomonas* have been seen secondary to burn wounds in several snakes (Plate XIII-11). In humans *P. aeruginosa* colonizes 60% of burn patients by the fifth day after the burn.[22] Snakes are commonly burned from electrical heating pads used within their cages. The lesions consist of hemorrhagic body scales with edema and necrosis. The lesions most often involve ventral scales in areas of direct contact with heating devices. Large areas of skin may slough, exposing subcutaneous tissue. Severe cases of *Pseudomonas* skin disease can result in a pneumonic condition after inhalation of microorganisms being shed into the surrounding atmosphere from the lesion site. Snakes with extensive skin lesions need to be soaked in a dilute iodine solution followed by application of a burn ointment, such as mafenide acetate (Sulfamylon® Cream—Winthrop Pharmaceuticals). Systemic antibiotics, such as amikacin, should also be used.

Pseudomonas aeruginosa, as well as *Corynebacterium xerosis*, *Staphylococcus* spp., *Streptococcus* spp., and *Citrobacter freundii*, were isolated from a necrotizing skin lesion in a rattlesnake, *Crotalus mitchelli pyrrhus*.[23] A recently imported adult Indonesian blue tongue skink, *Tiliqua gigas*, which arrived with a multifocal *P. aeruginosa* dermatitis, died despite treatment with appropriate broad spectrum antibiotics and was found to have a large intracoelomic perihepatic abscess connected to the overlying skin lesion by a thin stalk.[24] A pure growth of *P. aeruginosa* was cultured from this lesion. I have seen similar lesions in turtles in which shell ulcerations were continuous with coelomic abscesses via fistulous tracts.

Pseudomonas, one of the most common bacterial organisms associated with oral and respiratory disease in snakes, in advanced cases may enter the vascular compartment and ultimately produce necrotizing lesions at multiple sites, including the skin. Coagulation necrosis of the dermis results in sloughing of the overlying epidermal layer.

A condition has been seen in boa constrictors, pythons, and other snakes in which obstipation, necrosis of the gastrointestinal tract, or infection of the reproductive tract in females results in loss of the stratum corneum of the epidermis.[25] The outer portions of each scale are seen to "flake off" (Plate XIII-12). At first only a few scales may be seen in the cage, but as the disease progresses almost the entire body can be involved. If the primary cause of the problem can be identified and corrected, the outer portions of the skin will be replaced at the next cycle of ecdysis.

Aeromonas hydrophila is a significant opportunistic pathogen of crocodilians. Die-offs of American alligators, *Alligator mississippiensis*, caused by *A. hydrophila* have been reported in the wild.[26] Deaths have also been seen in farm-reared alligators that have suffered from heat stress. Organisms from the intestinal tract enter the vascular compartment and invade multiple visceral structures. Peripherally, necrotizing hemorrhagic skin lesions are commonly seen. Because *Aeromonas* often cannot be cultured from skin lesions, it is thought that the lesions result from bacterial toxins released into the vascular compartment or thrombosis of subjacent vessels in the dermis.

Mycobacteriosis

Cutaneous disease caused by mycobacteria has been described in reptiles, either as a primary skin disease or secondary to systemic involvement.[27] The lesions appear as subcutaneous swellings and must be distinguished from other causes, such as bacterial abscesses, mycotic granulomas, and neoplasia. The skin over the granuloma may ulcerate. Organisms from the subcutaneous lesions can spread elsewhere. In a boa constrictor with primary subcutaneous mycobacteriosis, a proliferative ulcerating oral lesion developed from which a mycobacterium was isolated.[28]

Several species of atypical mycobacteria have been isolated from reptiles and include *Mycobacterium marinum*, *M. chelonei*, and *M. thamnopheos*. Acid-fast staining of granulomas is often diagnostic for the presence of mycobacteria. In many situations an abundance of organisms in tissue section makes identification easy. *M. thamnopheos*, however, is minimally acid-fast and may be difficult to demonstrate in tissue section.

There are no reports of treating reptiles with mycobacteriosis. Many of the reptile isolates are resistant to drugs used in mammals. Epizootics are seldom a problem in reptile collections; therefore, control should involve removal of infected animals and decontamination of the cage.

Dermatophilosis

Dermatophilus congolensis is one of two species within the family Dermatophilaceae. Members of this family are unique in forming filamentous structures that segment transversely as well as longitudinally to form coccoid cells that become motile spores. *D. congolensis* is gram-positive and is not acid-fast. It is the etiologic agent of dermatophilosis (formerly called streptothricosis), a disease that has been seen in a variety of mammals including ruminants, horses, primates, and carnivores. In reptiles it has been reported in Australian bearded lizards (*Amphibolurus barbatus*)[29] and marble lizards (*Calotes mystaceous*)[30] imported into the United States. It has also been seen in a captive bearded lizard in Australia.[31] I have seen an organism with microscopic characteristics of *D. congolensis* in skin lesions of six recently imported Senegal chameleons (*Chameleo senegalensis*), one green iguana (*Iguana iguana*), one collared lizard (*Crotophytus collaris*), and one boa constrictor; an organism consistent with *Dermatophilus* was cultured from the chameleons and iguana. In the lizards the lesions were seen as raised brown multifocal encrustations, scattered over the integument (Fig. 16-2). The boa constrictor was found to have multiple subcutaneous nodules that bulged the overlying skin. In those reptiles with epidermal involvement, the encrustations were found to consist of necrotic cellular debris, accumulations of keratin, and inflammatory cells; the underlying epidermis was necrotic. In hematoxylin and eosin–stained tissue sections, numerous basophilic coccoid structures were seen on the surface of the lesions; in sections stained by the Giemsa method, numerous branching filamentous structures with longitudinal and transverse divisions were observed in the encrusted material (Fig. 16-3). In the boa constrictor, similar-appearing organisms were seen within the caseated center of a subcutaneous nodule. Rough, dry, white-gray colonies developed from skin lesions of a chameleon and iguana cultured on trypticase soy agar. Gram-stained smears of these colonies demonstrated gram-positive filamentous rods consistent with *D. congolensis*.

Treatment for dermatophilosis includes removal of skin encrustations and topical application of a dilute iodine solution. Antibiotics of choice are amikacin and penicillin.

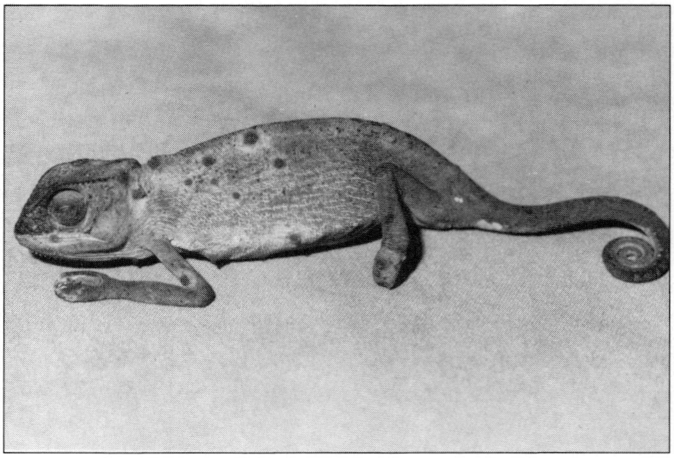

Figure 16-2. Multifocal raised, encrusted skin lesions in a Senegal chameleon. An organism resembling *Dermatophilus* was isolated from these lesions.

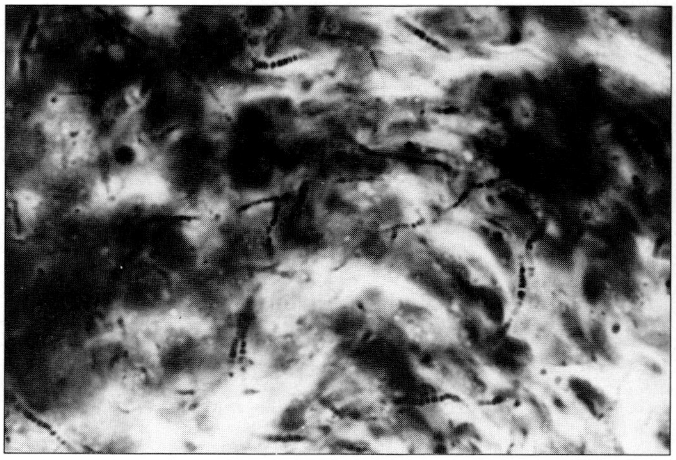

Figure 16-3. Photomicrograph of a skin lesion in a Senegal chameleon revealing a beaded filamentous organism resembling *Dermatophilus*. (Giemsa stain, x1000)

Drug Therapy for Bacterial Skin Disease

Bacterial disease problems in captive reptiles are caused most commonly by aerobic gram-negative microorganisms. Many of these organisms are secondary invaders, requiring predisposing problems before an infection begins. When treating these animals, one must not only isolate and identify the pathogen(s) but identify and correct the factors responsible for allowing the organism(s) to become established. For instance, reptiles kept at suboptimal environmental conditions are immunocompromised and are at risk for bacterial (and other pathogen) infections. In these cases treatment includes exposure to an appropriate ambient temperature regime.

The use of chemotherapeutics in reptile medicine has been discussed elsewhere[32] and is briefly reviewed here. In selecting the most appropriate antibiotic, ideally the causative agent needs to be identified and sensitivity patterns determined. Next, minimum inhibitory concentrations (MICs) of antibiotics should be determined. Because pharmacokinetic information is only available on a handful of antibiotics (in relatively few species of reptiles), scientifically treating these animals with appropriate antibiotics often narrows the range of drugs from which one can select. Pharmacokinetic data are available for chloromycetin, carbenicillin, ceftazadime, gentamicin, and amikacin. Dosages of antibiotics routinely used in treating reptiles with bacterial diseases(s) are listed in Table 16-1.

Many of the reptiles submitted with gram-negative sepsis are immunocompromised and thus bactericidal antibiotics would be more efficacious than bacteriostatic drugs. The health status of the reptile patient, the size of the patient, and the potential side effects of the drug should also be considered in selecting the most appropriate drug. In reptiles that are extremely dehydrated, the aminoglycosides should be avoided, at least until the animal is rehydrated. Ideally, reptiles that are being placed on a regimen of aminoglycoside administration (such as gentamicin and amikacin) should have a complete blood count (CBC) and serum chemical profile (including uric acid) performed before the initiation of therapy. For most reptiles normal uric acid levels should be below 14 mg/dl. If the reptile is administered an aminoglycoside, serum uric acid levels ideally should be monitored throughout the course of treatment and after treatment has ended. Isotonic saline at 20 ml/kg body weight

TABLE 16-1

Antibiotic Dosages for Reptiles

Antibiotic	*Trade Name*	*Dose (mg/kg)*	*Frequency*	*Duration*	*Route*
Chloramphenicol sodium succinate	Chloromycetin® sodium succinate (Parke-Davis)	40	Every 24 hours	5–14 days	SC
Chloramphenicol	Mychel-Vet Tevocin®	50	Every 12–72 hours depending on species	2 weeks	SC
Carbenicillin	Pyopen® (Beecham)	400	Every 48 hours in turtles Every 24 hours in snakes	2 weeks	IM IM
Ceftazadime	Fortaz®	20	Every 72 hours in snakes	2–3 weeks	IM
Gentamicin	Gentocin® (Schering-Plough Animal Health)	6	Every 72–96 hours in turtles	7–9 treatments	IM forelegs
		2.5	Every 72 hours in snakes	7–9 treatments	IM
		1.75	Every 96 hours in alligators	7–9 treatments	IM forelegs
Amikacin	Amiglyde® (Fort Dodge Laboratories)	5, 2.5	First dose; thereafter, every 72 hours in snakes	7–9 treatments	IM forelegs
		2.25	Every 96 hours in alligators	7–9 treatments	IM
Trimethoprim/ sulfadiazine	Tribrissen® (Coopers Animal Health)	30	First two doses 24 hours apart, then every other day	7–14 treatments	IM

(From Jacobson ER: Reptiles. *Vet Clin North Am [Small Anim Pract]* 17:1203–1225, 1987; with permission.)

should be administered subcutaneously, intraperitoneally, or orally on the days of treatment.

In general, oral administration of antibiotics to reptiles should be avoided. Few pharmacokinetic studies have been done on antibiotics administered orally in reptiles and uptake appears to be extremely variable and unpredictable. Many small species of lizards, however, have relatively small muscle masses and are extremely stressed when handled and injected. In such cases the medicament will have to be offered in the animal's food (if it is still feeding).

As a rule hind-leg muscles in quadrupedal reptiles and hind-body muscles in snakes should be avoided as injection sites because of the anatomy of the renal portal system. Such drugs as gentamicin and amikacin, if injected into the hind-leg musculature of a lizard, could go directly to the kidney, which, because these drugs are nephrotoxic, could be disastrous.

Ambient temperature has a marked effect on the uptake, distribution, and elimination of antibiotics in reptiles. As mentioned earlier, when ill reptiles are treated, they should be maintained at their preferred optimum temperature range. For many species a temperature range of 26 to 33 °C (78.8 to 91.4 °F) is ideal. At higher temperatures small species can dehydrate rapidly, and the clinician must constantly be aware of the hydration status of the patient.

Mycotic Diseases

Although at one time considered rare, mycotic diseases of the integumentary system are not uncommon in captive reptiles. I have also seen several cases of mycotic skin disease in free-ranging reptiles. The common dermatophytes, such as *Microsporum* and *Trichophyton*, are rarely recovered; instead, a variety of fungi, such as *Mucor, Fusarium, Trichosporon*, and *Geotrichum*, have been isolated from these lesions. While fungi are relatively easy to identify in tissue section, isolating the causative agent and making an accurate identification is extremely difficult. For ultimate identification the agent must be sent to an expert familiar with the genus of fungus isolated. Many new species of mycotic agents have been described in reptiles. In this section, mycotic diseases are reviewed by reptile group.

Mycotic Dermatitis of Chelonians

There are relatively few reports of cutaneous mycotic disease in chelonians. Mycotic dermatitis has been described in a radiated tortoise[33] and several other chelonians in a zoologic collection.[34] In the latter report, shell necrosis was associated with invasion of fungi in the order Mucorales with the plastron affected more often than the carapace. Six hatchling Florida softshell turtles (*Trionyx ferox*), representative of a group of approximately 400 with circular gray ulcerating lesions of the shell and skin (Plate XIII-13), were found on histopathology to have bacterial colonies and large numbers of branching nonseptate hyphae (Plate XIII-14).[35] *Mucor* spp., *Proteus* spp., *Escherichia coli*, and *Pseudomonas* were recovered from the lesions. The surviving turtles were immersed for 15 minutes in a solution of malachite green (0.15 mg/L) three times daily for one week. Turtles were thoroughly rinsed with fresh water after the immersion to reduce eye irritation. After one week of treatment, surviving turtles responded with regression of lesions. I have also seen fungal organisms in hatchling Ridley sea turtles (*Lepidochelys kempi*) with necrotizing palpebritis, in subcutaneous granulomas in the cervical region of an adult leopard tortoise (*Geochelone pardalis*), and in pitted shell lesions of hatchling Australian side-neck turtles (*Chelodina longicollis*).

Mycotic Skin Disease of Crocodilians

Relatively few cases of mycotic skin disease have been reported for this group of reptiles. In captivity crocodilians are often kept in cement pools and as a consequence, abrasions of the ventral integument are not uncommon. A bumblefoot-like condition of the footpads occurs and fungal organisms have been seen in these lesions. A *Trichophyton* sp. was isolated from one of these cases.[36]

Mycotic Skin Disease of Squamates (Lizards and Snakes)

Numerous cases of mycotic skin disease have been reported for this group of reptiles. The disease generally is seen as hyperkeratotic skin lesions, necrotizing skin lesions, or subcutaneous granulomas. I have seen numerous cases of mycotic skin disease in imported geckos. Recently a Madagascan day gecko (*Phelsuma madagascariensis*), representative of several species of recently imported *Phelsuma* that developed proliferative skin lesions, was examined. It was found to have raised circular proliferative lesions that became white in color as the lesions progressed. Ultimately there was a complete sloughing of the affected skin with development of a moist dermatitis. Examination of skin biopsy specimens revealed numerous branching septate hyphae throughout the tissue. I have also seen similar lesions in several species of recently imported West African ground geckos.

Trichosporonosis, caused by *Trichosporon beigelii* (*cutaneum*), has been isolated from a variety of lesions in reptiles including skin lesions of lizards.[36] I have isolated this fungus from subcutaneous hematomas in the American anole, *Anolis carolinensis* (Plate XIII-15). These lesions are a result of combat and biting by cagemates.

In snakes mycotic diseases of the integument include phycomycosis, penicillinosis, geotrichosis, fusariomycosis, and chromomycosis. In some cases the lesions are extremely necrotizing, as seen in a Burmese python (*Python molurus bivittatus*) with a *Fusarium* infection.[37] In other cases the lesions are proliferative and hyperkeratotic, such as in a *Trichoderma* infection in a ball python (*Python regius*) and *Penicillium* and *Oospora* infections in eastern king snakes (*Lampropeltis getulus*).[37] In a rosy rat snake (*Elaphe guttata rosacea*) with mycotic skin disease in addition to epidermal necrosis, there were well-developed dermal granulomas containing hyphae.[37] A case of dermal fibrosarcoma and chromomycosis was seen in a Mangrove snake (*Boiga dendrophila*), with the skin overlying the mass having several small deeply pigmented fistulous tracts extending into the fungal portion of the mass.[38]

In most cases epidermal skin lesions result in discoloration of the normal pigmentation of the skin. In snakes the scales appear thickened and have a yellow-orange-brown discoloration (Plate XIII-16). Once familiar with the gross appearance of these lesions the clinician will have little problem recognizing them. These are relatively common lesions in snakes that often are misdiagnosed.

Management/Treatment of Fungal Skin Disease

As in higher vertebrates, fungi in reptiles can be either primary or secondary invaders.[36] In my experience, they are more often secondary invaders with a multitude of predisposing factors being involved. In aquatic turtles, poor water quality is contributory. Lower environmental temperature results in immunosuppression in reptiles and may allow secondary agents to become invasive. In one study skin lesions in carpet pythons were associated with high humidity in the cage that may have reduced the capacity of the skin to resist infection.[39] Cages that are not kept clean promote the growth of numerous fungal organisms. In additional, fungal disease may follow a primary viral and/or bacterial skin infection.

Relatively few reports discuss treatment of reptiles with fungal skin disease. Localized mycotic infections of scales and subcutaneous mycotic granulomas are best treated by surgical removal. Several cases of mycotic skin disease have been treated successfully by soaking in a dilute organic iodine solution twice daily followed by the topical application of an antifungal ointment such as tolnaftate (Tinactin® —Schering-Plough) or miconazole nitrate (Monistat-Derm™—Ortho Pharmaceutical Corp.). As mentioned earlier, malachite green has been used for treating aquatic turtles with mycotic shell disease. Two cage-mate ball pythons (*P. regius*) diagnosed with a *Trichoderma* spp. dermatitis were unsuccessfully treated with oral griseofulvin at 20 and 40 mg/kg body weight, respectively, every 3 days for five treatments. Ketoconazole (Nizoral® —Janssen Pharmaceutica) has also been administered to reptiles with fungal skin disease. In a pharmacokinetic study in the gopher tortoise (*Gopherus polyphemus*), oral administration of 30 mg/kg body weight resulted in therapeutic plasma concentrations (> 1 μg/ml) from 4 to 32 hours after dosing.[40]

Parasitic Diseases

Pseudophyllidean Cestodes

Spirometra is a pseudophyllidean cestode that is widely distributed in different species of snakes, which serve as intermediate or paratenic hosts. Each egg releases a larva (coracidium) which, when ingested by a copepod, develops into a procercoid. Upon ingestion of the latter stage by a second intermediate host (reptile), procercoids develop into plerocercoids, which are known as spargana when they are present in skeletal muscle. When present subcutaneously, spargana can cause soft swellings of the overlying skin. Edema and hemorrhage of soft tissues may be found associated with this stage. The definitive host is generally a mammalian carnivore (most often a felid), although reptiles and birds can also serve as final hosts. In some parts of the world, human sparganosis is a common disease, and some cases result from the consumption of raw snake meat.

Mesocercariae Infections

Trematode mesocercariae of the genera *Alaria* and *Fibricola* have been identified in subcutaneous locations in a Texas indigo snake (*Drymarchon corais erebennus*) and red-sided garter snakes (*Thamnophis sirtalis parietalis*).[41] In the indigo snake, the trematodes were found within gelatinous subcutaneous masses in the intermandibular region and tail.

Spirorchidiasis

Adult members of the family Spirorchidae inhabit the circulatory system of susceptible reptiles. Turtles appear to be the most commonly infected reptilian host. Adult parasites generally are found within the great vessels leaving the heart or within the heart chambers, where focal endothelial hyperplasia has been seen. These lesions generally range in intensity from minimal to mild and show no clinical signs of illness that can be attributed directly to their presence.

The most significant lesions resulting from these parasites are a consequence of eggs released within the vascular compartment. Eggs ultimately become trapped within terminal vessels almost anywhere in the animal's body; at these places a severe granulomatous response often is elicited. Infected turtles have been seen with shell lesions ranging from focal to coalescing and ulcerative on the plastron and carapace. Edema of the limbs can also be seen and results from vascular occlusion.

Control of these parasites involves identification and elimination of the snail intermediate host. Transmission should be self-limiting in captivity, provided that no snails are present. Praziquantel (Droncit® —Mobay Corp.) at 8 mg/kg body weight given intramuscularly has been used in treating spirorchid infections of green turtles.

Filariasis

Filarial nematodes have been described for all major groups of reptiles. Some of the more important genera include *Oswaldofilaria*, *Foleyella*, and *Macdonaldius*. Limited studies have shown that there seems to be a low degree of host specificity for these genera. As adults all members of this group are found at extraintestinal sites (lungs, circulatory system, subcutaneous areas); these nematodes are either ovoviviparous or viviparous. Microfilariae are released into the circulatory system and transmission is achieved through blood-sucking arthropods, usually ticks and mosquitos.

Most reptilian filarial infections are diagnosed at necropsy. There are relatively few reports documenting clinical signs and gross lesions associated with infection. Several reticulated pythons in a zoologic collection developed cutaneous lesions; the transmission was presumably from boa constrictors kept in the same exhibit.[42] An argasid tick served as the vector. Lesions consisted of a necrotizing dermatitis; numerous parasites were found in the mesenteric arteries and obstruction of peripheral capillaries by microfilariae resulted in ischemic necrosis of the skin. The death of a bull snake (*Pituophis catenifer*) was attributed to the obstruction of the portal vein with *Macdonaldius seetae*.[43] In this case no signs of illness were seen before death.

Diagnosis depends on demonstration of adult parasites (most commonly found in the portal vein) at necropsy or identification of microfilariae in a blood sample. There are no reports describing the use of chemotherapeutic drugs. Telford found that an ambient temperature regime of 35 to 37 °C (95 to 98.6 °F) for 24 to 48 hours resulted in the death of adult parasites.[44] Care must be taken to carefully monitor snakes at this temperature regime and to ensure that the critical thermal maximum for the species is not exceeded.

Dracunculiasis

Several species of snakes with multifocal raised pustular lesions scattered over the body surface were found to contain myriads of nematode larvae within these lesions.[45] Larger slender nematodes in various stages of degeneration were associated with these lesions and were identified as a member of the superfamily Dracunculoidea. Dracunculoidea larvae develop in *Cyclops* sp. (a copepod) and tadpoles have been used as experimental transfer hosts. The intermediate host(s) is unknown.

Spiruridiasis

Larvae of the spirurid *Eustrongylides* have been reported to cause dermal lesions in red-sided garter snakes (*Thamnophis sirtalis parietalis*).[46] In addition to subcutaneous sites, larvae also were encountered in the lungs and free within the coelomic cavity. Intermediate hosts include fish and frogs. Adult parasites are located in the mucosa of the esophagus or the proventriculus or in the intestine of fish-eating birds.

Pentastomiasis

These primitive-appearing parasites are now placed in their own phylum. The adults are worm-like and superficially segmented; they range in size from 0.5 to 12 cm. All require intermediate hosts for completion of their life cycle. The most important genera infecting reptiles include *Sebekia* (in crocodilians), *Raillietiella* (in lizards and snakes), and *Kiricephalus*, *Porocephalus*, and *Armillifer* (in snakes). Mammals serve as intermediate hosts and several species within the genus *Armillifer* can infect humans. Most of the reports on human infection involve cases in Africa and Southeast Asia.

Ingested larvae migrate through the intestinal tract and may undergo extensive visceral migration before they reach maturity either in the lung and air sac or in subcutaneous tissues. Parasites distributed in subcutaneous sites may cause bulging of the overlying skin. Pentastomes are known to exit through lesions in the skin of newly captured wild reptiles.

Acarids

Mites. Most free-ranging reptiles are infested with mites. Some species of mites show a high degree of host specificity, whereas others are rather nonspecific in their predilection for a particular host. Because of their small size, mites may be overlooked in the recently acquired reptile.

The most commonly reported mite of reptiles is the snake mite (*Ophionyssus natricis*). This mite has a worldwide distribution and although it is only occasionally found on wild snakes, severe burdens are commonly encountered in recently imported snakes maintained under crowded, filthy conditions. The entire life cycle requires approximately 10 to 32 days, and a single female can lay up to 80 eggs. Eggs are deposited off the host in the immediate environment of the snake.

Severe infestations of *Ophionyssus* can result in a debilitated, anemic snake. Mites are often found in the axes between scales and in the sulcus formed between the spectacle and the periocular scales. The conjunctiva may become swollen and edematous. In addition, *Ophionyssus* is capable of transmitting the gram-negative bacteria *Aeromonas hydrophila*. Some strains of this bacteria are extremely pathogenic and can result in fatal septicemia. Under unusual conditions mites are capable of infesting humans, who may develop focal skin lesions.

Although mites are easy to overlook in light infestations, they appear almost to consume the host in severe cases. Mites generally are first noticed at the bottom of water bowls, where they fall off while the snake is drinking.

Ticks. Reptiles, including several marine species, are commonly infested by ticks. The more important hard-bodied genera infesting reptiles include *Amblyomma*, *Aponomma*, and *Hyalomma*. The most common soft-bodied tick is *Ornithidoros*. Even under captive conditions ticks rarely reach the burdens achieved by mites; still, they are significant potential pathogens causing anemia, producing focal ulcerating skin lesions, or acting as vectors for the transmission of other pathogens, such as *Macdonaldius* and rickettsiae.

Diptera. Numerous species of the order Diptera are known to feed upon reptiles and many are responsible for transmitting infectious agents. Several species of flies are known to parasitize reptiles directly in the larval (maggot) stages. Most cases of myiasis involve terrestrial chelonians; a few examples have been seen in debilitated crocodilians. Of turtles, box turtles (*Terrapene carolina*) and gopher tortoises (*Gopherus polyphemus*) in the southeastern United States appear particularly prone to infestation with *Cistudinamyia cistudinis*. In severe infestations maggots can be found at almost any subcutaneous site. Gopher tortoises have been found with focal lesions adjacent to the cloaca containing up to three dozen maggots. These fly larvae are incapable of penetrating intact skin but can utilize small openings, such as those caused by tick bites.

NONINFECTIOUS DISEASES

Environmentally Associated Skin Diseases

Trauma

Various traumatic injuries have been identified in captive reptiles, including abrasions, bite wounds, crushing injuries to turtle shells, damaged mouthparts (especially in turtles), and thermal burns.

Because reptiles are ectotherms, ultimately dependent upon environmental infrared radiation as a heat source, high wattage infrared and incandescent light bulbs are often used as heat sources in captivity. Often the bulb is placed within the cage where the animal can make direct contact, or too "hot" a bulb is used resulting in thermal burns to the animal. Captive reptiles ideally should be exposed to a gradient of temperature that spans the preferred optimum range for the species. Heat sources should originate outside the cage or at a distance where contact cannot be made. Reptiles receiving thermal burns will develop epidermal vesicles followed by necrosis.

Electric heating pads used to provide heat for captive reptiles often develop hot spots and result in ventral burning of the reptile's integument. As discussed earlier, severe necrotizing burn lesions often become invaded with *Pseudomonas* spp. and further add to the problems. Such animals require intensive chronic treatment with broad spectrum injectable antibiotics in addition to organic iodine soaks and topical application of organic iodine ointments.

Trauma in captive reptiles can result from direct aggression between cage-mates or indirectly when reptiles come together at feeding time. With snakes, when an animal is fed a prey species, a feeding frenzy often is elicited whereby anything smelling of the prey species will be attacked. Two snakes feeding upon the same rodent or fish may result in the larger snake inflicting cutaneous lacerations on the smaller snake. Depending upon the temperament of the animals, separation of cage-mates at feeding time may be necessary.

It is recommended that prey items be killed before feeding them to carnivorous reptiles, especially when food items are rodents. Live mice and rats can inflict serious bites upon their reptile predator. Snakes have been seen that have had large areas of skin and underlying musculature removed by prey rodent species left in the cage overnight. As discussed earlier, subcutaneous abscesses can develop several weeks or months after a rodent bite.

Dysecydysis

Humidity is an important environmental consideration when keeping reptiles in captivity. A relative humidity of 50 to 60% is used for many reptile species; however, some species will do better at lower relative humidities while others will thrive at higher relative humidities. In snakes and lizards, if the relative humidity is too low for the species, it may not be able to shed its old skin normally. If a snake's skin is retained for one day beyond the normal time of shedding, the integument will have the appearance of being dehydrated because of the drying of the retained skin. Spectacles also can be retained. If a snake has not molted properly, it should be soaked in a container having just enough water to cover the body. Retained spectacles can be gently removed with forceps or rubbed free with moistened cotton.

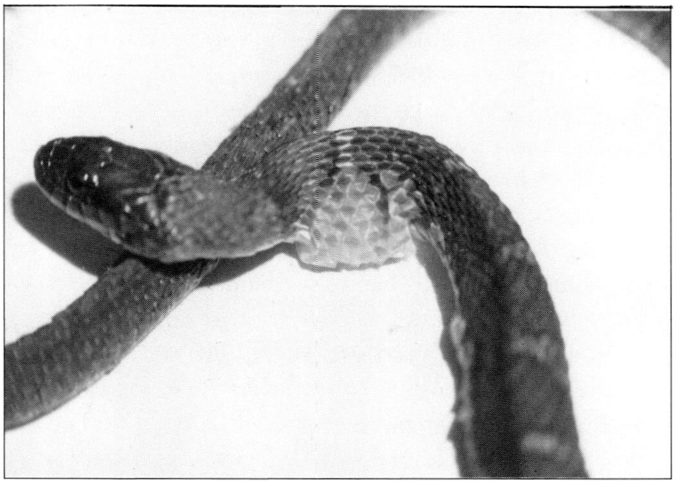

Figure 16-4. Blister disease in a northern water snake. (From Jacobson ER: Diseases of reptiles, Part I. Noninfectious diseases. *Compend Contin Educ Pract Vet* 3:122–126, 1981, with permission)

Blister Disease

For some species of lizards and snakes excess humidity can cause problems. Some of the fungal skin diseases have been seen in reptiles kept in cages with excess humidity. Another disease that has been described in snakes, although its pathogenesis is not understood, is blister disease. This disease is seen commonly in water snakes, garter snakes, and king snakes that are maintained under excessively moist conditions (Fig. 16-4). It is perplexing as to why this disease develops in water snakes, a species spending most of its time in or around water. Air exchange in the cage may be important in the development of the disease as many of the snakes developing this disease are in cages that have poor air circulation. Stagnant air of high relative humidity in some way may initiate pathologic changes in the skin resulting in cleft formation and accumulation of fluid in the epidermis. The pathogenesis of this disease needs to be elucidated.

Nutritional Deficiency–Associated Skin Diseases

Vitamin A Deficiency

Vitamin A is essential for the maintenance of epithelial integrity. Many cases of vitamin A deficiency in reptiles are epithelial-related problems, particularly disease of the adnexal structures of the eye in aquatic turtles. Turtles often are presented with palpebral edema, anasarca, hyperkeratosis of the skin, and overgrowth of the mandibular and maxillary horny mouthparts. Classic histopathologic changes seen are squamous metaplasia and hyperkeratosis of lacrimal and Harderian gland tubules.

Therapy should include treatment of the immediate problem and improvement of the deficient diet. In severe cases in which the animal's palpebrae are swollen and closed, injectable vitamin A can be administered intramuscularly at 2000 units/kg body weight every 3 days for 2 weeks. The commercial diet ReptoMin® (Tetra-Werke—West Germany), which is available in most pet stores selling reptiles, appears to be nutritionally complete and is readily accepted by most aquatic chelonians.

Collagen Disorders

A very interesting disease of collagen has been seen by the author in several recently imported reticulated pythons (*Python reticulatus*). The snakes were submitted with the epidermis detached from the dermis. The skin would tear after minimal abrasions or manual restraint. Fluid accumulated between the epidermis and dermis and in one snake moved as a column from the head to tail after tilting. One snake also regurgitated after feeding and after euthanasia, necropsy revealed that the gastric mucosa had separated from the submucosa and formed a balloon-like structure over the pylorus. Histologically, collagen in the dermis and submucosa was poorly organized and poorly developed. Chronic malnutrition (that is, protein deficiency) may have been instrumental in initiating this problem. Further, because some species of snakes are known to synthesize vitamin C in their kidney,[47] malnourished snakes may not produce enough vitamin C for adequate formation of collagen.

Neoplastic Skin Diseases

Neoplastic diseases are common in older captive reptiles whereas relatively uncommon in young reptiles. Several populations of free-ranging green turtles have been identified with cutaneous fibropapillomas, with both juvenile and adult green turtles equally represented. In crocodilians few neoplasms have been reported for any age group. This is especially surprising because crocodilians are long-lived reptiles (many live for 100 years) and are commonly kept in zoologic collections. The major neoplasms of the integument are discussed below.

Squamous Cell Carcinoma

Squamous cell carcinomas have been reported from the foot of a Ceylonese terrapin (*Geoemyda trijuga*)[48] and from the foot of a common tegu (*Tupinambis teguixin*).[49] In the latter report, the tumor measured 3 cm in diameter and almost destroyed the metacarpus as well as the proximal two phalanges of the fifth right digit. The tumor consisted of neoplastic epithelial cells and pearl formation with large areas of necrosis. Although squamous cell carcinoma has been described for the oral cavity and cloaca of snakes, few cases of cutaneous squamous cell carcinoma have been reported. A water moccasin (*Agkistrodon piscivores*) with a 1-cm spherical mass attached to the lower left mandible was histologically diagnosed as having a squamous cell carcinoma.[50]

Papillomas and Fibropapillomas

Papillomas, fibromas, and fibropapillomas were first described in captured adult green turtles (*Chelonia mydas*) 50 years ago.[51,52] Fibropapillomas are distributed over the dorsal cervical region, axillary regions of the hind legs, eyelids, and conjunctivae (Plate XIII-17). These lesions ranged from papillary projections of hyperplastic keratinized epithelium supported by a fibrous core to smooth round fibrous tumors composed of dense connective tissue covered by thickened epithelium. Today fibropapillomas are well established in populations of green turtles in the Indian River lagoon system of east central Florida, the Florida Keys, and the Hawaiian Islands. Although detailed pathologic studies have been done no specific agent has been incriminated.[53] From a comparative standpoint a viral agent seems most likely. Occasionally, particles with electron-dense centers and measuring 155 to 190 nm were observed in intracytoplasmic vacuoles in epidermal cells of the stratum basale. Their identity remains unknown.

As discussed in the section Viral Skin Diseases, cutaneous papillomas have been commonly seen in the European emerald lizard (*Lacerta viridis*) and several types of viral particles have been found in these lesions. Cutaneous papillomas have also been described for the sand lizard (*Lacerta agilis*) and the European wall lizard (*Lacerta muralis*). Relatively few cases of cutaneous papillomas have been described in snakes.

Pigment Cell Tumors

At least four varieties of pigment cells are found in the integument of reptiles: two kinds of melanophores containing melanin; xanthophores or erythrophores containing pteridines and carotenoids; and iridophores (guanophores) containing reflecting platelets of guanine, adenine, hypoxanthine, and uric acid. Three of these pigment cell types are uniquely located in the dermis, and it is only the epidermal melanophore (melanocyte) that is found in the epidermis.

A variety of pigment cell tumors have been described for snakes. Multiple skin melanomas were reported for each of two reticulated pythons (*Python reticulatus*),[54] and a malignant melanoma was described in each of a caged pair of pine snakes (*Pituophis melanoleucus*).[55] A new neoplasm, a chromatophoroma, was described in a western terrestrial garter snake (*Thamnophis elegans terrestris*),[56] and a malignant chromatophoroma consisting of mosaic chromatophores with pigment particles typical of more than one type of chromatophore was reported for a gopher snake (*Pituophis catenifer sayi*).[57] Combined iridophoroma and melanophoroma was recently described in a northern pine snake (*P. melanoleucus melanoleucus*) with metastases of malignant iridophores to multiple visceral sites.[58]

Fibrosarcoma

I have seen several cases of fibrosarcoma involving the integumentary system of snakes. These neoplasms generally appear as subcutaneous swellings with or without necrosis of the overlying skin, and often spread into surrounding tissues making it difficult to determine the tumor margins. Histologically, fibrosarcomas range from populations of undifferentiated anaplastic to well-differentiated cells producing abundant collagen.

Treatment/Management of Neoplastic Conditions

Treatment depends on many factors, including the age, species, and physical condition of the individual; type of neoplasm; system affected; and usually the cost of the procedure. Early diagnosis is necessary for the best success. Any unusual skin lesions and internal masses should be biopsied as soon as identified. Once a neoplasm has metastasized the prognosis is grave. Often these metastatic lesions are only diagnosed at necropsy. Although a variety of treatment regimens have been developed for the various cutaneous neoplasms found in mammals, there are few reports of their use in reptiles. The most successful treatment is that of surgical removal. In green turtles with cutaneous fibropapillomas, early lesions that were surgically removed did not recur at the surgical site. Such neoplasms as melanomas and chromatophoromas should have wide surgical margins because they often diffusely infiltrate surrounding tissue. After removal neoplasms should be submitted for histopathology to determine if neoplastic cells extend to the margins of the incised mass.

Congenital Abnormalities

A variety of congenital skin anomalies are described for reptiles. Various abnormalities with regard to coloration have been reported for all groups of reptiles. As mentioned earlier, most reptiles have an array of different pigment cells in the dermis, the various combinations of which give each species its distinctive coloration. Albinism, melanism, and other coloration anomalies have been seen (Plate XIII-18). Many private breeders of snakes are selecting for various colors and patterns that are in demand by the pet trade. The more unusual the color and pattern, the greater the price for the animals. Turtles with above-normal numbers of scutes on their carapace and plastron and scaleless snakes have been reported. Snakes with scales pointing rostrally instead of the normal caudal orientation have also been seen.

Many of the congenital defects in reptiles have been attributed to improper incubation conditions of eggs. Incubation temperatures above or below optimum may result in malformations in the developing embryo. Many of the color and pattern anomalies, however, have a genetic basis, and reptiles can be selectively bred for these traits.

DERMATOLOGIC DIAGNOSTIC TECHNIQUES

The key to evaluating skin lesions of reptiles is collecting and properly evaluating a good biopsy specimen for histologic evaluation, cytology, and microbial culture. Microbial culture by itself is often misleading, however, because many microbes often secondarily colonize skin lesions.

Chelonians

Of all the reptiles, chelonians present the greatest challenge for biopsy, especially when lesions involve the shell. As mentioned earlier, the reptile shell is a very hard biologic structure that makes biopsy somewhat difficult. A rotary power saw (Dremel Mototool® —Dremel Mfg. Co.) can be used to cut a wedge out of the shell. For anesthesia ketamine hydrochloride can be administered at 20 to 40 mg/kg body weight given intramuscularly in a forelimb. Ideally, the biopsy should include normal tissue along with the diseased component. A piece should be fixed in neutral buffered 10% formalin for histopathologic evaluation and a piece (with the most superficial contaminated portion removed) submitted for microbial culture. The defect created in the shell should be filled with calcium hydroxide dental paste (RootCal® —Ellman International Mfg.) and covered over with a methacrylate resin (Cyanoveneer® —Ellman International Mfg.). This technique is routinely used in repair of the chelonian shell.

For biopsy of soft tissue a 2% xylocaine block is satisfactory and can be infiltrated around the biopsy site. A biopsy punch can be used for collecting the sample. After biopsy the skin may require a single suture for closure. Monofilament nylon is routinely used.

Crocodilians and Lizards

A full-thickness biopsy may be difficult in those areas of the crocodilian integument having osteoderms. Small crocodilians and most lizards can be manually restrained, whereas large crocodilians and large monitors must be chemically immobilized. The area around the biopsy site should be infiltrated with 2% xylocaine and a full-thickness skin incision taken with a biopsy punch. As with chelonians at least two biopsies should be taken, one for histopathology and one for microbiology. For microbial culture the lesions should be ground in a sterile mortar and pestle and samples applied to the appropriate media. This appears to be particularly important for isolation of fungi from reptile skin lesions.

Snakes

Snakes are ideally suited for skin biopsy. Harmless species can be manually restrained, and poisonous species can be guided into a Plexiglas tube for restraint. Affected scales can be removed with a scalpel blade, or a sterilized one-hole paper punch can be used for biopsies of individual scales. In certain skin diseases, such as vesiculating skin lesions, larger samples may be needed. In such cases the area around the lesion should be infiltrated with 2% xylocaine hydrochloride and the skin sutured after removal of the specimen. Similarly, for sampling subcutaneous masses 2% xylocaine can be infiltrated subcutaneously around the mass. Once removed the mass should be split in half for both histologic evaluation and microbial culture.

ACKNOWLEDGMENTS

Sections of this chapter were taken from Jacobson ER: Parasitic diseases of reptiles. In: Fowler ME (ed): *Zoo and Wild Animal Medicine*. Philadelphia, WB Saunders Co, 1986, pp 162–181; and Jacobson ER: Reptiles. *Vet Clin North Am [Small Anim Pract]* 17:1203–1225, 1987, with permission.

REFERENCES

1. Zangerl R: The turtle shell. In: Gans C (ed): *Biology of the Reptilia*, vol 1. New York, Academic Press, 1969, pp 311–346.
2. Magliola L: The effects of estrogen on skeletal calcium metabolism and on plasma parameters of vitellogenesis in the male, three-toed box turtle (*Terrapene carolina triunguis*). *Gen Comp Endocrinol* 54:162–170, 1983.
3. Rainey WE: *Guide to Sea Turtle Visceral Anatomy*. NOAA Technical Memorandum, NMFS-SEFC-82, 1981.
4. Matoltsy AG, Huszar T: Keratinization of the reptilian epidermis: An ultrastructural study of the turtle skin. *J Ultrastruct Res* 38:87–101, 1972.
5. Maderson PFA: Histological changes in the epidermis of snakes during the sloughing cycle. *J Zool* 146:98–113, 1965.
6. Maderson PFA: Some developmental problems of the reptilian integument. In: Gans C, Billet F, Maderson PFA (eds): *Biology of the Reptilia*. New York, John Wiley and Sons, 1985, pp 523–598.
7. Rebell HA, Rywlin A, Haines H: A herpesvirus-type agent associated with skin lesions of green sea turtles in aquaculture. *Am J Vet Res* 36:1221–1224, 1975.
8. Haines H, Kleese WC: Effect of water temperature on a herpesvirus infection of sea turtles. *Infect Immun* 15:756–759, 1977.
9. Jacobson ER, Popp J, Shields RP, et al: Pox-like virus associated with skin lesions in captive caimans. *JAVMA* 175:937–940, 1979.
10. Foggin CM: Diseases and disease control on crocodile farms in Zimbabwe. In: Webb GJW, Manolis SC, Whitehead PJ (eds): *Wildlife Management, Crocodiles and Alligators*. New South Wales, Australia, Surrey Beatty and Sons Pty Limited, 1987, pp 351–362.
11. Horner RE: Poxvirus in farmed Nile crocodiles. *Vet Rec* 7:459–461, 1988.
12. Frye FL: *Biomedical and Surgical Aspects of Captive Reptile Husbandry*. Edwardsville, KS, Veterinary Medicine Publishing Co, 1981, p 167.
13. Jacobson ER, Gaskin JM, Clubb SL: Papilloma-like virus infection in Bolivian side-neck turtles. *JAVMA* 181:1325–1328, 1982.
14. Raynaud MMA, Adrian M: Lesions cutanees a structure papillomateuse associees a des virus chez le lizard (*Lacerta viridis* Laur). *CR Acad Sci Paris* 283:845–847, 1976.
15. Jackson CG, Fulton M: A turtle colony epizootic apparently of microbial origin. *J Wildl Dis* 6:446–468, 1970.
16. Wallach JD: The pathogenesis and etiology of ulcerative shell disease in turtles. *J Zoo Anim Med* 6:11–13, 1972.
17. Jackson CG Jr, Fulton M, Jackson MM: Cranial asymmetry with massive infection in a box turtle. *J Wildl Dis* 8:275–277, 1972.
18. Duran-Reynals F, Clausen HJ: A contagious tumor-like condition in the lizard (*Anolis equestris*) as induced by a new bacterial species, *Serratia anolium* (Sp.N.). *J Bacteriol* 33:369–379, 1937.
19. Boam GW, Sanger VL, Cowan DF, Vaughan DP: Subcutaneous abscesses in iguanid lizards. *JAVMA* 157:617–619, 1975.
20. Plowman CA, Montali RJ, Phillips LJ, et al: Septicemia and chronic abscesses in iguanas (*Cyclura cornuta* and *Iguana iguana*) associated with *Neisseria* species. *J Zoo Anim Med* 18:86–93, 1987.
21. Stewart JS: Anaerobic bacterial infections in reptiles. In: *Proceedings of the American Association of Zoo Veterinarians Annual Meeting*, Greensboro, North Carolina, 1989, p 173.
22. Dogget RG: Microbiology of *Pseudomonas aeruginosa*. In: Dogget RG (ed): *Pseudomona aeruginosa: Clinical Manifestations of Infection and Current Therapy*. New York, Academic Press, 1979, pp 1–7.
23. Murphy JB, Armstrong BL: *Maintenance of Rattlesnakes in Captivity*. Lawrence, KS, University of Kansas Publications, Museum of Natural History, 1978.
24. Jacobson ER: *Pseudomonas*. In: Hoff GL, Frye FL, Jacobson ER (eds): *Diseases of Amphibians and Reptiles*. New York, Plenum Press, 1984, pp 37–47.
25. Jacobson ER, Ingling AL: Pyloroduodenal resection in a Burmese python. *JAVMA* 169:985–987, 1976.
26. Shotts EB, Gaines JL, Martin C, Prestwood AK: *Aeromonas* induced death among fish and reptiles in a eutrophic inland lake. *JAVMA* 161:603–607, 1972.
27. Brownstein DG: Mycobacteriosis. In: Hoff GL, Frye FL, Jacobson ER (eds): *Diseases of Amphibians and Reptiles*. New York, Plenum Press, 1984, pp 1–23.
28. Quesenberry KE, Jacobson ER, Allen JL, Cooley AJ: Ulcerative stomatitis and subcutaneous granulomas caused by *Mycobacterium chelonei* in a boa constrictor. *JAVMA* 189:1131–1132, 1986.
29. Montali FJ, Smith EE, Davenport M, Bush M: Dermatophilosis in Australian bearded lizards. *JAVMA* 167:553–555, 1975.
30. Anver MR, Park JS, Rush HG: Dermatophilosis in the marble lizard (*Calotes mystaceus*). *Lab Anim Sci* 26:817–823, 1976.

31. Simmons GC, Sullivan ND, Green PE: Dermatophilosis in a lizard (*Amphibolurus barbatus*). *Aust Vet J* 48:465–467, 1972.
32. Jacobson ER: Use of chemotherapeutics in reptile medicine. In: Jacobson ER, Kollias GV (eds): *Exotic Animals*. New York, Churchill Livingstone, 1988, pp 35–48.
33. Frank W: Mycotic infections in amphibians and reptiles. In: Page LA (ed): *Wildlife Diseases*. New York, Plenum Press, 1976, pp 73–88.
34. Hunt TJ: Notes on diseases and mortality in testudines. *Herpetologica* 13:19–23, 1957.
35. Jacobson ER, Calderwood MB, Clubb SL: Mucormycosis in hatchling Florida softshell turtles. *JAVMA* 177:835–837, 1980.
36. Migaki G, Jacobson ER, Casey HW: Fungal diseases in reptiles. In: Hoff GL, Frye RL, Jacobson ER (eds): *Diseases of Amphibians and Reptiles*. New York, Plenum Press, 1984, pp 183–204.
37. Jacobson ER: Necrotizing mycotic dermatitis in snakes: Clinical and pathologic features. *JAVMA* 177:838–841, 1980.
38. Jacobson ER: Chromomycosis and fibrosarcoma in a mangrove snake. *JAVMA* 185:1428–1430, 1984.
39. McKenzie RA, Green PE: Mycotic dermatitis in carpet snakes. *J Wildl Dis* 12:405–408, 1976.
40. Page CD, Mautino M, Meyer JR, Mechlinski W: Preliminary pharmacokinetics of ketoconazole in gopher tortoises (*Gopherus polyphemus*). In: *Proceedings of Joint Conference, American Association of Zoo Veterinarians and American Association of Wildlife Veterinarians*, Toronto, Ontario, Canada, 1988, p 63.
41. Wright K, Tousignant A, Overstreet R, et al: *Mesocercariae* infections in a Texas indigo snake and red-sided garter snakes. In: *Third International Colloquium on the Pathology of Reptiles and Amphibians*, Orlando, Florida, 1989, p 54.
42. Frank W: Die pathogenen Wirkungen von *Macdonaldius oschei* Chaubaud et Frank 1961 (Filaroidea, Onchocercidae) bei ver schiedenen arten von schlangen (Reptilia, Ophidia). *Z Parasitenkd* 24:249, 1964.
43. Hull RW, Camin JH: *Macdonaldius seetae* Khanna, 1933 in captive snakes. *Trans Am Micros Soc* 78:323, 1959.
44. Telford SR Jr: Some observations on the effects of varying ambient temperatures in vivo on filarial worms of snakes. *Jpn J Exp Med* 35:291, 1965.
45. Jacobson ER, Greiner EC, Clubb SL, Harvey-Clarke C: Pustular dermatitis caused by subcutaneous dracunculiasis in snakes. *JAVMA* 189:1133–1134, 1986.
46. Lichtenfels JR, Lavies B: Mortality in red-sided garter snakes, *Thamnophis sirtalis parietalis*, due to larval nematode, *Eustrongylus* sp. *Lab Anim Sci* 26:465, 1976.
47. Vosburgh KM, Brady PS, Ullrey DE: Ascorbic acid requirements of garter snakes: Plains (*Thamnophis radix*) and eastern (*T. sirtalis sirtalis*). *J Zoo Anim Med* 13:38–42, 1982.
48. Cowen DF: Diseases of captive reptiles. *JAVMA* 153:848–859, 1968.
49. Schwarz E: Ueber swei geschwuelste bei kaltbluetern. *Z Krebsforsch* 20:353–357, 1923.
50. Wadworth JR: Tumors and tumor-like lesions in snakes. *JAVMA* 137:419–420, 1960.
51. Lucke B: Studies on tumors in cold-blooded vertebrates. *Ann Tortugas Lab* (Carnegie Institute, Washington, DC), 1938.
52. Smith GM, Coates C: Fibro-epithelial growths of the skin in large marine turtles, *Chelonia mydas* (Linnaeus). *Zoologica (New York)* 24:379–382, 1938.
53. Jacobson ER, Mansell JL, Sundberg JP, et al: Cutaneous fibropapillomas of green turtles (*Chelonia mydas*). *J Comp Pathol* 101:39–52, 1989.
54. Schlumberger HG, Lucke B: Tumors of fishes, amphibians and reptiles. *Cancer Res* 8:657–753, 1948.
55. Ball HA: Melanosarcoma and rhabdomyoma in two pine snakes (*Pituophis melanoleucus*). *Cancer Res* 6:134–138, 1946.
56. Frye FL, Carney J, Harshbarger J, Zeigel R: Malignant chromatophoroma in a western garter snake. *JAVMA* 167:557–558, 1975.
57. Ryan MJ, Hill DL, Whitney CD: Malignant chomatophoroma in a gopher snake. *Vet Pathol* 18:827–829, 1981.
58. Jacobson ER, Ferris W, Bagnara JT, Iverson WO: Chromatophoromas in a pine snake. *Pigment Cell Res* 2:26–33, 1989.

INDEX